P9-DEB-692

ORGANIZATIONAL BEHAVIOR, THEORY, AND DESIGN IN HEALTH CARE

Nancy Borkowski, DBA, CPA, FACHE

Department of Health Policy and Management
Robert Stempel School of Public Health
Florida International University

JONES AND BARTLETT PUBLISHERS

Sudbury, Massachusetts

BOSTON   TORONTO   LONDON   SINGAPORE

World Headquarters

Jones and Bartlett Publishers
40 Tall Pine Drive
Sudbury, MA 01776
978-443-5000
info@jbpub.com
www.jbpub.com

Jones and Bartlett Publishers
Canada
6339 Ormindale Way
Mississauga, Ontario L5V 1J2
Canada

Jones and Bartlett Publishers
International
Barb House, Barb Mews
London W6 7PA
United Kingdom

Jones and Bartlett's books and products are available through most bookstores and online booksellers. To contact Jones and Bartlett Publishers directly, call 800-832-0034, fax 978-443-8000, or visit our website www.jbpub.com.

Substantial discounts on bulk quantities of Jones and Bartlett's publications are available to corporations, professional associations, and other qualified organizations. For details and specific discount information, contact the special sales department at Jones and Bartlett via the above contact information or send an email to specialsales@jbpub.com.

Copyright © 2009 by Jones and Bartlett Publishers, LLC

All rights reserved. No part of the material protected by this copyright may be reproduced or utilized in any form, electronic or mechanical, including photocopying, recording, or by any information storage and retrieval system, without written permission from the copyright owner.

This publication is designed to provide accurate and authoritative information in regard to the Subject Matter covered. It is sold with the understanding that the publisher is not engaged in rendering legal, accounting, or other professional service. If legal advice or other expert assistance is required, the service of a competent professional person should be sought.

Production Credits
Publisher: Michael Brown
Production Director: Amy Rose
Associate Editor: Katey Birtcher
Editorial Assistant: Catie Heverling
Production Editor: Tracey Chapman
Marketing Manager: Sophie Fleck
Marketing Associate: Courtney Fleishman
Manufacturing and Inventory Control Supervisor: Amy Bacus
Composition: Cape Cod Compositors, Inc.
Illustrator: Accurate Art, Inc.
Cover Design: Brian Moore
Printing and Binding: Malloy, Inc.
Cover Printing: Malloy, Inc.

Library of Congress Cataloging-in-Publication Data
Borkowski, Nancy.
   Organizational behavior, theory, and design in health care / Nancy Borkowski.
      p. ; cm.
   Includes bibliographical references and index.
   ISBN-13: 978-0-7637-4285-0 (pbk.)
   ISBN-10: 0-7637-4285-6 (pbk.)
   1. Organizational behavior.   2. Health services administration.   I. Title.
   [DNLM: 1. Health Services Administration.   2. Group Processes.   3. Health Personnel—
   psychology.   4. Organizational Culture.   5. Personnel Management.   W 84.1 B734o 2009]
   RA971.B835   2009
   362.1068—dc22

                                                                        2008020465

6048

Printed in the United States of America
12   11   10   09   08   10   9   8   7   6   5   4   3   2   1

To my husband.

Contents

Preface

In 2005, I authored my first book, *Organizational Behavior in Health Care*, and in the Preface I wrote, "the U.S. healthcare industry has grown and changed dramatically over the past twenty-five years." That was an understatement! In the past three years, the industry has experienced dynamic changes. The Institute of Medicine issued its follow-up report *Crossing the Quality Chasm* that made an urgent call to redesign the U.S. healthcare system to close the "quality gap." Pay-for-performance is now a reality firmly ensconced in the payment systems of both public and private insurers. These new initiatives are being used to promote transparency and value-driven health care in the future. Health systems, insurers, and organizations in the public sector are moving forward and adopting various quality improvement programs. Healthcare managers are quickly learning what worked in the past may not (and probably won't) work in the future. This was my compelling reason for writing this book. I wish to assist those who are on the frontline everyday, healthcare managers who must motivate and lead others in, and adapt their organizations to, a complex and constantly changing environment. This is not an easy task, which I know firsthand. Before joining the academic world, I held the positions of chief operating officer, chief financial officer, and administrator for various healthcare organizations.

The purpose of this book is to provide health services administration students, managers, and other professionals with an in-depth analysis of the theories and concepts of organizational behavior and organization theory while embracing the uniqueness and complexity of the healthcare industry. Although health care is similar to other industries in various aspects, it is also very different. It is the nation's largest industry, employing over 15 million people. It is the most complex, with its numerous interrelated and interdependent segments. Healthcare managers need to deal with and attempt to balance numerous competing issues on a daily basis (i.e., providing care for the uninsured while controlling costs, providing quality care while experiencing labor shortages, providing market wages with declining reimbursements, etc.).

Using an applied focus, this book provides a clear and concise overview of the essential topics in organizational behavior and organization theory from the healthcare manager's perspective. It is my goal that after you have read this book, you will develop a greater understanding of why individuals and/or groups behave the way they do in the workplace and how organizations behave in relationship to their environments and an understanding of how organizations are affected by individuals' behaviors and how organizations affect individuals' behaviors. With this knowledge you will be able to better predict and thus effectively influence the behavior of those you lead, and ensure that the organization's structure in its environment is designed to facilitate success. Please let me know if I have accomplished my goal! You may reach me at *Nancy.Borkowski@fiu.edu* or by phone at (305) 348-0434. I tried to ensure that I referenced all the individuals whose works contributed to the development of this book. If by chance I failed to give credit to someone along the way, please contact me so that I may make the necessary correction.

At this time I wish to acknowledge the individuals without whose efforts and support I would not have been able to complete this book. First, I wish to thank my colleagues and contributors, Jean Gordon, Gloria Deckard, Judy Bachay, Lorrie Jones, Paul Harvey, Mark Martinko, Ray Kulzick, Kristina Guo, Yesenia Sanchez, and Paul Maxwell. Second, I want to thank my friend and colleague, Bob Amann, who provides me with his assistance whenever asked. As always, I am very thankful and appreciative for my husband and children, who over the years have given up much (and continue to) so I may pursue my goals. Finally, I wish to thank the many wonderful people employed throughout the healthcare industry that I have had and will have the opportunity to work with. My life continues to be blessed by these dedicated individuals!

Thank you for purchasing (and reading) my book. I welcome your comments and suggestions.

With personal regards,

Nancy M. Borkowski, DBA, CPA, FACHE

Contributors

Judith Bachay, PhD
Professor
Department of Social Sciences and
  Counseling
St. Thomas University
Miami, FL

Gloria Deckard, PhD
Associate Professor
Chair, Department of Health Policy
  and Management
Robert Stempel School of Public
  Health
Florida International University
Miami, FL

Jean Gordon, RN, DBA
Healthcare Consultant
Hollywood, FL

Kristina L. Guo, PhD
Associate Professor, Health Care
  Administration Program
Department of Public
  Administration
University of Hawai'i–West O'ahu
Pearl City, HI

Paul Harvey, PhD
Assistant Professor of Management
Whittemore School of Business and
  Economics
University of New Hampshire
Durham, NH

Lorrie Jones, PhD
Organizational Development /
  Human Resources Specialist
Hollywood, FL

Raymond Kulzick, DBA, CPA, CFE,
  FCPA
Professor
School of Business
St. Thomas University
Miami, FL

Mark Martinko, PhD
Bank of America Professor of
  Management
College of Business
Florida State University
Tallahassee, FL

Paul Maxwell, EdD
Associate Professor
School of Business
St. Thomas University
Miami, FL

Yesenia Sanchez, MPH
Senior Client Manager
CIGNA Healthcare
Ft. Lauderdale, FL

About the Author

Nancy Borkowski, DBA, CPA, FACHE is a visiting faculty member in the Department of Health Policy and Management at Florida International University's Robert Stempel School of Public Health. She earned her Doctorate of Business Administration in Health Services from Nova Southeastern University. Prior to her transition into academia in 1997, Dr. Borkowski held various healthcare executive positions. She is a past recipient of the American College of Healthcare Executive's Southern Florida Senior Career Healthcare Executive Award.

Dr. Borkowski is a Fellow of the American College of Healthcare Executives and has served on the editorial boards of the *Journal of Healthcare Management* and the *Journal of Healthcare Administration Education*. Dr. Borkowski served on the executive committee for the Academy of Management's Healthcare Management Division and is a member of the division's Practice Committee.

Her work has been published in *Organizational Behavior and Human Decision Processes, Health Care Management Review, Journal of Healthcare Administration Education, Journal of Health and Human Services Administration, International Journal of Public Administration, Hospital Topics*, and the *Journal of Healthcare Marketing*. Her book, *Organizational Behavior in Health Care*, won the 2005 AJN Book of the Year Award in the category of nursing leadership and management.

Dr. Borkowski teaches organizational behavior, leadership, and management. She is a past recipient of the American College of Healthcare Executives' "Excellence in Teaching" award and the "Developing Healthcare Leaders" award from Jackson Memorial Medical Center's School of Radiologic Sciences.

Dr. Borkowski continues to consult with and serve on many healthcare companies' boards. Dr. Borkowski is Past President of the South Florida Healthcare Executive Forum and the Women's Healthcare Executive Network of South Florida. She also serves on the American College of Healthcare Executive's Southern Florida Regent's Advisory Council and the TreasureCoast Healthcare Executive Network's Board of Directors.

Foreword

There are very few textbooks that address the joint topics of organizational behavior and organization theory (i.e., organizational studies) in the healthcare industry with an applied focus. There are even fewer that attempt to integrate the two so that health management students, managers, and other professionals can learn how organizations are affected by individuals' behaviors and how organizations affect individuals' behaviors. Such integration is known as the "meso perspective." The book discusses and integrates five interactive meso elements (drivers of change, alignment, processes, leadership, and people) that have been identified as critical for the successful transformation of healthcare organizations. This is the market niche that Professor Borkowski's book very ably fills.

This book is highly recommended for organizational studies courses in health care offered in both graduate and undergraduate programs in health administration, nursing, public health, and other health professions. It is very comprehensive, very readable, and very applied.

An understanding of individuals' behaviors and group dynamics and how these impact the healthcare organization is a critical part of the present and future success of healthcare executives. These executives need to be able to diagnose and understand the root causes of behavioral workplace problems such as poor communication, lack of employer motivation, poor performance, high turnover, conflict, and stress. In addition, they have to understand how the structure of the organization impacts each of these areas. With this background, these executives will be better able to influence the behavior of staff members to achieve organizational success through increased job satisfaction and productivity.

Professor Borkowski's previous book, *Organizational Behavior in Health Care*, won the American Journal of Nursing (AJN) Book of the Year Award in 2005 in the category of nursing management and leadership. The present book updates her previous book's chapters, adds a new micro chapter on "Attribution Theory and Motivation," and adds four new macro-level organization theory chapters. All of the new chapters present case studies and practitioner applications from the "real world" to illustrate and help students understand each of the concepts.

Among the topics covered are: individual perceptions and attitudes, diversity, communication, attribution theory, motivation, leadership, power, stress, conflict and conflict management, negotiations, group dynamics, team building, managing organizational change, overview of organization theory, strategy and structure, organization structures, and organization design. In addition to the usual and expected learning objectives, summaries, and case studies, other types of applied activities such as self-assessment exercises and evaluation instruments are also provided. These are intended as ways for the reader to gain a deeper understanding of how the many theories and concepts presented are successfully applied in the healthcare industry.

The book draws deeply on research and case studies published in a wide variety of healthcare management journals. This helps the reader to understand the relevance of the theory and empirical research to the types of problems and challenges currently facing today's healthcare executives. This book has a number of strengths. First, it is extremely comprehensive. All of the topics one might expect to find in such an organizational studies book (and more) are found in this book. Second, the book has a very applied focus so that students or practitioners are offered many applications and examples in each chapter that illustrate the concepts, which brings them down to varying practical levels.

Professor Borkowski is particularly well suited to write this book because she combines her academic qualifications with an extensive and successful background as a healthcare executive. She has held executive positions in physician practice management and managed care and is a past recipient of the ACHE Southern Florida Senior Career Healthcare Executive Award. Since joining the faculty at Florida International University, she has continued to consult with and serve on the boards of many healthcare organizations. In sum, Professor Borkowski has utilized all of her background and produced a unique and outstanding contribution to the field of healthcare administration.

Myron D. Fottler, PhD
University of Central Florida

Opening Remarks

Organizational behavior (OB) is the study of individual and group dynamics within an organization setting (micro level of analysis), whereas organization theory (OT) is the study of the organization as a whole (macro level of analysis).

This book integrates the study of organizational behavior and organization theory to provide the reader with an understanding of how organizations are affected by individuals' behaviors and how organizations affect individuals' behaviors. House, Rousseau and Thomas-Hunt (1995) pointed out:

> Individuals and groups affect the organization and the organization in return influences individuals and groups. To thrive in organizations, managers and employees need to understand multiple levels [within organizations] simultaneously. For example, research may show that employee diversity enhances innovation. To facilitate innovation, managers need to understand how structure and context (organization theory) are related to interactions among diverse employees (organizational behavior) to foster innovation, because both macro and micro variables account for innovation.

For example, Miller and Droge, as cited in House, et al. (1995, p. 81), found that small companies' organizational form could partially be explained by the degree to which the entities' CEOs were achievement-oriented (see Chapter 5, McClelland's 3-Needs Theory). CEO achievement orientation was associated with a more centralized organizational form (see Chapter 21—Organizational Structures), which reflected the CEO's desire to be closely involved in critical decision making (see Chapter 13—Decision Making).

Today's healthcare managers are being challenged to redesign the industry due to its complexity and the many problems associated with the overuse, underuse, or misuse of health services. As such, managers need to understand the interrelationship between organizational behavior and organization theory to successfully lead the transformation of their organizations to meet the needs and demands of society. For example, in 1999 the Institute of Medicine (IOM) Committee on Quality of Health Care in America published *To Err is Human: Building a Safer Health System*, which implied, on the basis of previously published research findings, that 44,000 to 98,000 individuals die each year as a result of medical errors that could have been avoided. The major points made by the IOM report were that the cause of medical errors is not an issue of clinicians' competence or incompetence but due to faulty system factors, such as "unrealistic reliance on human memory, poor communication systems, unrealistic demands on human vigilance, too little respect for the consequences of fatigue, reliance on handwriting in a computer age, and so on" (Berwick, 2002, p. 84). IOM related that these systems must be redesigned and patient safety must become a national priority.

Less than two years later, the IOM committee followed up with a more comprehensive report, *Crossing the Quality Chasm: A New Health System for the Twenty-first Century*, which analyzed the needed changes in the U.S. healthcare system at four different levels: the experience of the patient (i.e., patient-centered care), the functioning of the small units of care, such as a cardiac surgical team, the night shift in an emergency department, etc. ("microsystem"), the functioning of the organizations that support the microsystems ("macrosystems"), and the external environment that affects the operations of the macrosystem (i.e., policy, payment systems, regulations, accreditation, etc.) (Berwick, 2002, p. 84). The IOM (2001) identified six aims or goals for improvement of the U.S. healthcare system:

1. *Safe:* avoiding injuries to patients from the care that is intended to help them.
2. *Effective:* providing services based on scientific knowledge to all who could benefit, and refraining from providing services to those not likely to benefit.
3. *Patient-centered:* providing care that is respectful of and responsive to individual patient preferences, needs, and values, and ensuring that patient values guide all clinical decisions.
4. *Timely:* reducing waits and sometimes harmful delays for both those who receive and those who give care.
5. *Efficient:* avoiding waste, including waste of equipment, supplies, ideas, and energy.
6. *Equitable:* providing care that does not vary in quality because of personal characteristics such as gender, ethnicity, geographic location, and socioeconomic status.

If asked, I'm confident we would all agree that the changes called for in the *Quality Chasm* report will be difficult to accomplish in the short- and long-terms. However, some organizations have begun the process of transformation. For example, VanDeusen Lukas and colleagues (2007) examined twelve healthcare systems that are in process of transforming their organizations to deliver high-quality patient-centered care. The healthcare systems studied were either participants in the Robert Wood Johnson Foundation's *Pursuing Perfection Program* or have existing reputations for long-standing commitments to improvement and high-quality care. The researchers identified five interactive elements as critical for the successful transformation of a healthcare organization to deliver high-quality patient care (see Figure I–1).

The five elements identified by VanDeusen Lukas, et al. were:

1. *Strong impetus to change*—Impetus to change can be external or internal to the organization. In most cases, external pressure for change was

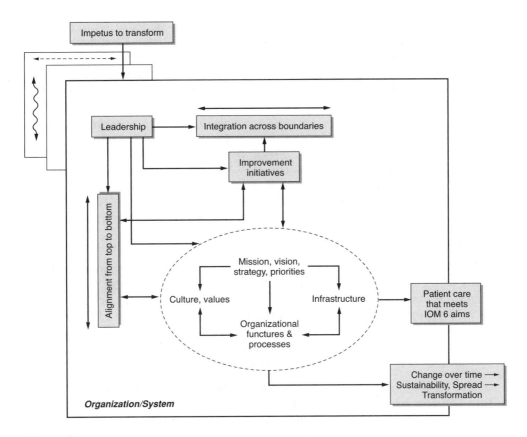

Figure I–1
Source: VanDeusen Lukas, C., Holmes, S.K., Cohen, A.B., Restuccia, J., Cramer, I.E., Shwartz, M., & Charns, M.P. (2007). Transformational change in health care systems: an organizational model. *Health Care Management Review, 32*, 4, p. 314.

the strongest (i.e., political, IOM reports, changes in reimbursement schemes, etc.).

2. *Leadership commitment to quality*—Leadership is a critical element for organizational transformation. Leaders must demonstrate authentic passion for and commitment to quality and steer the change through the organization's structures and processes to maintain urgency, set a consistent direction, reinforce expectations, and provide resources and accountability to support the change.

3. *Improvement initiatives that actively engage staff in meaningful problem solving*—Improvement initiatives must actively engage staff across disciplines and hierarchical levels in problem solving around objective, meaningful, urgent problems (i.e., surgical infections). These initiatives, such as clinical redesign and improved operations, must be built into routine work new practices that are visible, easier to perform, more reliable, and more efficient than old practices.

4. *Alignment to achieve consistency of organization goals with resource allocation and actions at all levels of the organization*—Changes must be aligned with the organizational mission and strategic direction. As such, changes need to be consistent with plans, processes, information, resource decisions, actions, results, and analysis to support key organization-wide goals.

5. *Integration to bridge traditional intraorganizational boundaries among individual components*—For the organization to succeed, change initiatives must be integrated across intraorganizational boundaries to improve coordination and continuity of care (i.e., patient flow, case management, electronic health records). Extensive integration is needed to break down barriers between departmental silos so that the system operates as a fully interconnected unit to support organization-wide goals.

VanDeusen Lukas and colleagues (2007) stated that,

> These [five] elements drive change by affecting the components of the complex health care organization in which they operate: (1) *Mission*, *vision*, and *strategies* that set forth its direction and priorities; (2) *Culture* that reflects its informal values and norms; (3) *Operational functions* and *processes* that embody the work done in patient care; (4) *Infrastructure* such as information technology and human resources that support the delivery of patient care.

In this book's twenty-two chapters, we examine these four elements in detail within the context of numerous OB and OT theories and concepts. In Section One, our focus will be the micro level of analysis: individuals and groups. Within Section One's eighteen chapters, you will gain an understanding of how and why people and groups behave the way they do in the workplace. With this understanding, managers are better able to predict behavior responses and, as a result, manage the resulting outcomes. Section Two focuses on the macro level of analysis: the organization. Within Section Two's four chapters, we will discuss the theories and concepts related to the structure and design of organizations to achieve effectiveness (i.e., doing the right thing—delivering high-quality patient care) and efficiency (i.e., doing it the right way).

By definition, an organization is a collection of people working together under a defined structure to achieve predetermined outcomes. Therefore, it makes sense that we examine both organizational behavior and organization theory simultaneously since organizations affect individuals' behaviors and individuals' behaviors affect organizations!

REFERENCES

Berwick, D. M. (2002). A user's manual for the IOM's 'Quality Chasm' report. *Health Affairs, 21,* 3, 80–90.

House, R., Rousseau, D. M., & Thomas-Hunt, M. (1995). The Meso Paradigm: A framework for the integration of micro and macro organizational behavior. *Research in Organizational Behavior, 17,* 71–114.

Institute of Medicine. (2001). *Crossing the quality chasm: a new health system for the twenty-first century.* Washington, DC: National Academy Press.

Kohn, L. T., Corrigan, J. M., & Donaldson, M. S. (1999). *To err is human: building a safer health system.* Washington, DC: National Academy Press.

Miller, D., & Droge, C. (1986). Psychological and traditional determinants of structure. *Administrative Science Quarterly, 31*, 539–560.

VanDeusen Lukas, C., Holmes, S. K., Cohen, A. B., Restuccia, J., Cramer, I. E., Shwartz, M., & Charns, M. P. (2007). Transformational change in health care systems: An organizational model. *Health Care Management Review, 32*, 4, 309–320.

OTHER SUGGESTED READINGS

Hackman, J. R. (2003). Learning more by crossing levels: Evidence from airplanes, hospitals, and orchestra. *Journal of Organizational Behavior, 24*, 905–922.

Hearld, L. R., Alexander, J. A., Fraser, I., & Jiang, H. J. (2008). How do hospital organizational structure and processes affect quality of care? *Medical Care Research and Review, 65*, 3, 259–299.

Hoff, T., Jameson, L., Hannan, E., & Flink, E. (2004). A review of the literature examining linkages between organizational factors, medical errors, and patient safety. *Medical Care Research and Review, 61*, 1, 3–37.

Mitchell, P. H., & Shortell, S. M. (1997). Adverse outcomes and variations in organization of care delivery. *Medical Care, 53*, 11 Supplement, NS19–NS32.

SECTION ONE

Microlevel—"The Individual"

Introduction

Part I includes four different but related topics. In Chapter 1, the history of organizational behavior and its importance to today's healthcare managers are discussed. Chapter 2 describes the changing environment in which healthcare managers find themselves. The chapter examines the numerous issues that have emerged within the healthcare industry because of the nation's changing demographics. Chapter 3 deals with attitudes and perceptions, which are the "backbone" to understanding organizational behavior. You will find the terms attitude and perception frequently referred to within the various organizational behavior theories. Finally, Chapter 4 discusses the importance of communications. It is said that 90 percent of the world's problems are due to ineffective or the lack of communication. No wonder communication skills are considered one of the top five skills necessary for today's healthcare leader.

CHAPTER 1

Overview and History of Organizational Behavior

Nancy Borkowski, DBA, CPA, FACHE

LEARNING OUTCOMES

After completing this chapter, the student should understand:

- ☛ The definition of organizational behavior.
- ☛ The major challenges facing today's and tomorrow's healthcare organizations and healthcare managers.
- ☛ The importance of the Hawthorne Studies to the study of organizational behavior.
- ☛ The importance of McGregor's Theory X and Theory Y to the study of organizational behavior.
- ☛ The difference between organizational behavioral, organization theory, organizational development, and human resources management.

OVERVIEW

Organizational behavior (OB) is an applied behavioral science that emerged from the disciplines of psychology, sociology, anthropology, political science, and economics. OB is the study of individual and group dynamics within an organization setting. Whenever people work together, numerous and complex factors interact. The discipline of OB attempts to understand these interactions so that managers can predict behavioral responses and, as a result, manage the resulting outcomes.

According to Ott (1996, p. 1), OB asks the following questions:

1. Why do people behave the way they do when they are in organizations?
2. Under what circumstances will people's behavior in organizations change?
3. What impacts do organizations have on the behavior of individuals, formal groups (such as departments), and informal groups (such as people from several departments who meet regularly in the company's lunchroom)?
4. Why do different groups in the same organization develop different behavior norms?

There are three goals of OB. First, OB attempts to explain why individuals and groups behave the way they do within the organizational setting. Second, OB tries to predict how individuals and groups will behave on the basis of internal and external factors. Third, OB provides managers with tools to assist in the management of individuals' and groups' behaviors so that they willingly put forth their best effort to accomplish organizational goals. In the healthcare industry, OB has become more important because people with diverse backgrounds and cultural values have to work together effectively and efficiently.

WHY STUDY ORGANIZATIONAL BEHAVIOR IN HEALTH CARE?

The largest US industry is health care, which currently employs over 14 million individuals with an expected growth of approximately 22 percent through 2016. This growth will be 11 percent faster than all other industries (Bureau of Labor Statistics, 2008).

Each segment of the healthcare industry (e.g., hospitals, home health, rehabilitation facilities) employs a different mix of health-related occupations ranging from highly skilled licensed professionals, such as physicians and nurses, to those with on-the-job training. Furthermore, each segment of the industry has various economic structures (e.g., for-profit, not-for-profit, governmental). As such, today's healthcare managers need to possess the skills to communicate effectively with, motivate, and lead diverse groups of people within a large, dynamic, and complex industry. Communication, motivation, and leadership are all concepts within the discipline of OB. Furthermore, managers need to understand the causes of workplace problems, such as low performance, turnover, conflict, and stress, so that they may be proactive and avoid these unnecessary negative outcomes. With a greater understanding of OB, managers are better able to predict and, thus, influence the behavior of employees to achieve organizational goals.

Given the service-related intensity of the industry, the understanding of individuals' behavior and group dynamics within health service organizations is critical to a healthcare manager's success. Research indicates that the primary reasons managers fail stem from difficulty in handling change, not being able to work well in teams, and poor interpersonal relations.

THE HEALTHCARE INDUSTRY

Changes within the healthcare industry over the past 25 years have been powerful, far-reaching, and continuous. Since readers are probably familiar with most of these changes from either their own experiences or from a previous healthcare delivery system course, the discussion will address some of the trends or future concerns that will impact tomorrow's healthcare organization for the industry.

Past changes and future trends are interrelating forces that have or will shape tomorrow's healthcare organizations, whether they occur at the system level or the organizational level. Declining reimbursement for services has had, and will continue to have, one of the deepest impacts on the industry. Technology has also made a pervasive change in the industry. Biomedical and genetic research, along with advances in information technology, are producing rapid changes in treatment. In addition, the industry has experienced increased government mandates such as the Medicare Prescription Drug, Improvement and Modernization Act of 2003 and the Health Insurance Portability and Accountability Act of 1996. With an increased focus on disease management, patients are living longer and are requiring increased long-term and home health care now and in the future. Patients' and healthcare workers' characteristics are also changing. Both populations are becoming older and more diverse. Patients are better informed and, as such, have increasingly higher expectations of healthcare professionals. This trend has changed the way healthcare services are delivered, with a focus on patient satisfaction and quality of services. Physician–patient relationships have changed because patients are beginning to understand that much of the responsibility for wellness lies with them. The economics of health care is in a state of flux. For example, reimbursements are directly linking payments to hospitals with quality of care; therefore, we will see an increase in the use of evidence-based medicine. There are continuing shortages of staff, especially in the areas of nursing, imaging technicians, and pharmacists, leading to competition for well-qualified people. There are changes taking place in the disease environment. Many factors of modern life are contributing to the emergence of new diseases, reemergence of old ones, and evolution of pathogens immune to many of today's medications. In addition, because of terrorism attacks, healthcare providers are concerned with biodisaster preparedness. Finally, there continues to be the issue of caring for the uninsured that contributes to the overuse and misuse of hospital emergency departments.

To deal with these changes, we have seen a number of healthcare organizations restructure themselves into integrated delivery networks, which may be part of a local, regional, or national system. We have seen increased vertical, horizontal, and virtual integration. Vertical integration focuses on the development of a continuum of care services to meet the patient's full range of healthcare needs. This integration model, in which a single entity owns and operates all the segments providing care, may include preventive services, specialized and primary ambulatory care, acute care, subacute care, long-term care, and home health care, as well as a health plan. Horizontal integration usually occurs through mergers, acquisitions, and/or consolidation within one segment of the industry. For example, during the 1990s we saw numerous hospital acquisitions by the large, for-profit, privately, and publicly held hospital chains of HCA/Columbia, Tenet Healthcare System, or Health Management Association. In addition, not-for-profit hospitals have merged with for-profit health systems as a result of competition. Virtual integration, which emphasizes coordination of healthcare services through patient-management agreements, provider incentives, and/or information systems, has increased. This virtual integration has evolved to meet the need for better technology and information infrastructures that allow for information sharing, patient care management, and cost control.

Because of the dramatic changes and the future trends in the healthcare industry, most managers have been required to change the way they and their employees carry out their job responsibilities. These changes have been forced upon the industry by the need to increase productivity due to decreasing reimbursement and increasing competition. At the same time, healthcare providers must continue to demonstrate high-quality patient care. These are not easy tasks! As a result, many healthcare providers are breaking down their traditional hierarchical structures and moving toward team-managed environments (Sovie, 1992). Employees are finding themselves in new roles with new responsibilities. All of these changes cause disruptions in the workplace. The study of OB will assist healthcare managers to minimize the negative effects (such as stress and conflict) of this "new" environment and maximize their ability to motivate staff and effectively lead their organizations. [For a discussion of changing organization structures, see Part VII—Organization Theory and Design.]

HISTORY OF ORGANIZATIONAL BEHAVIOR

The beginnings of OB can be found within the human relations/behavioral management movement, which emerged during the 1920s as a response to the traditional or classic management approach. Beginning in the late 1700s, the Industrial Revolution was the driving force for the development of large factories employing many workers. Managers at that time were concerned "about how to design and manage work in order to increase productivity and help organizations attain maximum efficiency" (Daft, 2004, p. 24). This traditional approach included Frederick Taylor's (1911) well-known framework of scientific management, or "Taylorism," as it is now labeled. Taylor believed that efficiency was achieved by creating jobs that economized time, human energy, and other productive resources. Through his time-and-motion studies, Taylor scientifically divided manufacturing processes into small efficient units of work. Through Taylor's work, productivity greatly increased. For example, Henry Ford developed his assembly line according to the principles of Taylorism and was able to churn out Model Ts at a remarkable and economical pace (Benjamin, 2003).

Although the classic approach to management focused on efficiency within organizations (see Chapter 19), Taylor did attempt to address a human relations aspect in the workplace. In his book, *The Principles of Scientific Management*, Taylor stated that:

> in order to have any hope of obtaining the initiative (i.e., best endeavors, hard work, skills and knowledge, ingenuity, and good-will) of his workmen the manager must give some special incentive to his men beyond that which is given to the average of the trade. This incentive can be given in several different ways, as, for example, the hope of rapid promotion or advancement; higher wages, either in the form of generous piecework prices or of a premium or bonus of some kind for good and rapid work; shorter hours of labor; better surroundings and working conditions than are ordinarily given, etc., and, above all, this special incentive should be accompanied by that personal consideration for, and friendly contact with, his workmen which comes only from a genuine and kindly interest in the welfare of those under him. It is only by giving a special inducement or incentive of this kind that the employer can hope even approximately to get the initiative of his workmen.

Although Taylor discussed a concern for workers within the scientific management approach, the human relations or behavioral movement of management did not begin until after the landmark Hawthorne Studies.

THE HAWTHORNE STUDIES

Elton Mayo, Frederick Roethlisberger, and their colleagues from Harvard Business School conducted a number of experiments from 1924 to 1933 at the Hawthorne Plant of the Western Electric Company in Cicero, Illinois. The Hawthorne Studies were significant to the development of OB because they demonstrated the important influence of human factors on worker productivity. It was through these experiments that the Hawthorne Effect was identified. The Hawthorne Effect is the bias that occurs when people know that they are being studied. Roethlisberger and Dickson (1939) in their book *Management and the Worker* and Homans (1950) in his book *The Human Group* provided a comprehensive account of the Hawthorne Studies. There were four phases to the Hawthorne Studies: the illumination experiments, the relay-assembly group experiments, the interviewing program, and the bank-wiring observation-room group studies. The intent of these studies was to determine the effect of working conditions on productivity.

The illumination experiments were conducted to determine whether increasing or decreasing lighting would lead to changes in productivity. The researchers were surprised to learn that productivity increased by both the control group (no change in lighting) and the experimental group (lighting alternated upward and downward). The researchers determined it was not the lighting that caused the increased productivity, but that it resulted from the attention received by the group.

In the relay-assembly group experiments, productivity of a segregated group of workers was studied as they were subjected to different working conditions. The researchers and management closely observed the group for five years. During the first part of the experiment, the working conditions of employees were improved by extending their rest periods, decreasing the length of their workday, and providing them a "free" day and lunches. In addition, the workers were consulted before any changes were made, because their agreement had to be obtained before the change would be implemented. The workers of the group were given the freedom to interact with one another during the workday. Furthermore, one researcher also served as their supervisor who, during the experiment, expressed concern about their physical health and well-being. The researchers eagerly sought the employees' opinions, hopes, and fears during the experiment. During the improved-conditions period, the workers' productivity increased. Part two of the experiment called for the original working conditions to be restored. Again, the researchers were surprised to see that the employees' productivity remained at the previous high level (when they had the improved working conditions). This result was attributed to group dynamics in that the group was allowed to develop socially with a common purpose.

The bank-wiring observation-room experiment was similar to the relay-assembly experiment. A group of workers were segregated so their productivity and group dynamics could be studied. The workers were paid with a piecework rate that reflected both group and individual efforts. The researchers found that the wage incentive did not work. The group had developed its own standard as to what constituted a "proper day's work." As such, the group's level of productivity remained constant because they did not want management to know that they could produce at a higher level. If a member of the group produced more than the agreed-upon level, the other members influenced the "rate buster" to return his productivity level to the group's norm. In addition, if a member of the group failed to produce the required level of output, the other members traded jobs to ensure the group's output level remained constant. The results of the bank-wiring experiment mirrored the relay-assembly experiment results. The researchers concluded that there was no cause-and-effect relationship between working conditions and productivity and that any increase or decrease in productivity was attributed to group dynamics. (See Chapter 13 for a detailed discussion of group dynamics.)

As a result of the bank-wiring experiment, researchers became very interested in exploring informal employee groups and the social functions that occur within the group and that influence the behavior of the individual group members. As part of the Hawthorne Studies, the researchers conducted extensive interviews with the employees. Over 21,000 interviews were conducted to determine the employees' attitudes toward the company and their jobs. A major outcome of these interviews was that the researchers discovered that workers were not isolated, unrelated individuals; they were social beings and their attitudes toward change in the workplace were based upon (1) the personal social conditioning (values, hopes, fears, expectations, etc.) they brought to the workplace, formed from their previous family or group associations, and (2) the human satisfaction the employee derived from his or her social participation with coworkers and supervisors. As such, the researchers learned that an employee's expression of dissatisfaction may be a symptom of an underlying problem on the job, at home, or in the person's past.

THEORY X AND Y

Another significant impact in the development of OB came from Douglas McGregor (1957, 1960) when he proposed two theories by which managers motivated their employees: Theory X and Theory Y. However, as Ott (1996, p. 28) points out, McGregor's Theory X and Theory Y is about much more than the motivation of people at work. "In its totality, it is a cogent articulation of the basic assumptions of the organizational behavior perspective. . . ." Theory X and Theory Y are ways of seeing and thinking about people, which, in turn, affect their behavior.

Theory X states that employees are unintelligent and lazy. They dislike work, avoiding it whenever possible. In addition, employees should be closely controlled because they have little desire for responsibility, have little aptitude for creativity in solving organizational problems, and will resist change. In contrast, Theory Y states that employees are creative and competent; they want meaningful work; they want to contribute; and they want to participate in decision-making and leadership functions.

Borrowing from Maslow's *Hierarchy of Needs* (see Chapter 5 for a full discussion of this motivation theory), McGregor stated that the autocratic, or Theory X managers were no longer effective in the workplace because they relied on an employee's lower needs for motivation (physiological concerns and safety), but in modern society those needs were mostly satisfied and thus no longer acted as a motivator for the employee. For example, managers would ask, "Why aren't people more productive? We pay good wages, provide good working conditions, have excellent fringe benefits and steady employment. Yet people do not seem to be willing to put forth more than minimum efforts." The answers to these questions were embedded in Theory X's managerial assumptions of people. If managers believed that their employees had an inherent dislike for work and must be coerced, controlled, and directed to achieve organizational goals, the resulting behavior was nothing more than self-fulfilling prophesies. (See Chapter 3 for a discussion of the self-fulfilling prophecy–Pygmalion effect.) The manager's assumptions caused the staff's "unmotivated" behavior.

However, at the opposite end of the spectrum from Theory X, McGregor proposed Theory Y, where managers created opportunities, removed obstacles, and encouraged growth and learning for their employees. McGregor stated that participative, or Theory Y managers supported decentralization and delegation, job enlargement, and participative management because they allowed employees degrees of freedom to direct their own activities and to assume responsibility, thereby satisfying their higher-level needs (see Figure 1–1).

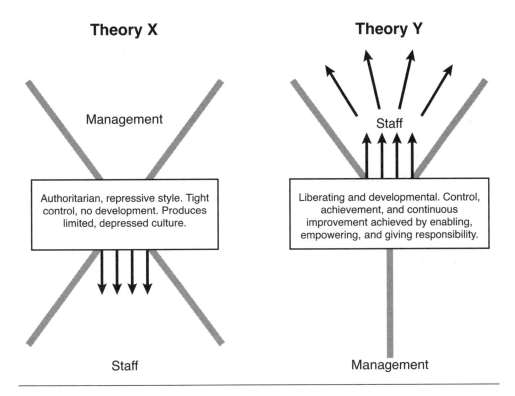

Figure 1–1 McGregor X-Y Theory Diagram (SOURCE: © Alan Chapman 2001–4, based on Douglas McGregor's X-Y Theory. Reprinted with permission.)

SUMMARY

Since 1960, a wealth of information has emerged within the study of OB, which will be addressed in this textbook. In Part I, the issues of diversity, perceptions and attitudes, and communication are discussed. Part II addresses motivation and individual behaviors. Part III examines the subject of leadership from four approaches—power and influence, behavioral, contingency, and transformational. Part IV emphasizes the importance of intrapersonal and interpersonal issues within the context of stress and conflict management. Part V examines group dynamics, working in groups, and teams and team-building. Part VI provides an overview of managing organizational change within the context of organizational development. Part VII changes our focus to a macro level of analysis, in which we examine the organization as a whole.

Before we conclude this chapter, I would like to explain the differences between OB and three other related fields—organization theory (OT), organizational development (OD), and human resources management (HRM). As noted previously, OB is the study of individual and group dynamics within an organization setting and, therefore, is a micro-approach. OT analyzes the entire organization and is a macro perspective, since the organization is the unit examined (see Part VII). The field of OD describes a planned process of change that is used throughout the organization, with the goal of improving the effectiveness of the organization (see Chapter 17). Since, like OT, OD involves the entire organization, it is a macro examination. Finally, HRM can be viewed as a micro-approach to "managing" people. The difference between HRM and OB is that the latter is theoretically based and the former is commonly viewed as a functional unit within organizations (Luthans, 2002).

END-OF-CHAPTER DISCUSSION QUESTIONS

1. Define organizational behavior.
2. What are some of the major challenges facing today's and tomorrow's healthcare organizations and healthcare managers? Why?
3. Why did the Hawthorne Studies have an impact on the study of organizational behavior?
4. Why did McGregor's Theory X and Theory Y have an impact on the study of organizational behavior?
5. Discuss the difference between organizational behavior, organization theory, organizational development, and human resources management.

X-Y THEORY QUESTIONNAIRE

Score the statements (5 = always, 4 = mostly, 3 = often, 2 = occasionally, 1 = rarely, 0 = never), to indicate whether the situation and management style is 'X' or 'Y':

SCORE

1. My boss asks me politely to do things, gives me reasons why, and invites my suggestions.　＿＿＿＿＿

2. I am encouraged to learn skills outside of my immediate area of responsibility.　＿＿＿＿＿

3. I am left to work without interference from my boss, but help is available if I want it.　＿＿＿＿＿

4. I am given credit and praise when I do good work or put in extra effort.　＿＿＿＿＿

5. People leaving the company are given an "exit interview" to hear their views on the organization.　＿＿＿＿＿

6. I am incentivized to work hard and well.　＿＿＿＿＿

7. If I want extra responsibility, my boss will find a way to give it to me.　＿＿＿＿＿

8. If I want extra training, my boss will help me find how to get it or will arrange it.　＿＿＿＿＿

9. I call my boss and my boss's boss by their first names.　＿＿＿＿＿

10. My boss is available for me to discuss my concerns or worries or suggestions.　＿＿＿＿＿

11. I know what the company's aims and targets are.　＿＿＿＿＿

12. I am told how the company is performing on a regular basis.　＿＿＿＿＿

13. I am given an opportunity to solve problems connected with my work.　＿＿＿＿＿

14. My boss tells me what is happening in the organization.　＿＿＿＿＿

15. I have regular meetings with my boss to discuss how I can improve and develop.　＿＿＿＿＿

TOTAL SCORE　＿＿＿＿＿

RESULTS:
60–75 = strong Y-Theory management (effective short- and long-term)
45–59 = generally Y-Theory management
16–44 = generally X-Theory management
　0–15 = strongly X-Theory management (autocratic, may be
　　　　　effective short-term, poor long-term)

(Continued)

Score the statements (5 = always, 4 = mostly, 3 = often, 2 = occasionally, 1 = rarely, 0 = never), to indicate whether the person prefers being managed by 'X' or 'Y' style

SCORE

1. I like to be involved and consulted by my boss about how I can best do my job. _____

2. I want to learn skills outside of my immediate area of responsibility. _____

3. I like to work without interference from my boss, but be able to ask for help if I need it. _____

4. I work best and most productively without pressure from my boss or the threat of losing my job. _____

5. When I leave the company, I would like an 'exit interview' to give my views on the organization. _____

6. I like to be incentivized and praised for working hard and well. _____

7. I want to increase my responsibility. _____

8. I want to be trained to do new things. _____

9. I prefer to be friendly with my boss and the management. _____

10. I want to be able to discuss my concerns, worries, or suggestions with my boss or another manager. _____

11. I like to know what the company's aims and targets are. _____

12. I like to be told how the company is performing on a regular basis. _____

13. I like to be given opportunities to solve problems connected with my work. _____

14. I like to be told by my boss what is happening in the organization. _____

15. I like to have regular meetings with my boss to discuss how I can improve and develop. _____

TOTAL SCORE _____

RESULTS:
60–75 = strongly prefers Y-theory management
45–59 = generally prefers Y-theory management
16–44 = generally prefers X-theory management
 0–15 = strongly prefers X-theory management

© Alan Chapman 2001–4, based on Douglas McGregor's X-Y Theory. Reprinted with permission.

Most people prefer 'Y-theory' management. These people are generally uncomfortable in 'X-theory' situations and are unlikely to be productive, especially long-term, and are likely to seek alternative situations. These short assessments provide a broad indication as to management style and individual preference, using the 'X-Y Theory' definitions.

REFERENCES

Benjamin, M. (2003, February 24). Fads for any and all eras. *U.S. News & World Report, 134,* 74–75.

Bureau of Labor Statistics, U.S. Department of Labor. (2008). Career guide to industries, 2008-09 edition, health care, on the Internet at http://www.bls.gov/oco/cg/cgs035.htm, last accessed February 11, 2008.

Daft, R. L. (2004). *Organization theory and design* (8th ed.). Mason, OH: Thomson South-Western.

Homans, G. C. (1950). *The human group.* New York: Harcourt, Brace and Company.

Luthans, F. (2002). *Organizational behavior* (9th ed.). New York: McGraw-Hill Book Company.

McGregor, D. M. (1957). The human side of enterprise. *Management Review, 46,* 22–28.

McGregor, D. M. (1960). *The human side of enterprise.* New York: McGraw-Hill Book Company.

Ott, J. S. (1996). *Classic readings in organizational behavior* (2nd ed.). Albany, NY: Wadsworth Publishing Company.

Roethlisberger, F. J., & Dickson, W. J. (1939). *Management and the worker.* Cambridge, MA: Harvard University Press.

Sovie, M. (1992). Care and service teams: A new imperative. *Nursing Economics, 10,* 94–100.

Taylor, F. W. (1911). *The principles of scientific management.* New York: Harper and Brothers.

CHAPTER 2

Diversity in Health Care

Jean Gordon, RN, DBA

LEARNING OUTCOMES

After completing this chapter, the student should be able to:

- Define diversity.
- Define cultural competency.
- Define diversity management.
- Understand why changes in US demographics affect the healthcare industry.

OVERVIEW

Demographics of the US population have changed dramatically in the last three decades. These changes directly impact the healthcare industry in regard to the patients we serve and our workforce. By 2050, the term "minority" will take on a new meaning. According to the US Census Bureau, by mid-century the white, non-Hispanic population will comprise less than 50 percent of the nation's population. As such, the healthcare industry needs to change and adopt new ways to meet the diverse needs of our current and future patients and employees.

The American Heritage Dictionary of the English Language (4th ed.) defines diversity as: "(1) the fact or quality of being diverse; difference, and (2) a point in which things differ." Dreachslin (1998) provided us with a more specific definition of diversity. She defined diversity as "the full range of human similarities and differences in group affiliation including gender, race/ethnicity, social class, role within an organization, age, religion, sexual orientation, physical ability, and other group identities" (p. 813). For our discussions, we will focus on the following diversity characteristics: (1) race/ethnicity, (2) age, and (3) gender.

This chapter is presented in three parts. First, we discuss the changing demographics of the nation's population. Second, we examine how these changes are affecting the delivery of health services from both the patient's and employee's perspectives. Because diversity challenges faced by the healthcare industry are not limited to quality-of-care and access-to-care issues, in the third part of our discussions we explore how these changes will affect the health services workforce, and more specifically the current and future leadership within the industry.

17

CHANGING UNITED STATES POPULATION

There is no doubt that the demographic profile of the US population has undergone significant changes within the past 10 years regarding age, gender, and ethnicity (see Table 2–1).

During the 1990s, the combined US population of black non-Hispanic, Native Americans, Asians, Pacific Islanders, and Hispanics/Latinos grew at 13 times the rate of the white non-Hispanic population (United States Department of Commerce, 2000). In addition, for the first time respondents to the 2000 US Census were allowed to choose more than one racial category. In fact, 1.6 percent of the US population (6.8 million people) did so by identifying with and choosing two or more races (United States Department of Commerce, 2003, p. 24). It is predicted that the number of Americans reporting themselves or their children as multiracial is expected to increase. In addition to the changing ethnic and racial composition of America, another issue is the aging population. According to the US Census Bureau, 35 million people (12.4

Table 2–1 Resident Population of the United States by Age, Gender, Race/Ethnicity, and Region

	1990		2000	
	Number	Percent	Number	Percent
Total population	248,709,873	100.0	281,421,906	100.0
Under age 18	63,604,432	25.6	72,293,812	25.7
Ages 18 to 64	153,863,610	61.9	174,136,341	61.9
Ages 65 and over	31,241,831	12.6	34,991,753	12.4
Males	121,239,418	48.7	138,053,563	49.1
Females	127,470,455	51.3	143,368,343	50.9
White, non-Hispanic[a]	188,128,296	75.6	194,552,774	69.1
Black, non-Hispanic[a]	29,216,293	11.7	33,947,837	12.1
Hispanic	22,354,059	9.0	35,305,818	12.5
Asian, non-Hispanic[a]	6,968,359	2.8	10,476,678	3.7
American Indian, non-Hispanic[a]	1,793,773	0.7	2,068,883	0.7
Some other race, non-Hispanic[a]	249,093	0.1	467,770	0.2
Two or more races, non-Hispanic	N/A	N/A	4,602,146	1.6

SOURCE: AmeriStat, August 2001.
CITATIONS:
U.S. Census Bureau, Census 2000 Redistricting Data (PL 94-171) Summary File for States, Tables PL1, PL2, PL3, and PL4, accessed at www.census.gov/population/www/cen2000/phc-t1.html (August 17, 2001); U.S. Census Bureau, "Table DP-1. Profile of General Demographic Characteristics for the United States: 2000," accessed at www.census.gov/Press-Release/www/2001/tables/dp_us_2000.xls (August 17, 2001); and U.S. Census Bureau, "Table DP-1. Profile of General Demographic Characteristics for the United States: 1990," accessed at www.census.gov/Press-Release/www/2001/tables/dp_us_1990.xls (August 17, 2001).
NOTE: N/A = Not Available.
[a]For 2000, excludes people who identified with two or more races.

percent of the US population) are 65 years of age or older. This is 3.8 million more people than in 1990 (see Figure 2–1).

Although this was the first time in the history of the census that the population aged 65 and over did not grow faster than the total population, it is predicted that the trend will reverse as the baby boomers (those born between 1946 and 1964) reach age 65 starting in 2011 (see Figure 2–2).

In addition to the increasingly older population, there is a declining number of young people in America. From 1950 to 2000, the percentage of the American population under the age of 18 fell from 31 percent to 26 percent (United States Department of Commerce, 2003, p. 23). This decline in America's younger population will have a direct effect on the industry's ability to recruit healthcare professionals to provide sufficient services in the future. Young people of all ethnicities must be attracted to the healthcare industry as a career choice in order to meet the healthcare needs of the country's growing population.

Although males and females are almost evenly divided, representing 50.9 percent and 49.1 percent, respectively, in the population under 25 years, males dominate females with 105 males for every 100 females. However, among older adults, the male–female ratio changes, with women outnumbering men. For people 55 to 64 years old, the male–female ratio is 92 to 100, but for those 85 and over, the ratio decreases to only 41 men for every 100 women (United States Department of Commerce, 2003).

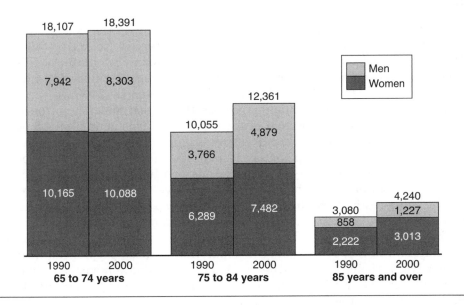

Figure 2–1 Population 65 Years and Over by Age and Sex: 1990 and 2000 (Numbers in thousands. For information on confidentiality protection, nonsampling error, and definitions, see www.census.gov/prod/cen2000/doc/sfl.pdf.) (Source: U.S. Census Bureau, Census 2000 Summary File I: 1990 Census of Population, General Population Characteristics, United States (1990 CP-1-1).)

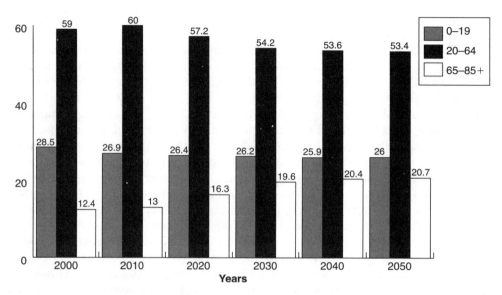

Figure 2–2 Projected Population of the United States by Age 2000–2050 (Source: U.S. Census Bureau, Population Division, Population Projections Branch. Last Revised May 18, 2004.)

Race/Ethnicity

The US population has continued to diversify during the last 30 years, as minority populations continue to increase at a faster rate than the white, non-Hispanic population. Although the white, non-Hispanic population still represents the largest group (69 percent) of the US population, this is down from 83 percent in 1970 (United States Department of Commerce, 2003).

In 2000, the Hispanic population became the largest minority in the United States, representing 12.5 percent of the population. This is up from 4.5 percent in 1970, the first census in which Hispanic origin was identified. The remaining population comprises approximately 12 percent black non-Hispanics, 4 percent Asians and Pacific Islanders, 1 percent American Indians and Alaska Natives, and 1.6 percent of those who identified themselves as belonging to more than one race. Interestingly, of the 6.8 million people reporting two or more races, 42 percent were under 18 (United States Department of Commerce, 2003).

The Asian population in the United States is increasing faster than the total population. From 1990 to 2000, the population of those people who identified themselves as being Asian (either alone or in combination with another race) grew 72 percent, while the total population grew only 13 percent (United States Department of Commerce, 2003).

Aging Population

According to the 2000 US Census, people aged 85 and over showed the highest percentage increase of the country's population. This group represented

9.9 percent in 1990 and increased to 12.2 percent of the "older" population in 2000. It is estimated that this group will represent 5 percent of the total US population by 2050 and will represent 31 percent of the older population.

One of the most striking characteristics of the older population is the change in the ratio of men to women as people age (United States Department of Commerce, 2003). In 2000, for the group aged 65 and over, there were 70 men for every 100 women, and 41 men for every 100 women in the group over 85. It is predicted that in 2050 men will represent 37 percent of the 85 and over group, and 46 percent of the 65 and over group. Therefore, in the future the elderly population will be 46 percent men and 54 percent women.

The elderly comprise a nonhomogeneous population. The racial composition of the older population differs from the racial composition of the US population as a whole. In 2000, the US population, as a whole, included 69 percent white non-Hispanic, 12 percent black non-Hispanic, 12 percent Hispanic, 4 percent Asian, and approximately 3 percent other races. A much higher proportion of the population over 65 is white non-Hispanic (more than 86 percent). Eight percent of the older population is black non-Hispanic and 5 percent is Hispanic. Asians make up just over two percent of this group, with other races forming the remainder. This racial composition will change over the next two decades. By 2030, it is predicted that black non-Hispanic, Hispanic, and Asian populations will show the greatest population increase (United States Department of Commerce, 2004).

Gender

As previously noted, according to the US Census Bureau, in 2000, 50.9 percent of the US population was female, and 49.1 percent was male. That translates to 96 men for every 100 women. However, the ratio of men to women varies significantly by age group. There were about 105 males for every 100 females under 25 in 2000, reflecting the fact that more boys than girls are born every year and that boys continue to outnumber girls through early childhood and young adulthood. However, the male–female ratio declines as people age. For men and women aged 25 to 54, the number of men for each 100 women in 2000 was 99. Among older adults, the male–female ratio continued to fall rapidly, as women increasingly outnumbered men. For people 55 to 64, the male–female ratio was 92 to 100, but for those 85 and over, there were only 41 men for every 100 women (United States Department of Commerce, 2003). These male/female ratios reflect a new trend occurring since 1980. From 1900 to 1940, there were more males. Beginning in 1950, there were increasingly more females due to reduced female mortality rates. This trend reversed between 1980 and 1990 as male death rates declined faster than female rates and as more men immigrated to the United States than women (United States Department of Commerce, 2003).

When we look at education, it appears that females are outpacing men. Among the population aged 25 and over, 84 percent of both men and women were high school graduates. However, in this age group, 28 percent of men had graduated from college as compared to 25 percent of women. But in the 25 to 29 age group, more college graduates are women than men, with 30 percent of women holding a bachelor's degree or higher, in comparison to 28 percent of men. However, even with college degrees, a high number of women continue to be employed in administrative support positions. Therefore, it is not surprising that only 5.5 percent of working women reported earnings of $75,000 or more, as compared to 15.8 percent for men.

Implications for the Healthcare Industry

The changing demographics of America's population affect the healthcare industry twofold. First, healthcare professionals need to have cultural competence to provide effective and efficient health services to diverse patient populations. However, before we continue our discussion, we need to define what is meant by cultural competence (see Hofstede's Cultural Dimensions, Exhibit 2–1). Although the literature provides many definitions of cultural competence, such as "ongoing commitment or institutionalism of appropriate practice and policies for diverse populations" (Brach & Fraser, 2000;

Exhibit 2–1 Hofstede's Cultural Dimensions

One of most extensive cross-cultural surveys ever conducted is Hofstede's (1983) study of the influence of national culture on organizational and managerial behaviors. National culture is deemed to be central to organizational studies, because national cultures incorporate political, sociological, and psychological components.

Hofstede's research was conducted over an 11-year period, with more than 116,000 respondents in more than 40 countries. The researcher collected data about "values" from the employees of a multinational corporation located in more than 50 countries. On the basis of his findings, Hofstede proposed that there are four dimensions of national culture, within which countries could be positioned, that are independent of one another. Hofstede's (1983, pp. 78–85) four dimensions of national culture were labeled and described as:

- *Individualism–Collectivism:* Individualism–collectivism measures culture along a self-interest versus group-interest scale. Individualism stands for a preference for a loosely knit social framework in society wherein individuals are supposed to take care of themselves and their immediate families only. Its opposite, collectivism, stands for a preference for a tightly knit social framework in which individuals can expect their relatives, clan, or other in-group to look after them in exchange for unquestioning loyalty. Hofstede (1983) suggested that self-interested cultures (e.g., individualism) are positively related to the wealth of a nation.

- *Power Distance:* Power distance is the measure of how a society deals with physical and intellectual inequalities, and how the culture applies power and wealth relative to its inequalities. People in large Power Distance societies accept hierarchical order in which everybody has a place, which needs no further justification. People in small Power Distance societies strive for power equalization and demand justification for power inequalities. Hofstede (1983) indicated that group interest cultures (e.g., Collectivism) have large Power Distance.

- *Uncertainty Avoidance:* Uncertainty avoidance reflects the degree to which members of a society feel uncomfortable with uncertainty and ambiguity. The scale runs from tolerance of different behaviors (i.e., a society in which there is a natural tendency to feel secure) to one in which the society creates institutions to create security and minimize risk. Strong Uncertainty Avoidance societies maintain rigid codes of belief and behavior and are intolerant toward deviant personalities and ideas.

- *Weak Uncertainty:* Avoidance societies maintain a more relaxed atmosphere in which practice counts more than principles and deviance is more easily tolerated.
- *Masculinity versus Femininity.* Masculinity versus femininity measures the division of roles between the genders. The masculine side of the scale is a society in which the gender differences are maximized (e.g., need for achievement, heroism, assertiveness, and material success). Feminine societies are ones in which there are preferences for relationships, modesty, caring for the weak, and the quality of life.

Hofstede proposed that the most important dimensions for organizational leadership are Individualism/Collectivism and Power Distance and the most important for decision making are Power Distance and Uncertainty Avoidance. Uncertainty Avoidance plays an integral part in a country's culture regarding change. For example, Nahavandi and Malekzadeh (1999, pp. 495–496) point out that countries such as Greece, Portugal, and Japan have national cultures that do not easily tolerate uncertainty and ambiguity. Therefore, the resultant behavior emphasizes the issue avoidance or the importance of planned and well-managed activities. Other countries such as Sweden, Canada, and the United States are able to tolerate change because of the potential for new opportunities that may come with change.

The question frequently asked is whether Hofstede's (1983) cultural dimensions are still applicable today? Patel (2003) found that the characteristics of Chinese, Indian, and Australian cultures corroborated Hofstede's study results. Patel's study of the relationship between business goals and culture, measured by correlating the relative importance attached to the various business goals with the national culture dimension scores from Hofstede's study, found that although the four cultural dimension scores were nearly 20 years old, they were validated in this large, cross-national survey. In a study that measured 1,800 managers and professionals in 15 countries, statistically significant correlations with the Hofstede indices validated the applicability of the first study's cultural dimension findings (Hofstede et al., 2002). The findings from these studies suggest that Hofstede's cultural dimensions continue to be robust and are still applicable measure components of national culture differences.

Note: Hofstede (1991) subsequently included an additional dimension based on Chinese values referred to "Confucian dynamism." Hofstede renamed this dimension as a long-term versus short-term orientation in life.

Weech-Maldonado et al., 2002), for our discussions we adopted the definition used by the Office of Minority Health (OMH) of the US Department of Health and Human Services, which defines cultural competence as a set of congruent behaviors, attitudes, and policies that come together in a system, in an agency, or among professionals and that enables effective work in cross-cultural situations. "Culture" refers to integrated patterns of human behavior that include the language, thoughts, communications, actions, customs, beliefs, values, and institutions of racial, ethnic, religious, or social groups. "Competence" implies having the capacity to function effectively as an individual and an organization within the context of the cultural beliefs, behaviors, and needs presented by consumers and their communities (HHS Office of Minority Health, 1999).

Second, because of the changing demographics of the nation's population, the healthcare industry needs to ensure that the healthcare workforce mirrors the patient population it serves, both clinically and managerially. As noted by Weech-Maldonado et al. (2002), healthcare organizations must develop policies and practices aimed at recruiting, retaining, and managing a diverse workforce in order to provide both culturally appropriate care and improved access to care for racial/ethnic minorities.

Diversity Issues within the Clinical Setting

Consider the following:

Scenario One: An insulin-dependent, indigent black non-Hispanic male was treated at a predominantly Hispanic border clinic. Later, he was brought back to the clinic in a diabetic coma. When he awoke, the nurse who had counseled him asked whether he had been following her instructions. "Exactly!" he replied. When the nurse asked him to show her, the monolingual Spanish-speaking nurse was startled when the patient proceeded to inject an orange and eat it.

Scenario Two: As Maria (an elderly, monolingual Hispanic female) was being prepared for surgery, which was not why she came to the hospital, her designated interpreter (a young female relative) is told by an English-speaking nurse to tell Maria that the surgeon is the best in his field and she'll get through this fine. The young interpreter translated, "the nurse says the doctor does best when he's in the field and when it's over you'll have to pay a fine!"

These may seem rather humorous misunderstandings, but real-life experiences such as these happen every day in the United States (Howard et al., 2001). For example, a recent survey by the Commonwealth Fund (2002) found that black non-Hispanics, Asian Americans, and Hispanics are more likely than white non-Hispanics to experience difficulty communicating with their physician, to feel that they are treated with disrespect when receiving health care, to experience barriers to access to care, such as lack of insurance or not having a regular physician, and to feel they would receive better care if they were of a different race or ethnicity. In addition, the survey found that Hispanics were more than twice as likely as white non-Hispanics (33% vs. 16%) to cite one or more communication problems such as not understanding the physician, not being listened to by the physician, or not asking questions they needed to ask. Twenty-seven percent of Asian Americans and 23 percent of black non-Hispanics experience similar communication difficulties.

Cultural differences between providers and patients affect the provider–patient relationship. For example, Fadiman (1998) related a true and poignant story of cultural misunderstanding within the healthcare profession. Fadiman described the story of a young female epileptic Hmong immigrant whose parents believed that their daughter's condition was caused by spirits called "dabs," which had caught her and made her fall down, hence the name of Fadiman's book *The Spirit Catches You and You Fall Down*. The patient's parents struggled to understand the prescribed medical care that only recognized the scientific necessities, but ignored their personal belief about the spirituality of one's soul in relationship to the universe. From a unique perspective, Fadiman examined the roles of the caregivers (physicians, nurses, and social workers) in the treatment of ill children. She studied the way the medical care system responded to its own perceptions that the family was refusing to comply with medical orders without understanding the meaning of those orders in the context of the Hmong culture, language, and beliefs.

Because of our increasingly diverse population, healthcare professionals need to be concerned about their cultural competency, which is more than just cultural awareness or sensitivity. Although formal cultural training has been found to improve the cultural competence of healthcare practitioners, a recent study found that only 8 percent of US medical schools and no Canadian medical schools had formal courses on cultural issues (Kundhal, 2003). However, changes are occurring within the industry to reduce the healthcare disparities among different minority groups (see Exhibit 2–2) by assisting healthcare practitioners in developing their cultural competences as they encounter more diverse patients.

One leader in this effort has been the Commonwealth Fund. The Commonwealth Fund (2003), in addition to funding initiatives regarding quality of care for underserved populations, has also initiated an educational program that assists healthcare practitioners in understanding the importance of communication between culturally diverse patients and their physicians, the tensions between modern medicine and cultural beliefs, and the ongoing problems of racial and ethnic discrimination. The goals of this program are for clinicians to:

1. Understand that patients and healthcare professionals often have different perspectives, values, and beliefs about health and illness that can lead to conflict, especially when communication is limited by language and cultural barriers.

2. Become familiar with the types of issues and challenges that are particularly important in caring for patients of different cultural backgrounds.

3. Think about each patient as an individual, with many different social, cultural, and personal influences, rather than using general stereotypes about cultural groups.

Exhibit 2–2 Unequal Treatment

A study in 2002 by the Institute of Medicine, entitled Unequal Treatment: Confronting Racial and Ethnic Disparities in Health Care, found that a consistent body of research demonstrates significant variation in the rates of medical procedures by race, even when insurance status, income, age, and severity of conditions are comparable. This research indicated that US racial and ethnic minorities receive even fewer, routine medical procedures and experience a lower quality of health services than the majority of the population. For example, minorities are less likely to be given appropriate cardiac medications or to undergo bypass surgery, and are less likely to receive kidney dialysis or transplants. By contrast, they are more likely to receive certain less desirable procedures, such as lower limb amputations for diabetes.

The study's recommendations for reducing racial and ethnic disparities in health care included increasing awareness about disparities among the general public, healthcare providers, insurance companies, and policymakers.

Source: *Unequal Treatment: Confronting Racial and Ethnic Disparities in Health Care* (p. 3), by B. D. Smedley, A. Y. Stitch, and A. R. Nelson (Eds.), 2002, Washington, DC: National Academy of Sciences, Institute of Medicine Committee on Understanding and Eliminating Racial and Ethnic Disparities in Health Care.

4. Understand how discrimination and mistrust affect the interaction of patients with physicians and the healthcare system.

5. Develop a greater sense of curiosity, empathy, and respect toward patients who are culturally different, and thus be encouraged to develop better communication and negotiation skills through ongoing instruction.

In addition to the Commonwealth Fund, the W.K. Kellogg Foundation has led efforts to lessen the recognized disparity of racial and ethnic minority groups' representation among the nation's health professionals. It was the Kellogg Foundation that requested the recent Institute of Medicine's (2004) study entitled *In the Nation's Compelling Interest: Ensuring Diversity in the Health Care Workforce*. The Institute of Medicine found that racial and ethnic diversity is important in the health professions because:

1. Racial and minority healthcare professionals are significantly more likely than their peers to serve minority and medically underserved communities, thereby helping to improve problems of limited minority access to care.

2. Minority patients who have a choice are more likely to select healthcare professionals of their own racial or ethnic background. Moreover, racial and ethnic minority patients are generally more satisfied with the care that they receive from minority professionals, and minority patients' ratings of the quality of their health care are generally higher in racially concordant than in racially discordant settings.

3. Diversity in healthcare training settings may assist in efforts to improve the cross-cultural training and competencies of all trainees.

In addition to the Commonwealth Fund and the W.K. Kellogg Foundation, other organizations have begun to bridge cultural differences in the attempt to lessen health disparities due to cultural differences. For example, the OMH has developed a list of 14 standards for Culturally and Linguistically Appropriate Services (CLAS), which healthcare organizations and practitioners should use to ensure equal access to quality health care by diverse populations. The 14 standards are:

1. Promote and support the attitudes, behaviors, knowledge, and skills necessary for staff to work respectfully and effectively with patients and one another in a culturally diverse work environment.

2. Have a comprehensive management strategy to address culturally and linguistically appropriate services, including strategic goals, plans, policies, procedures, and designated staff responsible for implementation.

3. Utilize formal mechanisms for community and consumer involvement in the design and execution of service delivery, including planning, policy-making, operations, evaluation, training, and, as appropriate, treatment planning.

4. Develop and implement a strategy to recruit, retain, and promote qualified, diverse, and culturally competent administrative, clinical, and support staff that are trained and qualified to address the needs of the racial and ethnic communities being served.

5. Require and arrange for ongoing education and training for administrative, clinical, and support staff in culturally and linguistically competent service delivery.

6. Provide all clients with Limited English Proficiency access to bilingual staff or interpretation services.

7. Provide oral and written notices, including translated signage at key points of contact, to clients in their primary language, informing them of their right to receive no-cost interpreter services.

8. Translate and make available signage and commonly used written patient educational material and other materials for members of the predominant language groups in service areas.

9. Ensure that interpreters and bilingual staff can demonstrate bilingual proficiency and receive training that includes the skills and ethics of interpreting, as well as knowledge in both languages of the terms and concepts relevant to clinical or nonclinical encounters. Family or friends are not considered adequate substitutes, because they usually lack these abilities.

10. Ensure that the clients' primary spoken language and self-identified race/ethnicity are included in the healthcare organization's management information system as well as any patient records used by provider staff.

11. Use a variety of methods to collect and utilize accurate demographic, cultural, epidemiological, and clinical-outcome data for racial and ethnic groups in the service area, and become informed about the ethnic/cultural needs, resources, and assets of the surrounding community.

12. Undertake ongoing organizational self-assessments of cultural and linguistic competence, and integrate measures of access, satisfaction, quality, and outcomes for CLAS into other organizational internal audits and performance-improvement programs.

13. Develop structures and procedures to address cross-cultural ethical and legal conflicts in healthcare delivery and complaints or grievances by patients and staff about unfair, culturally insensitive or discriminatory treatment, difficulty in accessing services, or denial of services.

14. Prepare an annual progress report documenting the organization's progress with implementing CLAS standards, including information on programs, staffing, and resources.

Aging Population

In addition to the changing ethnic and racial composition of America, another area of concern is the growing elderly population. Technology has given us the ability to enhance longevity; the challenge now is whether or not the healthcare profession can learn how to best serve this growing population of patients.

As our citizens grow older, more services are required for the treatment and management of both acute and chronic health conditions. The profession must devise strategies for caring for the elderly patient population. America's older citizens are often living on fixed incomes and have small or nonexistent support groups. While this may be considered an American infrastructure dilemma, the reality is that medical professionals must be able to understand and empathize with poor, sick, elderly people of all races, sexes, and creeds.

Ageism can be defined as "any attitude, action, or institutional structure, which subordinates a person or group because of age or any assignment of roles in society purely on the basis of age" (Traxler, 1980, p. 4). Healthcare professionals often make assumptions about their older patients on the basis of age rather than functional status. This may be due to the limited training physicians receive in the care and management of geriatric patients. For example, Warshaw (2002) related that only 10 percent of US medical schools require coursework or rotation in geriatric medicine. Although medical schools offer geriatric courses as electives, fewer than 3 percent of medical school graduates choose to take these courses. A report from the Alliance for Aging Research (2003) related that there continue to be shortcomings in medical training, prevention, screening, and treatment patterns that disadvantage older patients. The report outlined four key recommendations to safeguard against ageist bias:

1. Increase training and education of healthcare providers and research into aging. The training infrastructure needs to be enhanced so physicians, nurses, pharmacists, and allied health professionals receive appropriate exposure to geriatrics. Geriatrics competency and knowledge should be part of licensing and credentialing examinations wherever appropriate.

2. Include older patients in clinical trials. Older people are consistently excluded from clinical trials, even though they are the largest users of approved drugs.

3. Utilize appropriate screening and treatment methods. Older patients are less likely than younger people to receive preventative care and are less likely to be tested or screened for diseases and other health problems. As such, proven medical interventions for older patients are often ignored, leading to inappropriate or incomplete treatment.

4. Empower and educate older Americans. Older patients neglect to bring health problems to the attention of their care providers, contributing to the symptoms of old age.

Diversity Management

Diversity management is a challenge to all organizations. Diversity management is "a strategically driven process whose emphasis is on building skills and creating policies that will address the changing demographics of the workforce and patient population" (Svehla, 1994; Weech-Maldonado et al. 2002). A study by the National Urban League (2004) found that few American workers believed their companies had effective diversity programs. The two-year study, entitled Diversity Practices That Work: The American Worker

Speaks, surveyed more than 5,500 American workers regarding their views on diversity. Although 45 percent believed that diversity was part of the organization's corporate culture of their respective employers, only 32 percent believed that their company had an effective diversity initiative. The study found that workers tended to have more favorable perceptions of diversity initiatives at companies where:

1. Leaders demonstrated a personal commitment to diversity and held themselves and others accountable.
2. Diversity training increased diversity awareness and provided a link to improving business results.
3. There was an established track record for recruiting people of diverse backgrounds.
4. Employees earned rewards for their contributions in diversity.

Studies on diversity within the healthcare industry reflect that it has been slow to embrace diversity management. For example, a study by Motwani et al. (1995) found that only 27.7 percent of healthcare workers in six Midwest hospitals felt that their institutions had a program to improve employee skills in dealing with people of different cultures and only 38.9 percent felt that management realized that cultural factors were sometimes the cause of conflicts among employees. The healthcare industry may be slow to embrace diversity management because of the low percentage of demographic diversity in senior management positions.

Healthcare Leadership

The American College of Healthcare Executives (ACHE), the National Association of Health Services Executives (NAHSE), and the Institute for Diversity in Healthcare Management (IFD) released a study in 2003 that measured the representation of black non-Hispanics, Hispanics, women, and other minorities in healthcare executive leadership roles. This study was a follow-up to similar studies completed in 1992 and 1997. The study, completed in 2002, was based on a random-sample survey of 1,621 healthcare executives. Respondents worked in a variety of settings—hospitals, healthcare-provider organizations, government health agencies, and consulting and educational institutes (see Table 2–2).

Although the results of the 1997 study reflected improvements in diversity over the 1992 study, the 2002 results indicated that the healthcare industry did not do as well in promoting minorities and women in positions of chief executive officers, chief operating officers, and senior vice presidents as in subsequent years. In the 2002 ACHE study (see Table 2–3), only 23 percent of black non-Hispanic female respondents held senior management positions in 1997, as compared to 26 percent in 2002. Although white non-Hispanic female healthcare senior managers made progress, from 35 percent in 1997 to 40 percent in 2002 (see Table 2–4), the gap between white non-Hispanic males and females holding senior healthcare management positions widened from 16 percent in 1997 to 22 percent in 2002.

Table 2–2 American College of Healthcare Executives 2002 Diversity Study
Population, Sample, and Response Rates[a]

	1992		1997				2002				
	Black	White	Black	White	Hispanic	Asian	Black	White	Hispanic	Asian	Native American
Population	795	17,775	1,623[b]	16,096	662[c]	235	2,033[d]	13,601	449[e]	240	153[f]
Sample	517	966	767	802	662	2.5	1,573	1,608	449	24	153
Response	367	565	410	408	264	124526	779	215	118	68	
Response Rate (%)	46.2	58.5	53.5	50.9	39.9	52.8	33.4	48.4	47.9	49.2	44.4
Analyzed[a]	328	524	380	386	240	115497	742	204	114	64	
Males	165	242	177	192	154	76222	359	125	65	37	
%	50.3	46.2	46.6	49.7	64.2	66.1	44.7	48.4	61.3	57	57.8
Females	163	282	203	194	86	39275	383	79	49	27	
%	49.7	53.8	53.4	50.3	35.8	33.9	55.3	51.6	38.7	43	42.2

SOURCE: American College of Healthcare Executives. Reprinted with permission.

[a]Responses were analyzed if they were from employed healthcare executives who gave their gender.

[b]Composed of 603 ACHE members, 375 of whom were sampled, and 224 of whom responded,
and 1,020 NAHSE members, 625 of whom were sampled, and 186 of whom responded (233 having proved unlocatable).

[c]Composed of 296 ACHE members, 179 of whom responded, and 366 members and contacts of Association of Hispanic Healthcare Executives (AHHE), 85 of whom responded.

[d]Composed of 696 ACHE members, 539 of whom were sampled and 282 of whom responded, and 1337 NAHSE members, 1034 of whom were sampled and 244 of whom responded.

[e]Composed of 281 ACHE members, 159 of whom responded, and 168 AHHE members, 56 of whom responded.

[f]Composed of 51 ACHE members, 29 of whom responded, and 102 EDLP members, 39 of whom responded.

Table 2-3 American College of Healthcare Executives 2002 Diversity Study
Position by Race/Ethnicity and Year Males

	1992		1997				2002				
	Black	White	Black	White	Hispanic	Asian	Black	White	Hispanic	Asian	Native American
PCEO	23%	35%[a]	17%	26%	23%	16%	19%	37%	23%	11%	32%[b]
COO/Senior Vice President	48	65	43	51	47	36	44	62	47	34	46
Vice President	20	16	19	23	19	21	24	19	23	20	16
Department Head	20	10	27	13	21	28	22	10	20	31	30
Department Staff/Other	13	8	11	13	12	15	11	9	10	15	8
	100%[d]	100%[d]	100%	100%	100%[d]	100%	100%	100%	100%	100%	100%
n	(163)	(240)	(168)	(198)	(145)	(75)	(216)	(355)	(123)	(65)	(37)
Position Level in Hierarchy											
1 5 CEO	29	37[b]	17	26	24	18[c]	18	37	24	15	33[b]
2	20	24	17	26	15	13	17	26	16	22	21
3	22	26	19	22	20	29	25	20	14	20	21
4	13	8	24	14	23	26	15	13	20	18	15
51	17	5	22	13	18	13	24	4	26	25	9
	100%[d]	100%	100%[d]	100%[d]	100%	100%[d]	100%	100%	100%	100%	100%
n	(152)	(230)	(149)	(188)	(136)	(68)	(206)	(328)	(111)	(55)	(33)

SOURCE: American College of Healthcare Executive. Reprinted with permission.
[a]Chi-square significant P, .01.
[b]Chi-square significant P, .001.
[c]Chi-square significant P, .05
[d]Responses may not total to 100 because of rounding.

31

Table 2-4 American College of Healthcare Executives 2002 Diversity Study
Position by Race/Ethnicity and Year Females

	1992		1997				2002				
	Black	White	Black	White	Hispanic	Asian	Black	White	Hispanic	Asian	Native American
CEO	13%	9%[a]	9%	10%	6%	5%[a]	11%	13%	9%	9%	12%[b]
COO/Senior Vice President	31	34	23	35	26	15	26	40	25	24	28
Vice President	17	28	22	24	25	21	19	28	24	19	8
Department Head	20	14	33	25	33	23	39	19	32	34	44
Department Staff/Other	32	24	22	16	16	41	17	14	20	26	20
	100%	100%	100%	100%	100%	100%[d]	100%	100%	100%	100%	100%
n	(161)	(280)	(203)	(191)	(80)	(39)	(266)	(381)	(76)	(47)	(25)
Position Level in Hierarchy											
1 5 CEO	12	9[b]	10	12	7	6[c]	10	14	9	10	13[b]
2	15	25	8	23	15	22	14	28	15	15	9
3	23	35	28	31	32	13	21	28	31	18	52
4	30	18	23	21	26	28	23	18	22	25	13
51	20	13	31	14	20	31	33	12	22	32	13
	100%[d]	100%	100%[d]	100%[d]	100%	100%[d]	100%	100%	100%	100%	100%
n	(150)	(266)	(170)	(173)	(74)	(32)	(229)	(353)	(67)	(40)	(23)

SOURCE: American College of Healthcare Executive. Reprinted with permission.

[a]Chi-square significant P, .01.
[b]Chi-square significant P, .001.
[c]Chi-square significant P, .05
[d]Responses may not total to 100 because of rounding.

In 2003, the National Center for Healthcare Leadership (NCHL) commissioned a study to identify specific strategies to advance careers of women and racially/ethnically diverse individuals in healthcare management. Dreachslin and Curtis's (2004, p. 456) literature review confirmed the findings of the 2002 ACHE report that career advancement of women and racially/ethnically diverse individuals in healthcare management was characterized by: (1) underrepresentation, especially in senior-level management positions; (2) lower compensation, even controlling for education and experience; and (3) more negative perceptions of equity and opportunity in the workplace. The researchers identified three areas that are key organization-specific factors for shaping career outcomes for women and racially/ethnically diverse individuals: (1) leadership and strategic orientation (i.e., senior management's commitment for successful implementation of diversity initiatives), (2) organizational culture/climate (i.e., the depth and breadth of the organization's strategic commitment to diversity leadership and cultural competence), and (3) human resources practices (i.e., establishing best practices in advancing the management careers of women and racially/ethnically diverse individuals, such as formal mentoring programs, professional development, work/life balances, and flexible benefits).

On the basis of Dreachslin's and others' research, the NCHL, ACHE, IFD, and the American Hospital Association developed the Diversity and Cultural Proficiency Assessment Tool for Leaders (see Exhibit 2–3). The assessment tool begins the process of developing a cultural awareness for the organization's workforce. Going forward, managers will need to develop models that establish benchmarks for cultural competence to enable their organizations to develop competent interventions, thereby improving the quality of health care (Betancourt et al., 2002).

Exhibit 2–3 A Diversity and Cultural Proficiency Assessment Tool for Leaders

CHECKLIST		
As Diverse as the Community You Serve	YES	NO
• Do you monitor at least every three years the demographics of your community to track change in gender and racial and ethnic diversity?	___	___
• Do you actively use these data for strategic and outreach planning?	___	___
• Has your community relations team identified community organizations, schools, churches, businesses, and publications that serve racial and ethnic minorities for outreach and educational purposes?	___	___
• Do you have a strategy to partner with them to work on health issues important to them?	___	___
• Has a team from your hospital met with community leaders to gauge their perceptions of the hospital and to seek their advice on how you can better serve them, both in patient care and community outreach?	___	___
• Have you done focus groups and surveys within the past three years in your community to measure the public's perception of your hospital as being sensitive to diversity and cultural issues?	___	___
• Do you compare the results among diverse groups in your community and act on the information?	___	___

(Continued)

Exhibit 2–3 *(Continued)*

	YES	NO

- Are the individuals who represent your hospital in the community reflective of the diversity of the community and your organization?   ____ ____
- When your hospital partners with other organizations for community health initiatives or sponsors community events, do you have a strategy in place to be certain you work with organizations that relate to the diversity of your community?   ____ ____
- As a purchaser of goods and services in the community, does your hospital have a strategy to ensure that businesses in the minority community have an opportunity to serve you?   ____ ____
- Are your public communications, community reports, advertisements, health education materials, Web sites, etc. accessible to and reflective of the diverse community you serve?   ____ ____

Culturally Proficient Patient Care

- Do you regularly monitor the racial and ethnic diversity of the patients you serve?   ____ ____
- Do your organization's internal and external communications stress your commitment to culturally proficient care and give concrete examples of what you're doing?   ____ ____
- Do your patient satisfaction surveys take into account the diversity of your patients?   ____ ____
- Do you compare patient satisfaction ratings among diverse groups and act on the information?   ____ ____
- Have your patient representatives, social workers, discharge planners, financial counselors, and other key patient and family resources received special training in diversity issues?   ____ ____
- Does your review of quality assurance data take into account the diversity of your patients in order to detect and eliminate disparities?   ____ ____
- Has your hospital developed a "language resource," identifying qualified people inside and outside your organization who could help your staff communicate with patients and families from a wide variety of nationalities and ethnic backgrounds?   ____ ____
- Are your written communications with patients and families available in a variety of languages that reflects the ethnic and cultural fabric of your community?   ____ ____
- Depending on the racial and ethnic diversity of the patients you serve, do you educate your staff at orientation and on a continuing basis on cultural issues important to your patients?   ____ ____
- Are core services in your hospital . . . such as signage, food service, chaplaincy services, patient information, and communications attuned to the diversity of the patients you care for?   ____ ____
- Does your hospital account for complementary and alternative treatments in planning care for your patients?   ____ ____

Strengthening Your Workforce Diversity

- Do your recruitment efforts include strategies to reach out to the racial and ethnic minorities in your community?   ____ ____
- Does the team that leads your workforce recruitment initiatives reflect the diversity you need in your organization?   ____ ____
- Do your policies about time off for holidays and religious observances take into account the diversity of your workforce?   ____ ____

	YES	NO

- Do you acknowledge and honor diversity in your employee communications, awards programs, and other internal celebrations?
- Have you done employee surveys or focus groups to measure their perceptions of your hospital's policies and practices on diversity and to surface potential problems?
- Do you compare the results among diverse groups in your workforce? Do you communicate and act on the information?
- Have you made diversity awareness and sensitivity training available to your employees?
- Is the diversity of your workforce taken into account in your performance evaluation system?
- Does your human resources department have a system in place to measure diversity progress and report it to you and your board?
- Do you have a mechanism in place to look at employee turnover rates for variances according to diverse groups?
- Do you ensure that changes in job design, workforce size, hours, and other changes do not affect diverse groups disproportionately?

Expanding the Diversity of Your Leadership Team

- Has your Board of Trustees discussed the issue of the diversity of the hospital's board? Its workforce? Its management team?
- Is there a Board-approved policy encouraging diversity across the organization?
- Is your policy reflected in your mission and values statement? Is it visible on documents seen by your employees and the public?
- Have you told your management team that you are personally committed to achieving and maintaining diversity across your organization?
- Does your strategic plan emphasize the importance of diversity at all levels of your workforce?
- Has your board set goals on organizational diversity, culturally proficient care, and eliminating disparities in care to diverse groups as part of your strategic plan?
- Does your organization have a process in place to ensure diversity reflecting your community on your Board and subsidiary and advisory boards?
- Have you designated a high-ranking member of your staff to be responsible for coordinating and implementing your diversity strategy?
- Have sufficient funds been allocated to achieve your diversity goals?
- Is diversity awareness and cultural proficiency training mandatory for all senior leadership, management, and staff?
- Have you made diversity awareness part of your management and board retreat agendas?
- Is your management team's compensation linked to achieving your diversity goals?
- Does your organization have a mentoring program in place to help develop your best talent, regardless of gender, race, or ethnicity?
- Do you provide tuition reimbursement to encourage employees to further their education?
- Do you have a succession/advancement plan for your management team linked to your overall diversity goals?
- Are search firms required to present a mix of candidates reflecting your community's diversity?

SOURCE: Institute for Diversity in Health Management. (2004). Reprinted with permission.

In order to best serve their patient base, healthcare organizations and providers must be willing to invest the time, money, and effort needed to educate all their employees. Educating senior staff is important, but so is educating the entire healthcare workforce. For healthcare managers to transform their organizations into an inclusive culture where all employees feel the opportunity to reach their full potential, Guillory (2004, pp. 25–30) recommended a ten-step process:

1. Development of a customized business case for diversity for your organization. In other words, how does diversity relate to the overall success of the organization?

2. Education and training for your staff to develop an understanding of diversity, its importance to your organization's success, and diversity skills to apply on a daily basis.

3. Establishment of a baseline by conducting a comprehensive cultural survey that integrates performance, inclusion, climate, and work/life balance.

4. Selection and prioritization of the issues that lead to the greatest breakthrough in transforming the culture.

5. Creation of a three- to five-year diversity strategic plan that is tied to organizational strategic business objectives.

6. Leadership's endorsement of and financial commitment to the plan.

7. Establishment of measurable leadership and management objectives to hold managers accountable to top leadership for achieving these objectives.

8. Implementation of the plan, recognizing that surprises and setbacks will occur along the way.

9. Continued training in concert with the skills and competencies necessary to successfully achieve the diversity action plan.

10. Survey one to one-and-a-half years after initiation of the plan to determine how inclusion has changed.

The Future Workforce

As part of diversity management, healthcare managers need to devise strategies for attracting younger workers to enter the healthcare field while maintaining positive relationships with older workers. For example, Barney (2002, p. 83) points out Generation-X workers (individuals born between 1965 and 1976) want "managers who listen, consider their ideas, and treat them as peers. They want to be part of the decision-making process and want flexibility in their work environment because they value their time and freedom."

What about Generation-Y workers, sometimes referred to as the echo boomers and millennials? Generation-Y, individuals born from 1977 to 1995, are beginning to enter the workforce. Generation-Y will be the fastest-growing segment of the workforce—growing from 14% of the workforce to 21% over the past four years to nearly 32 million workers (Armour, 2005). Although it is impossible to generalize about the wants and needs of millions of people in each generation, workplace experts tend to use the following characteristics to describe Generation-Y (Martin & Tulgan, 2006):

- *High expectations of self:* They aim to work faster and better than other workers.
- *High expectations of employers:* They want fair and direct managers who are highly engaged in their professional development.
- *Ongoing learning:* They seek out creative challenges and view colleagues as vast resources from whom to gain knowledge.
- *Immediate responsibility:* They want to make an important impact on day one.
- *Goal-oriented:* They want small goals with tight deadlines so they can build up ownership of tasks.

In addition to the younger workers, healthcare managers must also consider the needs of older workers. For example, in a recent Robert Wood Johnson Foundation study, Hatcher and colleagues (2006) suggested that hospitals seeking to recruit and retain older nurses needed to implement strategies, such as flexible work hours, increased benefits, newly created professional roles, and an atmosphere of respect for nurses.

Generational diversity poses challenges for today's and tomorrow's employers. Younger workers have a strong need for immediate feedback, workers now in their 30s and 40s demand greater work–life balance and flexibility, and older workers expect increased benefits and professionalism. With a multigenerational workforce, employers will need to develop age-diversity training programs for their managers so they can better understand the needs and expectations of each generation (Martin & Tulgan, 2006).

SUMMARY

Healthcare organizations need to be flexible to change to meet diversity challenges. The greatest barrier to the industry's success may be its inability to understand and appreciate the increasing diversity within our population, whether relating to patients or employees.

END-OF-CHAPTER DISCUSSION QUESTIONS

1. Discuss what the term diversity means.
2. Explain the meaning of cultural competency.
3. What do we mean when we say "diversity management"?
4. Explain why and how changes in US demographics affect the healthcare industry.

EXERCISE 2–1

You have been asked to join the hospital's task force for developing a plan to increase the organization's workforce diversity from its current 10 percent level to 30 percent over the next five years. What recommendations would you make as a member of the task force?

EXERCISE 2–2

Interview a healthcare professional who was born and raised in a country other than your own. Focus on the following topics:

- Family background
- Cultural background
- Educational background
- Community
- Religious background

Analysis: List some of the major differences between your background and the interviewee. What are some of the similarities? Discuss what you believe some of the major challenges are to raising healthcare professionals' awareness of diversity.

EXERCISE 2–3

In December 2006, the American College of Healthcare Executives released its fourth report in a series of research surveys designed to compare the career attainments of men and women healthcare executives. View this report, titled A Comparison of the Career Attainments of Men and Women Healthcare Executives, December 2006, at www.ache.org. In small groups, discuss the changes regarding women advancing to senior leadership positions that have occurred in the healthcare industry since the previous report in 2000.

REFERENCES

Alliance for Aging Research. (2003). Ageism: How healthcare fails the elderly. Last accessed January 28, 2008 from http://www.agingresearch.org.

American College of Healthcare Executives. (2002). A race/ethnic comparison of career attainments in healthcare management, Summary Report—2002. Last accessed February 11, 2008 from http://www.ache.org.

Armour, S (2005, November 6). Generation Y: They arrived at work with an attitude. *USA Today*. Retrieved January 15, 2008 from http://www.usatoday.com/money/workplace/2005-11-06-gen-y_x.htm.

Barney, S. M. (2002). A changing workforce calls for twenty-first century strategies. *Journal of Healthcare Management, 47*(2), 61–65.

Betancourt, J., Green, A.R., & Carrillo, E. (2002). Cultural competence in health care: Emerging frameworks and practical approaches. The Commonwealth Fund. Available at: http://www.commonwealthfund.org/usr_doc/betancourt_culturalcompetence_576.pdf?section=4039.

Brach, C., & Fraser, I. (2000). Can cultural competency reduce racial and ethnic racial health disparities? A review and conceptual model. *Medical Care Review, 57*(Suppl. 1), , 181–217.

Commonwealth Fund. (2003). Worlds apart: A film series on cross-cultural health care, Last accessed April 20, 2004 from http://www.cmwf.org.

Commonwealth Fund. (2002). International health policy survey of adults with health problems, Last accessed April 20, 2004 from http://www.cmwf.org.

Dreachslin, J. L. (1998). Conducting effective focus groups in the context of diversity: Theoretical underpinnings and practical implications. *Qualitative Health Research, 8*(6), 813–820.

Dreachslin, J. L., & Curtis, E. F. (2004). Study of factors affecting the career advancement of women and racially/ethnically diverse individuals in healthcare management. *The Journal of Health Administration Education, 21*(4), 441–484.

Fadiman, A. (1998). The spirit catches you and you fall down. New York: Farrar, Straus and Giroux.

Guillory, W. A. (2004). The roadmap to diversity, inclusion, and high performance. *Healthcare Executive, 19*(4), 24–30.

Hatcher, B., Bleich, M. R., Connolly, C., Davis, K., O'Neill Hewlett, P., & Stokley Hill, K. (2006). Wisdom at work: The importance of the older and experienced nurse in the workplace. Princeton, NJ: The Robert Wood Johnson Foundation. Available at: http://www.rwjf.org/files/publications/other/wisdomatwork.pdf

HHS Office of Minority Health. (1999). Assuring cultural competence in healthcare: Recommendations for national standards and outcomes-focused research agenda, Last accessed January 20, 2008 from http://www.omhrc.gov/CLAS.

Hofstede, G. (1983). The cultural relativity of organizational practices and theories. *Journal of International Business Studies, 14*(2), 75–89.

Hofstede, G., Van Deusen, C. A., Mueller, C. B., & Charles, T. A. (2002). What goals do business leaders pursue? A study in fifteen countries. *Journal of International Business Studies, 33*(4), 785–803.

Howard, C., Andrade, S. J., & Byrd, T. (2001). The ethical dimensions of cultural competence in border healthcare settings. *Family and Community Health, 23*(4), 36–49.

Institute for Diversity in Health Management. (2004). Strategies for leadership: Does your hospital reflect the community it serves? Last accessed February 11, 2008 from http://www.diversityconnection.org.

Institute of Medicine. (2004). In the nation's compelling interest: Ensuring diversity in the health care workforce. Washington, DC: National Academy Press.

Kundhal, K. K. (2003). Cultural diversity: An evolving challenge to physician-patient communication. *Journal of the American Medical Association, 289*(1), 94.

Martin, C. & Tulgan, B. (2006). Managing the generation mix, 2nd edition. Armhurst, MA: HRD Press.

Motwani, J., Hodge, J., & Crampton, S. (1995). Managing diversity in the healthcare industry. *The Healthcare Supervisor, 13*(3), 16–25.

Nahavandi, A., & Malekzadeh, A. R. (1999). Organizational behavior: The person-organization fit. Upper Saddle River, NJ: Prentice Hall.

National Urban League (2004). Diversity practices that work: The American worker speaks, Last accessed January 18, 2008 from http://www.nul.org.

Patel, C. (2003). Some cross-cultural evidence on whistle-blowing as an internal control mechanism. *Journal of International Accounting Research, 2,* 69–96.

Svehla, T. (1994). Diversity management; key to future success. *Frontiers of Health Services Management, 11*(2), 3–33.

Traxler, A. J. (1980). Let's get gerontologized: Developing a sensitivity to aging. The multi-purpose senior center concept: A training manual for practitioners working with the aging. Springfield, IL: Illinois Department of Aging.

United States Department of Commerce, Bureau of the Census. (2000). Current population reports: Population projections of the United States by age, sex, race, and Hispanic origin: 1995 to 2050, Last accessed January 18, 2008 from http://www.npg.org/facts/us_pop_projections.htm.

United States Department of Commerce, Bureau of the Census. (2003). Chartbook on trends in the health of Americans. Retrieved March 21, 2004 from InfoTrac on-line database.

United States Department of Commerce, Bureau of the Census. (2004). US interim projections by age, sex, race, and Hispanic origin, Last accessed February 9, 2008 from http://www.census.gov/ipc/www/usinterimproj/, Internet Release Date: March 18, 2004.

Warshaw, G. A. (2002). Academic geriatrics programs in US allopathic and osteopathic medical schools. *Journal of the American Medical Association, 288,* 2313–2319.

Weech-Maldonado, R., Dreachslin, J. L., Dansky, K. H., DeSouza, G., & Gatto, M. (2002). Racial/ethnic diversity management and cultural competency: the case of Pennsylvania hospitals. *Journal of Healthcare Management, 47*(2), 111–124.

OTHER SUGGESTED READING

The Institute of Medicine's 2004 Report: In the Nation's Compelling Interest: Ensuring Diversity in the Healthcare Workforce. A copy of the full text of the study can be found at: www.nap.edu/catalog/10885.html.

A full list of reference texts discussing cultural beliefs and influences, issues, and how to identify/develop materials can be found on the National Center for Cultural Healing, at: www.culturalhealing.com/patientedu.htm.

Information relating to Anne Fadiman's book, *The Spirit Catches You and You Fall Down*, may be viewed at: www.spiritcatchesyou.com.

Learn more about how language and culture affect the delivery of quality services to ethnically diverse populations at: www.diversityrx.org.

CHAPTER 3

Attitudes and Perceptions

Nancy Borkowski, DBA, CPA, FACHE*

LEARNING OUTCOMES

After completing this chapter, the student should be able to:

- ☛ Appreciate the importance of attitudes to understanding behavior.
- ☛ Understand the three components of attitude.
- ☛ Understand how attitudes can be changed.
- ☛ Understand how perceptions allow individuals to simplify their worlds.
- ☛ Understand the four stages of the perception process.
- ☛ Understand social perception and the various subgroups.
- ☛ Understand the importance of using objective methods for employee selection.

OVERVIEW

This chapter explains how understanding the psychology of attitudes and perceptions can help us better manage the employees of the health services organizations in which we work. Psychological principles, when applied to organizational behavior issues, can assist healthcare managers to deal with staff fairly, make jobs interesting and satisfying, and motivate employees to higher levels of productivity. By the end of this chapter, you will gain some key insights into attitudes and perception and how they relate to human behavior.

ATTITUDES

What is an attitude? Allport (1935) defined an attitude as a mental or neural state of readiness, organized through experience, exerting a directive or dynamic influence on the individual's response to all objects and situations to which it is related. A simpler definition of attitude is a mind-set or a tendency to act in a particular way toward an object or entity (i.e., person, place, or thing) due to both an individual's experience and temperament.

Typically, when we refer to a person's attitudes, we are attempting to explain his or her behavior. Attitudes are a complex combination of an individual's personality, beliefs, values, behaviors, and motivations. As an example, we understand when someone says, "She has a positive attitude toward work" versus "She has a poor work attitude." When we speak of someone's attitude,

*I wish to acknowledge and thank Dr. Jeffrey Pickens, who was a contributing author of an earlier version of this chapter, which appeared in *Organizational Behavior in Health Care* (2005), Jones and Bartlett Publishers.

we are referring to the person's emotions and behaviors. A person's attitude toward preventive medicine encompasses his or her point of view about the topic (e.g., thought) and how he or she feels about this topic (e.g., emotion), as well as the actions (e.g., behaviors) he or she engages in as a result of attitude to preventing health problems. This is the tri-component model of attitudes (see Figure 3–1). An attitude includes three components: an affect (a feeling), cognition (a thought or belief), and behavior (an action).

Attitudes help us define how we see situations, as well as define how we behave toward the situation or object. As illustrated in the tri-component model, attitudes include feelings, thoughts, and actions. Attitudes may simply be an enduring evaluation of a person or object (e.g., "I like John best of my coworkers") or other emotional reactions to objects and to people (e.g., "I dislike working on the department's annual budget" or "Jane makes me angry"). Attitudes also provide us with internal cognitions or beliefs and thoughts about people and objects (e.g., "Jane should work harder" or "Sam does not like working in this department"). Attitudes cause us to behave in a particular way toward an object or person (e.g., "I write clearly in patients' charts because it upsets me when I can't read others' handwriting"). Although the feeling and belief components of attitudes are internal to a person, we can view a person's attitude from his or her resulting behavior.

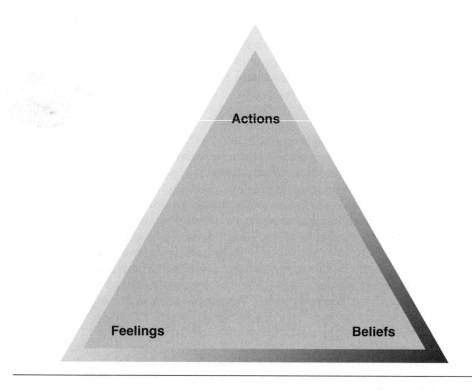

Figure 3–1 Tri-component Model of Attitudes

COGNITIVE DISSONANCE

Alfred Adler (1870–1937), a Viennese physician who developed the theory of Individual Psychology, emphasized that a person's attitude toward the environment had a significant influence on his or her behavior. Adler suggested that a person's thoughts, feelings, and behaviors were transactions with one's physical and social surroundings and that the direction of influence flowed both ways—our attitudes are influenced by the social world and our social world is influenced by our attitudes. These interactions, however, may cause a conflict between a person's attitude and behavior. This conflict is referred to as cognitive dissonance. Cognitive dissonance refers to any inconsistency that a person perceives between two or more of one's attitudes or between one's behavior and attitudes. Festinger (1957) stated that any form of inconsistency that is uncomfortable for the person will prompt the person to reduce the dissonance (conflict). As an example, Harry likes two coworkers, John and Mary, but John does not like Mary (i.e., inconsistency). Harry needs to eliminate the inconsistency. Harry may: (1) try to change John's feelings toward Mary, (2) change his feelings about either John or Mary, or (3) sever his relationship with either John or Mary (see Scott's Dilemma, Case Study 3–1).

Case Study 3–1 Scott's Dilemma

Scott is a licensed physical therapist who works for a national rehabilitation company. The rehabilitation facility in which Scott works is located in an urban Southwest city. He has worked at this facility for 4 years and, until, recently, was satisfied with his working environment and the interactions he shared with his coworkers. In addition, Scott received personal fulfillment from helping his patients recover from their disabilities and seeing them return to productive lives.

Last year the health system went through reorganization, with some new people being brought in and others being reassigned. Scott's new boss, George, was transferred from one of the system's Midwest facilities. Almost immediately upon taking his new position, George began finding fault with Scott's care plans, patient interactions, and so forth. Scott began feeling as if he couldn't do anything right. He was experiencing feelings of anxiety, stress, and self-blame. Although his previous performance evaluations had been above average, Scott was shocked by his first performance review under George's authority—it was an extremely low rating.

Scott began trying to work harder, thinking that by working harder he could exceed George's expectations. Despite the long hours and addressing George's critiques, George continued to find fault with Scott's work. Staff meetings began to be a great source of discomfort and stress because George would belittle Scott and single him out in front of his colleagues.

Scott began to feel alienated from his family, friends, and colleagues at work. His eating and sleeping habits were adversely affected as well. Scott's activities held no joy for him and the career that he had once loved and been respected in became a source of pain and stress. He began to call in sick more often and started visualizing himself confronting and even hurting George, which created even more guilt and anxiety for Scott.

As time went on, George encouraged Scott's coworkers to leave Scott alone to do his work. The perception of the coworkers became more sympathetic to George's point of view. Scott's coworkers mused that perhaps Scott really was a poor worker and that George knew better because of his position as the supervisor of the rehabilitation department. Eventually, Scott's coworkers began to distance themselves from him, in order to protect their own interests. They began to see Scott as a outsider, with whom it was unsafe to associate.

In an effort to resolve the situation, Scott spoke to George directly, stating his feelings and expressing an interest in how they might improve the situation. Rather than making the situation better, what George perceived as Scott's insubordination served to enrage George, and the personal attacks against Scott intensified. Feeling frustrated and helpless, Scott then decided to take his problem to the Human Resources Department (HRD). A human resources manager listened to Scott's complaints and suggested that Scott return with documented evidence of what Scott perceived to be George's mistreatment. In an effort to help ease the situation, the HRD manager discussed the issue with George, which only stirred the flames of George's anger and his negative behavior toward Scott.

As a last resort, Scott decided to go to George's boss, Rebecca. Rebecca met with George to get his side of the story. George portrayed Scott as an unproductive employee with no respect for authority. The result was a strong letter of reprimand in Scott's file for insubordination.

Discuss the cognitive dissonance reflected in Scott's Dilemma.

SOURCE: Case discussion: Workplace bully, by J. Pinto, M. Vecchione, and L. Howard, October 2004, presented at the 12th Annual International Conference of the Association on Employment Practices and Principles, Ft. Lauderdale, FL. Reprinted with permission.

Other approaches a person may use to reduce the inconsistency are:

• Eliminating his or her responsibility or control over an act or decision.
• Denying, distorting, or "selectively" forgetting the information.
• Minimizing the importance of the issue, decision, or act.
• Selecting new information that is consonant with an attitude or behavior.

For example, why do people continue to smoke when the hazards of smoking are known? Using the cognitive dissonance theory, Kassarjian and Cohen (1965) attempted to analyze how smokers rationalize their behavior. They found that smokers justify their continued smoking by: (1) eliminating their responsibility for their behavior ("I am unable to stop" or "it takes too great an effort to stop"); (2) denying, distorting, misperceiving, or minimizing the degree of health hazard involved ("many smokers live a long time" or "lots of things are hazardous"); and/or (3) selectively drawing out information that reduces the inconsistency of the smoker's behavior ("smoking is better than excessive eating or drinking" or "smoking is better than being a nervous wreck").

Although the theory of cognitive dissonance helps us understand how individuals try to make sense of the world they live in, it does not predict what an individual will do to reduce or eliminate the dissonance (as reflected in the previous Harry/John/Mary example). It only relates that the individual will be motivated to "do something" to bring attitudes and behaviors into balance. Cognitive dissonance theory has many practical managerial applications for motivating employees and is the theoretical basis for what are known as the equity theories of motivation (Ott, 1996). (See Chapter 6 for a discussion of Adam's Equity Theory.) Equity theory predicts that employees pursue a balance between their investments in and the rewards gained from their work, such that their own investment/reward ratio is the same as that of similar others. Disturbance of this balance results in behaviors to relieve the dissonance. For example, if an employee perceives that another employee is paid more for the same level of productivity, the employee will be motivated to ask for a raise, decrease his or her level of productivity, or seek another job.

FORMATION OF ATTITUDES

How are attitudes formed? Attitude formation is a result of learning, modeling others, and direct experiences with people and situations. Attitudes influence our decisions, guide our behavior, and impact what we selectively remember (not always the same as what we hear). Attitudes come in different strengths, and like most things that are learned or influenced through experience, they can be measured and they can be changed.

Measurement of Attitudes

Since the publication of Thurstone's procedure for attitude assessment in 1929 (Thurstone & Chave, 1929), employee surveys have been widely used in organizations to obtain information about workers' attitudes toward their environments. This information is helpful for healthcare managers to determine whether management is "doing the right things" for retaining and motivating employees. As an example, Lowe et al. (2003) found that workers who rated their work environments as "healthy" (task content, pay, work hours, career prospects, interpersonal relationships, security) reported higher job satisfaction, morale, and organizational commitment and lower absenteeism and intent to quit. Employee-attitude surveys are usually designed using 5-point Likert-type ("strongly agree–strongly disagree") or frequency ("never–very often") response formats. Questions typically asked are illustrated in Figure 3–2. However, as

---

Legend (check [X] the correct number that applies to each question):

1 = Strongly Disagree   2 = Disagree   3 = Neutral
4 = Agree   5 = Strongly Agree

	1	2	3	4	5
1. Do you feel that your salary reflects your worth to the organization?					
2. Do you feel appreciated for your work performance?					
3. Do you feel a sense of achievement for your work efforts?					
4. Are you provided the opportunity for growth/advancement to higher level tasks?					
5. Do you feel that you contribute to the overall success of the organization?					
6. Would you recommend the organization to family and friends?					
7. Are you given the opportunity to learn new skills through formal training?					
8. Do you feel the organization provides adequate resources to complete your work?					
9. Do you feel overwhelmed by your workload?					
10. Do you experience ongoing interests in your job/tasks?					

Figure 3–2 Employee Attitude Survey

Morrel-Samuels (2002) points out, organizations need to be cautious regarding the design of employee surveys to ensure that problem areas are not overlooked. Morrel-Samuels provided 16 guidelines for organizations to consider when designing an employee attitude survey (see Exhibit 3–1).

Effective managers continuously survey their employees so they can detect problem areas and implement the necessary measures for change.

Changing Attitudes

How do you change someone's attitude? To change a person's attitude you need to address the cognitive and emotional components. How would you con-

---

Exhibit 3–1 Guidelines to Help Companies Improve Their Workplace Surveys

Content

- Ask questions about observable behavior rather than thoughts or motives.
- Include some items that can be independently verified.
- Measure only behaviors that have a recognized link to your company's performance.

Format

- Keep sections of the survey unlabeled and uninterrupted by page breaks.
- Design sections to contain a similar number of items, and questions with a similar number of words.
- Place questions about respondent demographics last in employee surveys but first in performance appraisals.

Language

- Avoid terms that have strong associations.
- Change the wording in about one-third of questions so that the desired answer is negative.
- Avoid merging two disconnected topics into one question.

Measurement

- Create a response scale with numbers at regularly spaced intervals and words only at each end.
- If possible, use a response scale that asks respondents to estimate a frequency.
- Use only one response scale that offers an odd number of options.
- Avoid questions that require rankings.

Administration

- Make workplace surveys individually anonymous and demonstrate that they remain so.
- In large organizations, make the department the primary unit of analysis for company surveys.
- Make sure that employees can complete the survey in about 20 minutes.

SOURCE: Getting the truth into workplace surveys, by P. Morrel-Samuels, 2002, *Harvard Business Review, 80*(2), pp. 111–118.

vince another person to start an exercise program when the individual may say, "I don't have enough time" or "I'm just too busy"? One approach would be to challenge someone's behavior by providing new information. As an example, explain to the other person how you made time in your day and how, as a result, both your cholesterol level and blood pressure decreased. This is a cognitive approach when a person is presented with new information. Providing new information is one method for changing a person's attitude and therefore his or her behavior. Attitude transformation takes time, effort, and determination, but it can be done. It is important not to expect to change a person's attitudes quickly, as illustrated by the following story:

Gerd's cell phone rang.

"Hello Gerd, this is Tom. We can't meet tomorrow morning, I've got to go to my doctor."

"I hope it's nothing serious," Gerd replied.

"Only a colonoscopy," Tom reassured Gerd.

"Only? Do you have pain?" said Gerd.

"No," Tom replied, "my doctor said I need to have one, I'm forty-five. Don't worry, in my family, nobody ever had colon cancer."

Gerd said, "It can hurt. Did your doctor tell you what the possible benefits of a colonoscopy are?"

"No," Tom said, "he just said it's a routine test, recommended by medical organizations."

"Why don't we find out on the Internet?"

The men met later that day. Gerd and Tom first looked up the report of the U.S. Preventive Services Task Force. It said that there is insufficient evidence for or against routine screening with colonoscopy. Tom is Canadian and responded that he does not bank on everything American. So Gerd and Tom looked up the Canadian Task Force report, and it had the same result. Just to be sure, the men checked Bandolier at Oxford University in the United Kingdom, and once again they found the same result. No professional health association that the men looked up reported that people should have a routine colonoscopy—after all, a colonoscopy can be extremely unpleasant—but many recommended the simpler, cheaper, and noninvasive fecal occult blood test. What did Tom do? If you think that he canceled his doctor's appointment the next day, you are as wrong as Gerd was. Unable to bear the evidence, Tom got up and left, refusing to discuss the issue any further. Tom wanted to trust his doctor.

SOURCE: *Gut feelings: The intelligence of the unconscious*, by G. Gigerenzer, 2007, New York: Viking Penguin. Reprinted with permission.

Managers need to understand that attitude change takes time and should not set unrealistic expectations for rapid change (Moore, 2003). Attitudes are formed over a lifetime through an individual's socialization process. An individual's socialization process includes his or her formation of values and beliefs during childhood years, influenced not only by family, religion, and culture but also by socioeconomic factors. This socialization process affects a person's attitude toward work and his or her related behavior. (See Case Study 3–2: What Changed in the Housekeeping Department?)

Case Study 3–2 What Changed in the Housekeeping Department?[a]

Betty Smith, the newly assigned manager of the hospital's housekeeping department, could not understand why her employees never offered suggestions as to how their jobs could be performed more effectively and efficiently. Betty was of the opinion that she shouldn't have to tell her staff how to clean a floor or a patient's room; they should be telling her how they could do their jobs better. Finally, Sally, a 24-year-old recent Sierra Leone immigrant who had been employed in the hospital's housekeeping department for the past 5 years confided in Betty during her performance-evaluation conference, "I don't offer suggestions because I'm only a housekeeper with no formal education. I don't want to look stupid."

Betty immediately put into place a 3-month training program with the goals of giving her employees the skills to recognize problems and the self-confidence to bring them to her attention. The training program was designed to let employees know what is expected of them regarding performance, as well as how and where they "fit" in the overall organization. The training program helped the employees understand that their contributions make a difference to the organization achieving its goals.

After the employees had completed half of the training program, Betty started to hold staff meetings on Friday afternoons to discuss any problems that were encountered during the week. At the conclusion of a Friday's staff meeting, Betty asked, as she always did, if anyone had an item to discuss. Betty never received a reply, but she continued to ask the question in every staff meeting anyway. However, this Friday was different. Sally raised her hand and related that she "overheard" a physician talking to the emergency room manager about the delay of transferring his patients from the ER to the nursing floors. Sally thought that part of the delay might be related to patients' rooms not being cleaned in a timely fashion after a patient's discharge because the unit secretaries at the nurses' stations did not communicate when the patient was being discharged. Housekeepers were told after the fact—after the patient was discharged and after the ER called the nursing station secretaries informing them an ER patient needed to be transferred to the unit. Because of their other duties, sometimes a housekeeper could not get to the floor for cleaning for at least an hour or more. Sally asked, "Why can't the nursing station secretaries communicate with us before the patient is discharged so we can schedule our time appropriately?" Betty agreed with Sally. Why couldn't there be better communication between the nursing units and housekeeping? Betty told the group she would look into it.

Betty called the Vice President of Nursing, Mary Acton, and discussed her staff's observations regarding the turnaround time delay of a clean bed being made available for an ER patient transfer. Mary concurred with Betty, stating that administration had noticed that sometimes it took up to three hours from the time a bed became empty to the time the bed was reported clean and available for patient use.

A team was formed that included nurse managers, nursing supervisors, floor nurses, unit secretaries, and housekeeping staff, including Sally, to discuss the problem and develop a solution that was workable for everyone. The solution* was simple, low-cost and low-tech.

First, the nursing supervisors would e-mail a list of anticipated room discharges for the following day to housekeeping no later than midnight. The evening housekeeping staff would retrieve the e-mail and post the list for the morning shift so they could plan their daily job activities according to the anticipated discharges. Second, two jars were placed at the nurses' stations—one jar was marked for clean rooms and the other marked as dirty rooms. Third, once a patient was discharged, the nurse put a red slip of paper with the room number into the dirty-room jar. Fourth, when housekeeping finished cleaning and preparing the room for an incoming patient, they removed the red slip from the first jar and put a green slip with the same room number on it in the second jar. Fifth, the green slip in the jar served as a visible reminder to the unit secretary that an open bed was available and ready to be filled when he or she received the call from the ER.

---

[a]Portions of the solution were reported as being implemented by University Hospital of University Health System. See Blueprint at the Seams: Improving Patient Flow to Help America's Emergency Department. Available from the Robert Wood Johnson Foundation Urgent Matters Program. Reprinted with permission.

Mary Acton called Sally the following month to thank her for bringing her "proactive" observations to Betty's attention. Mary related that the new "communication" system had reduced the bed turnaround time from 3 hours to 30 minutes!

Betty related the news of the decreased turnaround time at her next Friday staff meeting, and she thanked Sally and everyone for participating in developing and implementing this new hospital procedure that had positively impacted both patient and physician satisfaction. When, she asked if anyone had anything else to discuss, Sally raised her hand and said, "Barry and I noticed that an excessive amount of paper towels are being used throughout the hospital, and we have a few suggestions that may save the hospital money." Joe interjected, "I've also noticed that the hospital is not taking advantage of recycling its paper waste, which could save money and reduce our workloads." Tina related, "I have a few suggestions regarding. . . ." Betty smiled as she listened to everyone's suggestions and recommendations.

Discuss why Sally and the other housekeeping staff's attitudes changed.

Healthcare managers may use techniques employed in the counseling and conflict-resolution fields to develop a step-by-step process for changing employees' attitudes when necessary (see Exhibit 3–2). Attitude assessment and change is serious business. One person with a consistently (and vocal) bad attitude can lower the morale of an entire workgroup in an otherwise "healthy" organization.

Exhibit 3–2 Step-by-Step Process for Changing Attitudes in the Workplace

1. Assessment of Attitudes
   (a) Identification—Recognize common workplace attitude problems
   (b) Environment—Identify challenges in the workplace environment
   Participants are introduced to common examples of "attitude-challenged" workers. Group activities help identify and role-play how to handle different types of attitude challenges. Focus is to assess the impact of negative attitudes on workers, management, and patients/customers and identify the causes of problems.

2. Adjusting Attitudes
   (a) How listening, coaching, and providing feedback are the tools for attitude change.
   (b) Role-play to practice how to use coaching and provide feedback with staff
   (c) Identify payoffs and rewards
   Participants learn how to use open-ended questions, active listening, and tactful confrontation to address attitude problems in the workplace.

3. Common Management Mistakes
   (a) How to be realistic and patient with attitude change
   (b) Why scolding employees does little to stop the problem
   (c) How to stop the culture of complaining and work to positively effect attitude change
       Group activities include examples of common management mistakes and exercises to practice more realistic and positive ways to provide employee feedback, facilitate group discussion, and role-play the best methods for confronting negative attitudes.

(Continued)

Exhibit 3–2 *(Continued)*

4. Resolving Conflict
   (a) The need to confront so that negative behaviors will not continue
   (b) Expectations and coping strategies of employees to stress and management directives
   (c) Recognizing personal conflict styles of workers and how to deal with them
   Exercises include ways to analyze communications to identify employee styles, planning the meeting and working collaboratively to discover win/win solutions.

5. How to Work with Problem Behaviors and Attitudes
   (a) Analyze the cause of the problem
   (b) Privately confront with a calm, nondefensive professional demeanor
   In this session, participants role-play with their preferred style for handling difficult employees. Managers and employees exchange roles and must reprimand or confront problem behaviors.

6. The Last Resort: Employee Termination and Legal Issues
   (a) Legal issues of employee terminations
   (b) Requirements, documentation, and procedure
   Exercises use case studies to work out remedial and probationary systems and to document fully intervention efforts prior to the need for termination or re-assignment.

7. Creating a Positive Work Environment
   (a) Evoke a positive, collaborative team environment
   (b) Top motivators include nonmonetary rewards
   (c) Characteristics of managing motivation in the workplace
   Exercises include engaging workers into teams, providing recognition awards for employees, and changing the climate by launching career development and advancement initiatives, leadership training, multicultural skills, and other positive incentive programs.

The first step in the change process is to identify the problem, followed by efforts to adjust attitudes, reduce conflict, and seek solutions (see Exhibit 3–3). Open communication creates environments where workers feel safe to dissent, and in which their opinions are respected. Everyone has attitudes, both positive and negative. To help workers realize their full potential requires ongoing efforts.

Exhibit 3–3 Facilitating an Attitude Workshop for Employees

Discussion groups are a great way to diagnose and treat attitude problems. Begin by stating the guidelines for the session to alleviate any anxiety and set a positive tone. Create a supportive atmosphere so that participants feel safe to examine their attitudes and beliefs.

The manager's role should be as facilitator versus guiding a question-and-answer session. One task of the effective facilitator is activating the group's resources to bring out the "best" of a group. For example, plan activities where people get involved with one another right off the bat (e.g., icebreaker type of exercise). Work with the energy of the group, use humor and laughter, and healthy competition. These interactions build trust and help people feel comfortable to share ideas and consider new options.

The second task of the facilitator is to activate participants' internal wisdom. Ask questions and then let people discover their own answers. You can assist participants by keeping the dialogue going to sort out their values and priorities, explore beliefs and assumptions, and encourage them to alter their work lives in ways that they choose.

The third task is to facilitate personal reflections by asking questions to help participants test the ideas that are developed against their own experiences. List issues, goals, problems, and solutions that come up in the group dialogue. Write the main ideas on a board, perhaps focusing on negative attitudes and things that may cause them in the workplace. Ask people to expand on these. Give personal examples and ask them how poor attitudes in others can make them feel.

Throughout the process, the facilitator's goal is to try to foster interpersonal support. By having participants share ideas and experiences, it initiates the process of each person supporting the other. Encourage team building and interpersonal support as part of creating a work atmosphere where negative attitudes are exposed and positive attitudes flourish.

At the end of each session it is important to provide a summary. This shows the participants that you have been actively listening and are prepared to offer a synthesis of the group's observations and insights. Begin by saying "What I have heard today is . . ." Offer participants a chance to compare notes with one another for feedback. You might also ask participants to jot down ideas and feelings about the attitude dialogue to bring to the next meeting. Always provide a "take home message" of commitment to change—everyone should leave with at least one clear idea about what they will do next.

Discussions to identify negative workplace attitudes can be very effective. These discussions lead to solutions and group commitment to improved morale.

Based, in part, on *Creative planning for the second half of life*, by B. Kreitlow and D. Kreitlow, 1997, New York: Whole Person Associates. Reprinted with permission.

PERCEPTION

Perception is closely related to attitudes. Perception is the process by which organisms interpret and organize sensation to produce a meaningful experience of the world (Lindsay & Norman, 1977). In other words, a person is confronted with a situation or stimuli. The person interprets the stimuli into something meaningful to him or her on the basis of prior experiences. However, what an individual interprets or perceives may be substantially different from reality.

The perception process follows four stages: stimulation, registration, organization, and interpretation (see Figure 3–3).

A person's awareness and acceptance of the stimuli play an important role in the perception process. Receptiveness to the stimuli is highly selective and may be limited by a person's existing beliefs, attitude, motivation, and personality (Assael, 1995). Individuals will select the stimuli that satisfy their immediate needs (perceptual vigilance) and may disregard stimuli that may cause psychological anxiety (perceptual defense).

Broadbent (1958) addressed the concept of perceptual vigilance with his filter model. Broadbent argued that, on the one hand, because of limited capacity, a person must process information selectively and, therefore, when presented with information from two different channels (i.e., methods of delivery such as visual and auditory), an individual's perceptual system processes only that which he or she believes to be most relevant. However, perceptual defense creates an internal barrier that limits the external stimuli passing through the

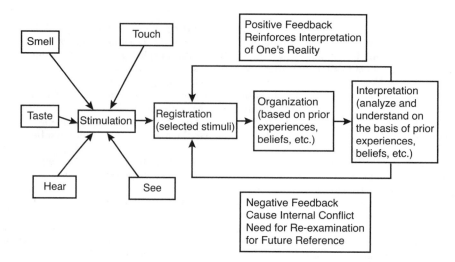

Figure 3–3 Perception Processing System

perception process when the stimuli is not congruent with the person's current beliefs, attitudes, motivation, and so on. This is referred to as selective perception. Selective perception occurs when an individual limits the processing of external stimuli by selectively interpreting what he or she sees on the basis of beliefs, experience, or attitudes (Sherif & Cantril, 1945).

Broadbent's filter theory has been updated in recent years. A "Selection-for-Action View" suggests that filtering is not just a consequence of capacity limitations but is driven by goal-directed actions (Allport, 1987, 1993; Neumann, 1987; Van der Heijden, 1992). The concept is that any action requires the selection of certain aspects of the environment that are action relevant and, at the same time, filtering other aspects that are action irrelevant. Therefore, when one is working toward a goal, one will skip over information that does not support one's plan. Recent studies of the brain have also led to new models, suggesting multiple channels of processing (Pashler, 1989) and selective perception as a result of activation of cortical maps and neural networks (Rizzolatti & Craighero, 1998). In any case, people are selective in what they perceive and tend to filter information on the basis of the capacity to absorb new data, combined with preconceived thoughts.

ATTRIBUTION THEORY

Since the 1950s, researchers have tried to understand and explain why people do what they do. Attribution theory was first introduced by Heidler (1958) as "naive psychology" to help explain the behaviors of others by describing ways in which people make casual explanations for their actions. Heidler believed that people have two behavioral motives: (1) the need to understand the world around them and (2) the need to control their environment. Heidler proposed that people act on the basis of their beliefs whether or not these beliefs are valid. Weiner (1979) suggested that individuals justify their performance decisions by cognitively constructing their reality in terms of internal–external, controllable–uncontrollable, and stable–unstable factors.

According to Weiner (1979), when one tries to describe the processes of explaining events and the relating behavior, external or internal attributions can be given. An external attribution assigns causality to an outside agent or force. An external attribution claims that some outside force motivated the event. By contrast, an internal attribution assigns causality to factors within the person. An internal attribution claims that the person was directly responsible for the event. Controllability refers to whether the person had the power to exert control over the events of the situation. Finally, stability of the cause relates to whether the behavior is consistent over time because of the individual's values and beliefs or because of outside elements such as rules or laws that would govern a person's behavior in the various situations.

Attribution theory is a concept from social psychology that allows people to offer explanations for why things happen and is more concerned with the individual's cognitive perceptions than the underlying reality of events (Daley 1996). As such, fundamental attribution error occurs when the influence of external factors is underestimated and the influence of internal factors is overestimated in regard to making judgments about behavior. Self-serving bias is the tendency for individuals to attribute their own successes to internal factors while putting the blame for failures on external factors.

When employees make attributions about a negative event that happened at work, they tend to underemphasize internal (dispositional) factors such as ability, motivation, or personality traits and overemphasize (external) situational factors. For example, some workers are "high achievers" because of their attributions. They approach rather than avoid tasks because they are confident of success due to their ability and effort. These high achievers persist when the work becomes more difficult rather than giving up because achieving their goals is self-rewarding and they will attribute their success to their personal drive and efforts. In contrast, the unmotivated "external" person will avoid or quit difficult tasks because he or she tends to doubt his or her ability and attributes success to luck or other factors out of his or her control. Such external persons have little drive or enthusiasm for work, because positive outcomes are not thought to be related to their direct effort.

Managers are often in a position where they make causal attributions regarding an employee's behavior or work pattern. Kelley's (1967, 1973) model of attribution theory incorporates three attributions: consensus, consistency, and distinctiveness (see Figure 3–4).

Consensus relates to whether an employee's performance is the same as or different from other employees. Consistency refers to whether the employee's behavior is the same in most situations. Whereas distinctiveness asks the question, "Does the employee act differently in other situations?" Managers will attribute an employee's behavior to external causes such as task difficulty if there is high consensus, low consistency, and high distinctiveness. As an example, the regional director of an international pharmaceutical company attributes her top salespersons' inabilities to reach their annual sales goals for

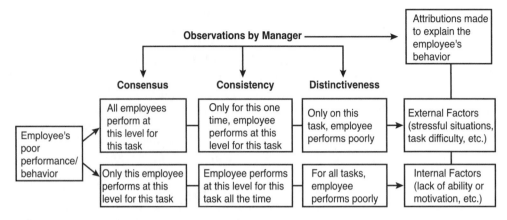

Figure 3–4 Kelley's Attribution Theory Model

a specific drug used to treat gastrointestinal conditions to recent negative media coverage of another, but similar drug's linkage to a high number of patients suffering strokes (e.g., adverse effects to the drug). Managers will attribute an employee's behavior to internal factors, such as lack of ability, if there is low consensus, high consistency, and low distinctiveness.

Mitchell et al. (1981, p. 199) gave the follow example to demonstrate the preceding: Suppose you are a physician, and you have asked a nurse to administer some medication to one of your patients. You check back later in the day, and you find that the medication was not given. Upon further discussions with the nurse, the supervisor, and other involved parties, you discover that (1) this nurse has failed to administer the proper medication on other occasions (low distinctiveness), and (2) this nurse has had difficulty on other tasks, such as charting or patient care (high consistency), and (3) none of the other nurses have failed to carry out a physician's order in the last three months (low consensus). The nurse has performed poorly on this task before; he or she has performed poorly on other tasks; and no one else seems to have this difficulty. In this case, the physician will most probably make a person attribution—the cause of the poor performance was some characteristic or trait of that particular nurse (e.g., lack of effort or ability).

Managers need to remember that there are many issues that factor into this process (i.e., explaining events and the relating behavior) and that organizational history, personal experiences, individual tendencies (toward internal versus external views of causality, intrinsic versus extrinsic motivations), and prior knowledge all impact perceptions of causes. Managers should avoid the "blame game" and focus on correcting workplace behavior (see Chapter 7 for a full discussion of attribution theory).

SOCIAL PERCEPTION

Social perception is how an individual "sees" others and how others perceive an individual. This is accomplished through various means, such as classifying an individual on the basis of a single characteristic (halo effect), evaluating a person's characteristics by comparison to others (contrast effect), perceiving others in ways that really reflect a perceiver's own attitudes and beliefs (projection), judging someone on the basis of one's perception of the group to which that person belongs (stereotyping), causing a person to act erroneously on the basis of another person's perception (Pygmalion effect), or controlling another person's perception of oneself (impression management).

Halo Effect

The halo effect occurs when an individual draws a general impression about another person based on a single characteristic, such as intelligence, sociability, or appearance. The perceiver may evaluate the other individual high on many traits because of his or her belief that the individual is high in one trait. For example, if an employee performs a difficult accounting task well because of the manager's belief of the employee's high intelligence, then the manager may also erroneously perceive the employee as having competencies in other areas such as management or technology.

The halo effect is applicable to individuals' perceptions of others and of organizations. For example, a hospital that is well known for its open-heart and cardiac programs may be perceived in the community as excellent in other clinical areas such as obstetrics or orthopedics whether proven that is to be true or not.

Opposite to the halo effect is the horn effect, whereby a person evaluates another as low on many traits because of a belief that the individual is low on one trait that is assumed to be critical (Thorndike, 1920). A study on obesity conducted with health professionals and researchers reflects the horn-effect concept. Study participants were asked to complete an Implicit Associations Test to assess overall implicit weight bias (associating "obese people" and "thin people" with "good" versus "bad") and three ranges of stereotypes: lazy–motivated, smart–stupid, and valuable–worthless. The study respondents were much quicker to pair "fat" with "lazy" and other negative traits and/or stereotypes (Schwartz et al., 2003).

Contrast Effects

Research has provided evidence that perceptions are also subject to what is termed perceptual contrast effects. Contrast effects relate to an individual's evaluation of another person's characteristics based on (or affected by) comparisons with other people who rank higher or lower on the same characteristics. For example, Wedell et al. (1987) found that, if compared to a highly attractive person, a target person of average attractiveness is judged less attractive than he or she would have been if rated on his or her own. When asked to contrast a target person with persons who were more physically attractive, ratings of attractiveness of the target were more negative, and when the target person was compared with those less attractive, it resulted in more positive evaluations (Thornton & Moore, 1993). In other words, the contrast effect relates to how an individual is perceived in relation to others around him or her. The contrast effect not only applies to the perception of attractiveness, but it has also been shown to influence self-esteem, public self-consciousness, and social anxiety (Thornton & Moore, 1993). It stands to reason that a worker's performance would be judged in contrast to the workers around him or her. However, managers need to be aware of this contrast-effect bias when interviewing job candidates or evaluating a worker's performance.

Projection

Whereas contrast effect is the perception of an individual based on the comparison to others, projection is the attribution of one's own attitudes and beliefs onto others. All of us are guilty of unconsciously projecting our own beliefs onto others. Sigmund Freud (1894/1966), along with his daughter Anna Freud (1936), suggested that projection was a defensive mechanism, where we attribute our own attitudes onto someone else as a defense against our feelings of anxiety or guilt. Projection can mean ascribing to others the negatives that we find inside ourselves, thereby protecting our self-esteem. Who has never blamed others for making them late to work, going off a diet, or being in a bad mood (when it was themselves at fault)? Projection is an interesting human tendency. Projection allows an individual to perceive others in ways that really reflect oneself, because, in general, people are in favor of those who are most like themselves.

Stereotyping

In 1798, printers invented a new way to permanently fix and reproduce visual images. This precursor to modern photographic printing processes was called stereotyping. Over time, this word came to apply not just to visual printed images, but also to how we fit attributes of ability, character, or behavior to groups and/or populations in order to make generalizations. As such, the term stereotype is defined to mean a conventional image applied to whole groups of people, and the treatment of groups according to a fixed set of generalized traits or characteristics.

Although stereotyping can be positive because it allows us to organize a very complex world, it may be considered negative if used as overly generalized views about groups of individuals. Researchers suggest that stereotypes wield a strong, covert influence on human behavior (even among those who do not agree with stereotypes). Social researchers have revealed that it is relatively easy for stereotypes to be activated across a wide range of contexts and situations, because of many factors, including race, gender, religion, physical appearances, disability, and occupation (see Bargh et al, 1996).

Stereotyping regarding race and ethnicity is problematic for healthcare professionals and health service organizations. The Institute of Medicine (2003) found that "racial and ethnic minorities tend to receive a lower quality of healthcare than non-minorities, even when access-related factors, such as patients' insurance status and income are controlled . . . and found evidence that stereotyping, biases, and uncertainty on the part of healthcare providers can contribute to unequal treatment" (p. 1).

In addition to stereotyping racial and ethnic minorities, healthcare professionals have a tendency to stereotype other groups, such as the elderly, homeless, disabled, and those suffering from obesity. The elderly are often stereotyped as infirm, inflexible, weak, deficient in vision and hearing, and being unable to advocate for themselves on health issues. Another example is the homeless or "skid row" population. There is a tendency to stereotype this group as either the elderly alcoholic male or perhaps the disheveled bag lady. However, homelessness affects families, children, and young people—groups that do not fit the typical stereotype of "homeless."

One of the most common forms of stereotyping is on the issue of gender and leadership. Women hold positions at all levels within healthcare organizations, but as noted in Chapter 2, only 40 percent hold senior healthcare management positions. The influence of gender stereotypes is one possible explanation of why it is sometimes difficult for people to accept women as leaders in the workplace. Traits often attached to leadership are "masculine" qualities such as courage, persuasiveness, and assertiveness. As such, an aggressive male leader may be viewed as "ambitious," compared with an assertive female leader who may be viewed as "pushy." This is, in part, because the assertive female leader's behavior violates a gender stereotype that women should be less authoritarian and more sensitive, gentle, and nurturing (see Exhibit 3–4).

Exhibit 3–4 Gender Stereotyping

In each culture, gender roles and gender stereotypes provide specific expectations of male and female behavior. When those expectations are violated (as in the case of a women acting assertively), it results in a negative label being applied to describe the person violating the expectation. This was at issue in Price Waterhouse v. Hopkins (1989), as cited in Lord & Maher (1991).

In the case of Ann Hopkins, she was a high-performing but masculine-acting prospective partner at Price Waterhouse. When she was denied a partnership at Price Waterhouse, she charged that gender stereotyping had played a role in the decision (Fiske et al., 1991). At the time of her eligibility/consideration for promotion to partner, Hopkins was the only woman among 88 candidates nominated for partnership. Her close colleagues submitted an evaluation noting her "outstanding performance" and strongly urged her admission to the partnership. When she was not accepted as a partner by the promotion board, she sued.

In response to the suit, Price Waterhouse countered that Ms. Hopkins had interpersonal problems and was considered too "macho" for the position. The person responsible for explaining the board's decision to Ms. Hopkins advised her that in order to improve her chances for partnership she "should walk more femininely, talk more femininely, dress more femininely, wear make-up, have her hair styled, and wear jewelry." In addition, another board member repeatedly commented that "he could not consider any woman seriously as a partnership candidate and believed that women were not even capable of functioning as partners." Ms. Hopkins brought her gender discrimination lawsuit all the way to the Supreme Court and won.

SOURCE: *Leadership and information processing: Linking perceptions and performance*, by R. G. Lord and K. J. Maher, 1991, Boston, MA: Unwin Hyman.

We all use stereotypes because it helps us simplify our world. However, most often we do not take the time to understand why we are perceiving groups in a certain way. We revert to our cognitive prototypes and ignore relevant information. These habits and biases are learned and, thus, can be unlearned. Training exercises can help to sensitize individuals to issues of bias, racism, sexism, ageism, and other biases. One goal of management is to assist staff in recognizing that stereotypes are illogical by challenging these faulty cognitions. The need to challenge gender and other stereotypes in the workplace is one of the reasons so much increased attention has been placed on managing diversity in organizations, as discussed in Chapter 2. It is important to be aware of how our perception of groups can influence our behavior, including our hiring and management practices and our interactions with workers. Stereotypes may lead to discrimination; therefore, it is important to discuss them and work toward destereotyping the workplace. Negative stereotypes can be problematic for any organization, and *proper* training can be effective in minimizing widely held false beliefs (see Exhibit 3–5). A recent study by Frank and his colleagues (2007) found that mandatory diversity training programs developed by companies to avoid liability in discrimination lawsuits were ineffective for increasing diversity in management. However, when diversity training is voluntary and undertaken to advance a company's business goals (and part of the organization's culture), it was associated with increased diversity in management. According to the study, it appears that employees don't react well when "sensitivity" training is forced on them!

Exhibit 3–5 Exercise to Identify Stereotypes within Our Organizations and Profession

---

Discussion: Have you seen any evidence of stereotypes in your workplace?

Which of the following positions are filled more by MEN or by WOMEN:

Physician _____	Pharmacist _____	Nurse _____
Computer Programmer _____	Nurses Aide _____	Chief of Staff_____
Medical Receptionist _____	Radiology Technician _____	

Statements:

Health Services Administrators need to be _____ to be effective.

The hospital cafeteria is staffed by people who are _____.

Disabled people that I have worked with are _____.

Pygmalion Effect

The Pygmalion effect, or self-fulfilling prophecy, describes a person's behavior that is consistent with another individual's perception whether or not it is accurate. In other words, once an expectation is made known by another person, an individual will have the tendency to behave in ways consistent with the expectation. This can have negative or positive results. If a manager sets high standards for a subordinate's performance, he or she will respond accordingly with high performance. If a manager sets low standards for a subordinate's performance because the subordinate is viewed as lacking in ability and/or motivation, the resulting work performance will be low. Therefore, managers' expectations directly influence subordinates' performance (see discussion of McGregor's Theory X and Theory Y in Chapter 1). In other words, what a manager communicates as the expectation is what will result. Livingston (1969) stated that what was critical in the communication of expectations was not what the manager said, so much as the way the manager behaved. Indifferent and noncommittal treatment, more often than not, was the kind of treatment that communicated low expectations and led to poor performance. Livingston related that managers were more effective at communicating low expectations to their subordinates than in communicating high expectations.

Closely related to the self-fulfilling prophecy is the "Galatea effect." This effect relates to the expectations we have for ourselves, rather than the expectations others have for us. To illustrate this concept, Livingston (1969) referred to the "Sweeney's Miracle." James Sweeney was an industrial management professor at Tulane University who wished to disprove the theory that a certain IQ level was needed to learn how to program computers. Sweeney trained a poorly educated janitor whose IQ indicated that he would be unable to learn to type, much less program. The janitor not only learned to program, but also eventually took charge of the computer room along with the responsibility of training new employees to program and operate the computers. As Livingston pointed out, Sweeney's expectations were based on what he believed about his teaching ability (internal expectations), not on the janitor's learning capabilities. Livingston related that, "the high expectations of superior managers are based primarily on what they think about themselves—about their own ability to select, train, and motivate their subordinates. What the manager believes about himself subtly influences what he believes about his subordinates, what he expects of them, and how he treats them" (Livingston, 1969).

Therefore, managers need to understand the effects of their own self-expectations and how these expectations interact with the expectations they hold and communicate regarding their subordinates' performance. Managers set the tone and culture of the workplace. By understanding the Pygmalion and Galatea effects, managers can set high (but realistic) performance expectations for their subordinates. If a manager rates subordinates as "excellent," they will continue their previous work behaviors. Managers can also have workers rate their own performance. Expectations about ourselves tend to be self-sustaining.

Impression Management

"You never get a second chance to make a first impression." This classic statement is all about impression management, where people try to shape another's impression of themselves. Impression management incorporates what we do, how we do it, what we say, and how we say it as we try to influence the perceptions others have of us. Individuals will try to present themselves in ways that will lead to positive evaluations by others by highlighting their achievements and avoiding the disclosure of failures. Giacalone and Rosenfeld (1989) point out that impression management is neither inherently good nor bad but rather is a fundamental part of our social and work lives, and we need to view it in the situations in which it is used. As an example, consider the concept of self-handicapping. Self-handicapping is where people place obstacles in their way, so if they do not succeed they can blame the obstacles or if successful, they can brag regarding their successful performance in spite of these barriers.

Schlenker and Weigold (1992) view impression management as a broad phenomenon in which we try to influence the perceptions and behaviors of others by controlling the information they receive. They relate that people actively carry out impression management in ways that help them achieve their objectives and goals, both individually and as part of groups and organizations. This can be done consciously and deliberately (i.e., perfecting job-interview skills), while other times it may be unconscious. At times, the impression that is managed serves to bolster or protect our own self-image (i.e., dressing for success); other times we manage impressions in hopes of pleasing significant audiences. Sometimes impression management is truthful and accurate. Other times it involves "false advertising" through the use of exaggeration, fabrication, deception, and falsehoods (Schlenker & Weigold, 1992) (see Exhibit 3–6).

EMPLOYEE SELECTION

Because perceptions determine our behavior toward and can cloud our judgments of others, one area that clearly benefits from using psychological principles has been the area of employee selection. The goals of selection are: (1) identify the knowledge, skills, abilities, and qualities necessary to perform a job well, (2) design tests to measure applicants' levels on those key job requirements, (3) administer and score the tests, and (4) determine the applicants most suitable for a given position, ensuring that the process is accurate and fair and does not discriminate against members of protected groups. The basis for this employee selection process is the ability to identify key invariant qualities of individuals (such as skills, character, motivation, attitude, leadership potential, and personality) that match up well with the demands of the position and the culture of the organization.

Psychometrics involves the measurement of human ability, potential, and attitude. This is most visible where employers use tests and special interview techniques in employee selection. Job analysis is designed to identify the skills, abilities, and attributes needed to perform well. Context-specific tests

Exhibit 3–6 The Liars Index

Twice a year, Jude M. Werra of Jude M. Werra & Associates, a headhunting firm in Brookfield, Wisconsin, reviews the hundreds of résumés he has seen in the previous six months—the elegant, triumphant CVs of CEOs and VPs—and he condenses them into a single statistic. "It's the number of people who've misrepresented their education divided by the number of people whose education we checked," Werra explained. Werra calls it the Liars Index—the percentage of people who invented a degree. The index, which has been published since 1995, was at its highest in the first half of 2000: 23.3 percent. It now stands at 11.2 percent.

If there is a case for regarding all résumés as adventures in narrative, it is one that should not be made to Mr. Werra. In his view, a lie is a lie, whether it is propagated by Ronald Zarrella, the chief executive of Bausch & Lomb, who confirmed two weeks ago that he did not, after all, have an MBA from NYU, or by Quincy Troupe, California's newly appointed poet laureate who, shortly after Zarrella's announcement, acknowledged that he had never received a degree from Grambling College in Louisiana, despite making that claim on his résumé. (Mr. Zarrella remains at his desk, backed by the Bausch & Lomb board; Mr. Troupe's resignation has been accepted by the California senate, presumably on the ground that the last thing a state needs is a poet who makes things up.) These embellished résumés, testing our taste for the legend of the self-made man (as well as Sir Philip Sidney's claim that "the poet . . . never lieth") can now be filed alongside those of Kenneth Lonchar, the former chief financial officer of Veritas Software (who gave himself a Stanford MBA), Sandy Baldwin, the former president of the U.S. Olympic Committee (doctorate in American literature), George O'Leary, the former Notre Dame football coach (master's degree in education), David Geffen, Miss Virginia 1995, and John Holmes (the porn star) who invented a degree in physical therapy from UCLA.

Werra, who has been in the business of "retained executive searches" for 25 years, used to interview candidates first and then do a background check. Now he checks first and interviews later, ever since an engaging interviewee said that they had been contemporaries at Marquette University in the mid-1960s. The man claimed to remember their graduation ceremony. Werra said, "I was talking about how President Johnson's daughter had attended, and about all the security, the metal detectors, and how the place was ringed with police and Secret Service and so on, and he was saying, 'Yeah, yeah, wasn't it amazing?' And he had never been there, of course."

Werra went on, "A few years ago, I spoke with a gentleman who claimed to have a degree from Fairleigh Dickinson. Let's call him John Martin. The university had no record of him, so I dropped him a note: 'Could you clarify this?' He wrote me back six weeks later: 'You know, I've accepted a job to be director of sales and marketing of your client's No. 1 competitor—just wanted to let you know. And, by the way, the reason you couldn't find information on my degree is that my name isn't really Martin, it's Martini, and my father was rubbed out by the Mob in New York years ago, and my mother got us into the witness-protection program, and when I went to Fairleigh Dickinson I got my degree under another name. But I have a special phone number—you can call it and whoever answers the phone will tell you I have a degree.'" Werra did not make that call.

Source: Department of Padding. *Dishonorable Degrees*, by I. Parker, November 4, 2002. *The New Yorker Magazine*. Reprinted with permission.

can measure applicants' skill levels on key job requirements, such as the operation of hardware and software. However, as with any tool, instruments used to measure human ability can be misused or misleading. Instruments that rely on self-report of personal information are subject to bias (such as impression management), and the interpretation of aptitude scores is also subject to bias (such as stereotypes and halo effects). Therefore, managers responsible for hiring and promoting should look for many sources of data from which to extract the qualities essential to the job, such as personality (see Exhibit 3–7).

One goal in this discussion is to help managers make accurate and fair assessments of staff or potential staff for various positions within their organizations. Who should function in positions of high contact with patients? Who is better off working with computers? Who is most able to direct a unit to promote the best clinical care? Who is most suited to manage the business office? How can we help those who are not ready to assume a leadership role develop the skills while still working comfortably in their current subordinate positions? These are the questions a manager or administrator must answer in personnel decisions. To do so requires a manager to perceive the unchanging qualities of a person across situations, or their key "traits" that underlie success in a job.

Many instruments used to assess personnel and management/leadership potential, such as the Campbell Interest and Skills Inventory, are trying to identify "constants" of personality and work style. The Campbell Interest and Skills Inventory compares employee-reported interests and skills to those of people

---

Exhibit 3–7 Five-factor Model of Personality

Personality traits are the regularities that we observe in someone's behavior, attitudes, and expressions. Prior research suggests that virtually all personality measures can be reduced or categorized under the Five-factor Model of Personality, also known as the "Big 5." The dimensionality of the Big 5 has been found to be applicable across all cultures.

The Big 5 is based on the concept that personality can be described and measured on five broad dimensions and/or traits: openness, conscientiousness, extraversion, agreeableness, and neuroticism.

Dimensions/Traits	Descriptions
Openness	imaginative, innovative, open-minded
Conscientiousness	competent, responsible, dependable, hardworking, goal oriented, self-disciplined
Extraversion	assertive, social, positive emotions
Agreeableness	trusting, straightforwardness, compliant, warmhearted, generous, modest
Neuroticism	emotional, insecure, self-consciousness, impulsiveness, vulnerability

SOURCE: An introduction to the five-factor model and its application, by R. R. McCrae and O. P. John, 1992, *Journal of Personality, 60,* 175–215.

who describe themselves as satisfied with their careers and highlights occupational areas to consider during career exploration. Here the invariant is a pattern of interests and work preferences that we carry from one job to another.

Another commonly used scale is the Myers-Briggs Type Indicator (MBTI), a personality instrument for measuring a person's preferences, using four opposing-pole dimensions (extraversion/introversion, sensate/intuitive, thinking/feeling, and judging/perceiving). How someone answers a series of questions forms a personality "type." Each personality type is suited for specific occupations. As an example, extroverts are better suited for sales positions and introverts do well with information technology positions. There are many pros and cons to using Myers-Briggs, or any instrument, as the sole selector of occupational areas based on "type." Nevertheless, these instruments pick up patterns (invariants) in self-reported behavioral characteristics and provide a categorization of types that may be useful in assessing certain qualities relevant to leadership and workplace issues.

SUMMARY

In this chapter, we reviewed several social psychology concepts that are important for managers to understand. These are factors that can influence and bias our perceptions, and therefore knowledge of these biases is needed to temper and inform our perceptions. In discussing attitudes and how to change them, we become more aware of those distinctly unique human qualities that complicate the workplace but also make it so interesting. Likewise, by understanding how workers "see" the world, we are in a better position to facilitate a productive workplace. Today's healthcare managers have many resources at their disposal, and this includes a wide-ranging scientific literature on organizational behavior, psychology, and human resource issues in the workplace. Hopefully, this chapter will encourage you to develop and use your own skills as a social perceiver, and give you some confidence that you can foster positive attitudes. We are always learning, improving, and building skills in social perception. In this way, we will continue to use our understanding of human behavior to create a positive and healthy workplace.

END-OF-CHAPTER DISCUSSION QUESTIONS

1. Define attitudes and provide examples.
2. What is meant by cognitive dissonance?
3. What are common methods to measure a person's attitude?
4. List and describe ways attitudes can be changed.
5. What is the difference between the halo effect and the horn effect?
6. Define the four stages of the perception process.
7. How does attribution theory allow managers to "justify" workers' behaviors?

8. Define social perception.

9. What is the difference between contrast effect and projection?

10. Is stereotyping negative or positive? Why?

11. Why is stereotyping so problematic for the healthcare industry?

12. What is the difference between the Pygmalion effect and the Galatea effect?

13. Is impression management negative or positive? Why?

14. Is employee selection an unbiased process? Why?

EXERCISE 3–1 Gender Stereotyping in Organizations

Role-play

Choose a male and a female volunteer. Each member of the pair will argue over a situation in the workplace, for example, departments negotiating over who gets to purchase a piece of new medical equipment (limited financial resources), or whether laptops or PCs are appropriate for the nursing stations, or which color to paint the hospital's hallways.

Designate one of the participants as the "influencer" who should try to "win" the argument. Designate the other as the "influencee" who should resist.

The influencer has a fixed amount of time, perhaps one minute, to persuade the influencee.

After you observe the interaction, break into groups for discussion of the influencer (i.e., leader) and make a list of adjectives used to describe the influencer. For example, was the leader "bossy" or "dominating" or "assertive"?

Have the male and female REVERSE roles with a new topic and repeat the discussion. Now discuss the two leadership influencers in both of the role-play episodes. Which one had more skill and fit your image of a "leader"? Record your responses.

Break into groups again and describe the influencer with an adjective list. Continue until several male–female dyads have role-played as influencers and influencees. Record the descriptive adjectives. Rate overall leadership of each influencer observed. Record responses.

Discussion Questions

Were differences in leader perceptions due to gender stereotypes or behavioral differences?

What social invariants ("constants" or "traits") can you identify as important for leadership positions?

Why are leadership perceptions important, and can attributions about leadership ability impact the behaviors of followers?

Debriefing

Research by Butler and Geis (1990) suggests that in role-play exercises, such as in the preceding discussion, the female leader was described differently in terms of her personality traits and was more likely to be the recipient of covert gender stereotyping compared to males.

EXERCISE 3–2 Free Birth Control for Teens

One organization's recent offer of free birth control pills to area teens has left some abstinence-only proponents outraged. The package of health services being offered at clinics by Plan Your Life includes the free birth control and a pelvic exam with a $50 health screening. The organization hopes the "special" encourages teens, ages 12 to 18, to talk about their sexual choices—and the repercussions of those choices—with medical professionals.

"We know we are helping the community because we see the need every day," said Mary Coleman, president of Plan Your Life. "Every day you hear a story about a young woman who is pregnant or infected with HIV or herpes or some other sexually transmitted infection and it's heartbreaking."

But in making the offer of free birth control to teens, Plan Your Life has stirred the controversy pot among those who favor abstinence only. "This is truly lowering the bar to the gutter for our children," said Susan Palmer, president of Take Charge of Your Life, an antiabortion, abstinence-based outreach organization. Terry Adams, executive director of Its Not About You, another antiabortion, abstinence-based outreach organization, echoed Palmer's disapproval. "It's like giving them a license to have sex," she said. "I have a hard time giving children something that can cause them harm."

Coleman countered their assessment. "Giving a contraceptive to a teen, either birth control pills or condoms, does not give them a license to have sex," she said. "Teaching about contraception does not encourage sexual behavior. The behavior is already there; it's up to parents and caregivers of teens to have open conversations about sexuality and contraception. When youth are educated, they make the right choices. When they're denied education, they have no choice but to make the wrong choice."

Carol Schmidt, a parent of a teenage daughter and son in college, said she's inclined to trust Plan Your Life's decision. "I certainly hope that most kids are able to talk to their parents about these issues, but I do think it's good for them to have a place to go if they can't," she said.

Coleman acknowledged her Plan Your Life affiliate has been getting calls from upset parents since announcing its special. But, she said, "We're also getting calls from parents who are thanking us!"

Palmer, however, is not convinced the new program benefits teens. "It's promoting promiscuity,' she said. "It's like an advertisement for sex."

Discuss why Mary Coleman, Susan Palmer, Terry Adams, and Carol Schmidt have different attitudes toward birth control.

EXERCISE 3–3 Only 15 Weeks to Thanksgiving!

SCENE I:

"I just hate the thought of going back to work," Mary told her brother Tom. It was the last night of her vacation, and Mary thought it had been much too short. "It's 15 weeks until Thanksgiving."

"Mary, I know you're miserable," Tom replied. "You've been increasingly unhappy in that job for the past five years. You're a totally different person when you're on vacation. I know we've discussed this a thousand times, but isn't there something else you can do?"

"Don't you think I'd do something else if I could?" Mary replied angrily. "I'm sorry, I know you're only trying to help, but I really think I'm trapped in this situation. With my diabetes and high blood pressure I can't afford to retire early because I need the health insurance. I could get Social Security at 62, but the healthcare coverage doesn't start until 65. A supplemental policy would be much too expensive, even if I could get one. I know that as soon as I go back to work my blood pressure and sugar will go up from the stress."

"Yes," commented Tom. "And you'll start counting the days until the weekend. You've already figured out how long it is until Thanksgiving! There's got to be some other solution to this, Mary."

"Sure! The Lottery!" Mary answered. "That's all I can think of!"

SCENE II:

Dan, the manager of the health information department of a large health system in South Florida, sighed as he finished his coffee. . . . "Mary will be back from vacation tomorrow. I keep hoping that she'll be less stressed out when she gets back, but it always seems to be the same. She has so much experience and she could be a great role model for the younger people at work, but I just can't seem to get her attitude turned around. I've tried everything I can think of—special projects outside the department, adjusted work schedule, more responsibility and authority on day-to-day stuff, advanced computer training—but she's my big failure as a boss."

"Oh, I think she's just jealous of you," his wife Sonia replied. "You've really worked hard on the old witch. I just don't think she's worth the effort. Why doesn't she just retire?"

"It's a good thing the Human Resources people didn't hear that!" Dan laughed. "Sonia, you're just plain wrong about Mary. She knows everything about the department. Without her help I couldn't have managed at all when I started there. I can't believe she's jealous of me; she's really been a lot of help. I just wish she weren't so unhappy. You know, I talked to Jean about her the other day. They started in the company together about 20 years ago. Jean said she wasn't sure what was going on with Mary because they haven't been very close lately, but she said that Mary's always been really independent. Stubborn, even. And quite outspoken about things she disagrees with. She's usu-

---

Author: Pidge Diehl, EdD. Reprinted with permission.

ally right, but sometimes it's tough for people to listen to her because of the way she puts things. I don't think she's kidding when she says that's part of her New England upbringing. Did you know she got thrown out of college for objecting to some policy? And then she forced them to reinstate her because they hadn't followed due process?"

"Oh, so she's always been a witch? From Salem, perhaps?" Sonia replied. "Come on, Dan, give it a rest. You don't need to figure Mary out until tomorrow! Don't you want to watch the Miami Dolphins beat the Tampa Bay Bucs? Can you imagine? They favor the Bucs to win!"

Question 1:

In SCENE I, what is Mary's attitude? Are you able to identify the three elements of an attitude in what she says?

Question 2:

In SCENE II, Dan and Sonia have very different perceptions about Mary. Why?

REFERENCES

Allport, D. A. (1987). Selection for action: Some behavioral and neurophysiological considerations of attention and action. In H. Heuer & F. Sanders (Eds.), *Perspectives on perception and action*. Hillsdale, NJ: Erlbaum.

Allport, D. A. (1993). Attention and control: Have we been asking the wrong questions? A critical review of twenty-five years. In D. E. Meyer & S. Kornblum (Eds.), *Attention and performance XIV* (pp. 183–218). Cambridge, MA: MIT Press.

Allport, G. W. (1935). Attitudes. In Murchison C. (Ed.), *Handbook of social psychology* (pp. 798–844). Worcester, MA: Clark University Press.

Assael, H. (1995). *Consumer behavior & marketing action* (5th ed.). London: PWS-Kent Publishing Company.

Bargh, J. A., Chen, M., & Burrows, L. (1996). Automaticity of social behavior: Direct effects of trait construct and stereotype activation on action. *Journal of Personality and Social Psychology, 71*(2), 230.

Broadbent, D. E. (1958). *Perception and communication*. New York: Pergamon Press.

Butler, D., & Geis, F. L. (1990). Nonverbal affect responses to male and female leaders: Implications for leadership evaluations. *Journal of Personality and Social Psychology, 58*, 48–59.

Daley, D. 1996. Attribution theory and the glass ceiling: Career development among federal employees. *Public Administration and Management: An Interactive Journal, 1*(1), Retrieved February 11, 2004 from http://www.pamij.com

Festinger, L. (1957). *A theory of cognitive dissonance*. Stanford, CA: Stanford University Press.

Fiske, S. T., Bersoff, D. N., Borgida, E., Deaux, K., & Heilman, M. E. (1991). Social science research on trial: Use of sex stereotyping research in Price Waterhouse v. Hopkins. *American Psychologist, 46*, 1049–1060.

Dobbin, F., Kalev, A., & Kelly, E. (2007). Diversity management in corporate America: Do America's costly diversity management programs work? Not always. *Contexts 6*(4), 21–27.

Freud, A. (1936). Ego & the mechanisms of defense (Vol. 2). In *The writings of Anna Freud*. New York: International Universities Press.

Freud, S. (1966). The neuro-psychoses of defense. In *The standard edition of the complete psychological works of Sigmund Freud*,(James Strachey, Trans.). (3rd ed., pp. 45–61). London: Hogarth Press. (Original work published 1923)

Giacalone, R. A., & Rosenfeld, P. (Eds.) (1989). *Impression management in the organization*. Hillsdale, NJ: Erlbaum.

Heidler, F. (1958). *The psychology of interpersonal relations*. New York: John Wiley & Sons.

Institute of Medicine. (2003). *Unequal treatment: Confronting racial and ethnic disparities in health care*. The National Academies Press, Retrieved April 30, 2004 from http://books.nap.edu/catalog/10260.html

Kassarjian, H. H., & Cohen, J. B. (1965). Cognitive dissonance and consumer behavior: Reactions to the Surgeon General's report on smoking and health. *California Management Review, 8*(1), 55–64.

Kelley, H. H. (1967). Attribution theory in social psychology. In D. Levine (Ed.), *Nebraska Symposium on Motivation* (Vol. 15, pp. 129–238). Lincoln: University of Nebraska Press.

Kelley, H. H. (1973). The process of causal attribution. *American Psychologist, 28,* 107–128.

Lindsay, P., & Norman, D. A. (1977). *Human information processing: An introduction to psychology*. New York: Harcourt Brace Jovanovich.

Livingston, J. S. (1969). Pygmalion in management. *Harvard Business Review, 81*(1), 97–106.

Lord, R. G., & Maher, K. J. (1991). *Leadership and information processing: Linking perceptions and performance*. Boston, MA: Unwin Hyman.

Lowe, G., Schellenberg, G., & Shannon, H. (2003). Correlates of employees' perceptions of a healthy work environment. *American Journal of Health Promotion, 17*(6), 390–399.

Mitchell, T. R., Green, S.G., & Wood, R.E. (1981). An attributional model of leadership and the poor performing subordinate. *Research in Organizational Behavior, 3,* 197–234.

Moore. M. (2003). How to improve staff morale using humor, appreciation and praise—Practical strategies to help you turn your workplace into a "Thank God it's Monday" type of organization, Retrieved January 18, 2004 from www.motivationalplus.com

Morrel-Samuels, P. (2002). Getting the truth into workplace surveys. *Harvard Business Review, 80*(2), 111–118.

Neumann, O. (1987). Beyond capacity: A functional view of attention. In H. Heuer & A. F. Sanders (Eds.), *Perspectives on perception and action* (pp. 361–394). Hillsdale, NJ: Erlbaum.

Ott, J. S. (1996). *Classic Readings in Organizational Behavior* (2nd ed.). Albany, NY: Wadsworth Publishing Company.

Pashler, H. (1989). Dissociations and dependencies between speed and accuracy: Evidence for a two-component theory of divided attention in simple tasks. *Cognitive Psychology, 21,* 469–514.

Price Waterhouse v. Hopkins, 109 S. Court 1775 (1989).

Rizzolatti, G., & Craighero, L. (1998). Spatial attention: Mechanisms and theories. In M. Sabourin, F. Craik, & M. Robert (Eds.), *Advances in psychological science (Vol. 2) Biological and cognitive aspects* (pp. 171–198). Hove, UK: Psychology Press.

Schlenker, B. R., & Weigold, M. F. (1992). Interpersonal processes involving impression regulation and management. *Annual Review of Psychology, 43,* 133–168.

Schwartz, M. B., Chambliss, H. O., Brownell, K. D., Blair, S. N., & Billington C. (2003). Weight bias among health professionals specializing in obesity. *Obesity Research, 11*(9), 1033–1039.

Sherif, M., & Cantril, H. (1945). The psychology of attitudes: I. *Psychology Review, 52,* 295–319.

Thorndike, E. L. (1920). A constant error on psychological rating. *Journal of Applied Psychology, IV,* 25–29.

Thornton, B., & Moore, S. (1993). Physical attractiveness contrast effect: Implications for self-esteem and evaluations of the social self. *Personality and Social Psychology Bulletin, 19,* 474–480.

Thurstone, L. L., & Chave E. J. (1929). *The measurement of attitude.* Chicago: University of Chicago Press.

Van der Heijden, A. H. C. (1992). *Selective attention in vision.* London: Routledge.

Wedell, D. H., Parducci, A., & Geiselman, R. E. (1987). A formal analysis of ratings of physical attractiveness: Successive contrast and simultaneous assimilation. *Journal of Experimental Social Psychology, 23,* 230–249.

Weiner, B. (1979). A theory of motivation for some classroom experiences. *Journal of Educational Psychology, 71,* 3–25.

OTHER SUGGESTED READING

Allport, G. W. (1937). *Personality: A psychological interpretation.* New York: Holt Rinehart & Winston.

Brief, A. P. (1998). *Attitudes in and around organizations.* Thousand Oaks, CA: Sage.

Barnes-Farrell, J. L., & Ratz, J. M. (1997). Accommodation in the workplace. *Human Resource Management Review, 7,* 77–107.

Briggs-Myers, I., & Briggs, K. C. (1980). *Myers-Briggs Type Indicator (MBTI). Gifts differing.* Palo Alto, CA: Consulting Psychologists Press.

Briggs-Myers, I., & McCaulley, M. H. (1985). *Manual: A guide to the development and use of the Myers Briggs Type Indicator.* Palo Alto, CA: Consulting Psychologists Press.

Butler, D., & Geis, F. L. (1990). Nonverbal affect responses to male and female leaders: Implications for leadership evaluations. *Journal of Personality and Social Psychology, 58,* 48–59.

Campbell, D. P. (1970). *Campbell Interest and Skill Survey–CISS*. Upper Saddle River, NJ: Pearson Assessments, Pearson Education, Last accessed December 28, 2003 from http://www.pearsonassessments.com

Della-Giustina, J. L., & Della-Giustina, D. E. (1989). Quality of work life programs and employee motivation. *Professional Safety, 34*(5), 24.

Denton, D. K., & Boyd, C. (1990). *Employee complaint handling tested techniques for human resources managers*. Westport, CT: Quorum Books.

Eagly, A., & Chaiken, S. (1993). *Psychology of attitudes*. New York: Harcourt, Brace Jovanovich.

Feingold, A. (1998). Gender stereotyping for sociability, dominance, character, and mental health: A meta-analysis of findings from the bogus stranger paradigm. *Genetic, Social, and General Psychology Monographs, 124*(3), 253–271.

Feingold, A. (1992). Good-looking people are not what we think. *Psychological Bulletin, 111*(2), 304.

Gibson, J. J. (1966). *The senses considered as perceptual systems*. Boston: Houghton Mifflin.

Hirsch, S. K. (1985). *Using the Myers-Briggs Type Indicator in organizations*. Palo Alto, CA: Consulting Psychological Press.

Kouzes, J. M., & Posner, B. (1997). *The leadership challenge: How to keep getting extraordinary things done in organizations*. San Francisco: Jossey-Bass.

Kouzes, J. M., & Posner, B. (1999). *Encouraging the heart: A leader's guide to rewarding and recognizing others*. San Francisco: Jossey-Bass.

McGuire, W. J. (1985). Attitudes and attitude change. In G. Lindzey & E. Aronson (Eds.), *Handbook of social psychology* (3rd ed., Vol. 2, pp. 136–314). Reading, MA: AddisonWesley.

Stern, M., & Karraker, K. H. (1992). Modifying the prematurity stereotype in mothers of premature and ill full-term infants. *Journal of Clinical Child Psychology, 21*(1), 76.

Sternberg, R. J., & Lubart, T. I. (1995). *Defying the crowd: Cultivating creativity in a culture of conformity*. New York: Free Press.

Stone, E. F., Stone, D. L., & Dipboye, R. L. (1992). Stigmas in organizations: Race, handicaps, and physical unattractiveness. In K. Kelly (Ed.), *Issues, theory, and research in industrial and organizational psychology* (pp. 385–457). New York: Elsevier Science.

Van Ryn, M., & Burke J. (2000). The effect of patient race and socio-economic status on physicians' perceptions of patients. *Social Sciences Medicine, 50*(6), 813–828.

Walsh, V., & Kulikowski, J. J. (1998). *Perceptual constancy: Why things look as they do*. Cambridge, UK: Cambridge University Press.

CHAPTER 4

Workplace Communication

Kristina L. Guo, PhD and Yesenia Sanchez, MPH

LEARNING OUTCOMES

After completing this chapter, the student should be able to:

- ☛ Describe the communication process.
- ☛ Understand the importance of feedback in the communication process.
- ☛ Understand various verbal and nonverbal methods of communication.
- ☛ Understand the common barriers to communication.
- ☛ Utilize various methods to overcome communication barriers.
- ☛ Discuss the elements of effective communication for knowledge management.
- ☛ Describe the various components for effective strategic communication.
- ☛ Understand the flow of intraorganizational communication.
- ☛ Understand the challenges of cross-cultural communication.
- ☛ Understand the flow of communication with external stakeholders and the public sector.

OVERVIEW

Fundamental and vital to all healthcare managerial functions, communication is a means of transmitting information and making oneself understood by another or others. Communication is a major challenge for managers because they are responsible for providing information, which results in efficient and effective performance in organizations. Every managerial function and activity involves some form of communication. Whether a manager is engaged in planning, organizing, directing, or leading, managers must communicate with and through others. Managerial decisions are only effective if they are communicated and understood by those responsible for enacting them. Furthermore, employee motivation and satisfaction are dependent on effective communication. Communication is essential to building and maintaining relationships in the workplace. Communication is the creation or exchange of thoughts, ideas, emotions, and understanding between sender(s) and receiver(s). Managers who understand this exchange can better analyze their communication patterns resulting in more effective communication within the workplace.

Although managers spend most of their time communicating (e.g., sending or receiving information), one cannot assume that meaningful communication occurs in all exchanges (Dunn, 2002). Once a memorandum, letter, fax, or e-mail has been sent, many are inclined to believe that communication has taken place. However, communication does not occur until information and understanding have passed between sender and the intended receiver.

To make oneself understood as intended is an important part of communication. A receiver may hear a sender but still not understand what the sender's message means. Being constantly engaged in encoding and decoding messages does not ensure that a manager is an expert in communication. Understanding is a personal matter between people, and different people may interpret messages differently. If the idea received is not the one intended, communication has not taken place; the sender has merely spoken or written.

COMMUNICATION PROCESS

Figure 4–1 illustrates the communication process. It shows that the sender is a person, department, or unit of an organization or system who originates the message. A sender uses words and symbols to put forth information into a message for the receiver, the individual(s) receiving the message. Messages are then received and decoded or interpreted by the receiver. Decoding is affected by the receiver's prior experiences and frames of reference. Accurate decoding of the message by the receiver is critical to effective communication. The closer the decoded message gets to the intent of the sender, the more effective the communication. However, environmental and personal barriers can hamper the communication process. Details on barriers are described in a later section of this chapter. For ensuring that messages are received as intended, feedback is a necessary component of the communication process. The receiver creates feedback to a message and encodes it before transmitting it back to the sender. The sender receives and decodes the feedback. Feedback is the destination's reaction to a message (Certo, 1992). It is an important element of communication since it allows for information to be shared between the receiver and sender in a two-way communication.

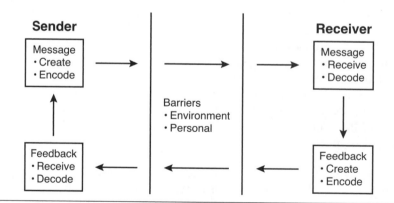

Figure 4–1 The Communication Process
SOURCE: Based on *Organizational behavior: Emerging realities for the workplace revolution* (2nd ed., 324), by S. L. McShane and M. A. Von Glinow, 2003, Boston, MA: McGraw-Hill Book Company.

FEEDBACK

Feedback is any information that individuals receive about their behavior. Feedback can be information related to the productivity of groups in an organization or the performance of a particular individual. For instance, a manager requires feedback to determine staff acceptance of his or her newly set policy, whereby staff must phone all patients to confirm their appointments 48 hours in advance of the appointments. Through the feedback process, senders and receivers may adjust their outputs as related to the transmitted information. In the absence of feedback, or in the case where the communication process does not allow for sufficient feedback to develop, or feedback is ignored, a certain amount of feedback will occur spontaneously and tends to take a negative form.

In one-way communication, a person sends a one-directional message without interaction. When a physician writes out a prescription and gives it to the nurse to hand to the patient, the physician's order is an example of one-way communication and does not provide the opportunity for the patient to ask questions directly. A negative feedback may occur if the patient expresses frustration or anger at the physician for not directly explaining the necessity and functions of the medication. However, the same patient could express satisfaction and appreciation toward the nurse who explains the purpose of the medication. In this case, the opportunity for feedback results in two-way communication between the patient and the nurse. Two-way communication is more accurate and information-rich when the message is complex, although one-way communication is more efficient, as in the case of the physician's written prescription.

To be effective, communication must allow opportunities for feedback. Feedback can take several forms, each with a different intent. Keyton (2002) describes three different forms of feedback: descriptive, evaluative, and prescriptive.

- *Descriptive Feedback:* Feedback that identifies or describes how a person communicates. For instance, Manager A asks Manager B to comment on her behavior at a staff meeting. B indicates that A was specific, clear, and instructive on introducing the staff to the computer database for managing patient accounts. B provides a descriptive feedback of A's behavior at the staff meeting.

- *Evaluative Feedback:* Feedback that provides an assessment of the person who communicates. In the preceding case, if Manager B evaluates Manager A's behavior and concludes that she is instructive and helpful, and that causes the staff to feel comfortable when going to A for help or asking questions, then B has provided positive evaluative feedback of A's interaction with the staff.

- *Prescriptive Feedback:* Feedback that provides advice about how one should behave or communicate. For example, Manager A asks Manager B how she could have made changes to better communicate her message to her staff. B suggests for A to be friendlier and more cooperative by giving the staff specific times that A is available for help with the new computer database. This type of advice is prescriptive feedback.

In addition to forms and intent, there are also four levels of feedback. Feedback can focus on a group or an individual working with specific tasks or procedures. It can also provide information about relationships within the group or individual behavior within a group (Keyton, 2002).

- *Task or Procedural Feedback:* Feedback at this level involves issues of effectiveness and appropriateness. Specific issues that relate to task feedback include the quantity or quality of a group's output. For instance, are patients satisfied with the new outpatient clinic? Did the group complete the project on time? Procedural feedback refers to whether a correct procedure was used appropriately at the time by the group.

- *Relational Feedback:* Feedback that provides information about interpersonal dynamics within a group. This level of feedback emphasizes how a group gets along while working together. It is effective when it is combined with the descriptive and prescriptive forms of feedback.

- *Individual Feedback:* Feedback that focuses on a particular individual in a group. For example, is an individual in the group knowledgeable? Does he or she have the skills helpful to this group? What attitudes does he or she have toward the group as they work together to accomplish their tasks? Is the individual able to plan and organize within a schedule that contributes to the group's goal attainment?

- *Group Feedback:* Feedback that focuses on how well the group is performing. Like the questions raised at the individual feedback level, similar questions are asked for the group. Do team members within the group have adequate knowledge to complete a task? Have they developed a communication network to facilitate their objectives?

Feedback can be in the form of questionnaires, surveys, and audio- or videotapes of group interaction. It can also occur in activities such as market research, client surveys, accreditation, and employee evaluations (Liebler & McConnell, 2004). Feedback should be used to help a group communicate more effectively by making group members identify with the group and increase its efficacy. Feedback should not be viewed as a negative process. Instead, it should be used as a strategy to enhance goals, awareness, and learning. As a managerial tool, feedback enables managers to anticipate and respond to changes. Structured feedback enhances managerial planning and controlling functions. Because of the value of feedback, managers should encourage feedback and evaluate it systematically.

The Johari Window

The process of feedback is also illustrated in the Johari Window, a useful model for understanding the communication process created by Joe Luft and Harry Ingham (hence the name "Johari") (Luft, 1984). The Johari Window model improves an individual's communication skills through identifying one's capabilities and limitations. As shown in Exhibit 4–1, windowpane 1 is the open area in which information about you is known both to you and to others. Tubbs (2001) described this area as the general cocktail party conversa-

Exhibit 4–1 The Johari Window

Feedback →

D
i
s
c
l
o
s
u
r
e ↓

| 1. Open Area (Known to self) (Known to others) | 2. Blind Area (Unknown to self) (Known to others) |
| 3. Hidden Area (Known to self) (Unknown to others) | 4. Unknown Area (Unknown to self) (Unknown to others) |

SOURCE: Based on *Group processes: An introduction to group dynamics* (3rd ed.), by J. Luft, 1984, Palo Alto, CA: Mayfield.

tion in which an individual willingly shares information with others. For instance, at an office party, you reveal to your coworkers that you do not drink alcohol because of health reasons. Windowpane 2 refers to a blind area in which others know information about you that you are either unaware of or that you do unknowingly. As an example, your colleagues know that you are a "close" talker, that you unconsciously stand too close to people while in conversation with them.

The third windowpane is the hidden area in which you have likes and dislikes that you are unwilling to share with others. This area includes all of your values, beliefs, fears, and past experiences that you would not wish to reveal. The last windowpane is the unknown. It is also an area of potential growth or self-actualization. It represents all the things that we have never tried, participated in, or experienced.

Increasing mutual understanding through feedback and disclosure allows an individual to increase the open area and reduce the blind, hidden, and unknown areas of oneself (McShane & Von Glinow, 2003). In the Johari Window, Luft (1984) argues for increasing the open area so that you and your coworkers are aware of your limitations. This is done by receiving more feedback from others and decreasing one's blind area (windowpane 2), and reducing the hidden area (windowpane 3) through disclosing more about oneself. The combination of feedback and disclosure may also help to produce more information in the unknown area (windowpane 4).

The Johari Window can be used for opening the channels of communication. Open communication is important for improving employee morale and increasing worker productivity. Open communication allows supervisors and subordinates to openly discuss organization-related issues such as goals and conflicts. Nevertheless, Luft (1984) is cautious on the use of the Johari Window for all situations. He offers several guidelines for the appropriateness of self-disclosure. He recommends that self-disclosure is a function of an ongoing relationship. Timing and extent of disclosure are critical. A competent communicator knows when, with whom, and how much to disclose.

COMMUNICATION CHANNELS

Another important component of the communication process is selecting the appropriate communication channel. It is the means by which messages are transmitted. There are two types of channels: verbal and nonverbal. The various channels of communication and the amount of information transmitted through each type are illustrated in Figure 4–2.

Verbal Communication

Verbal communication relies on spoken or written words to share information with others. Dialogue is a form of verbal communication. It is a discussion or conversation between people. It is a process in which participants are exposed to new information. The process involves a series of meetings of organizational members that represent different views on issues of mutual interest. According to Edgley and Robinson (1991), in order for dialogue to be successful, there are several fundamental principles: engage motivated people; use a facilitator and recorder to manage the process; have the group develop procedures and live by them; ensure confidentiality; let the process move at its own pace—don't try to rush it; focus on understanding the issue and not on developing an end product; and

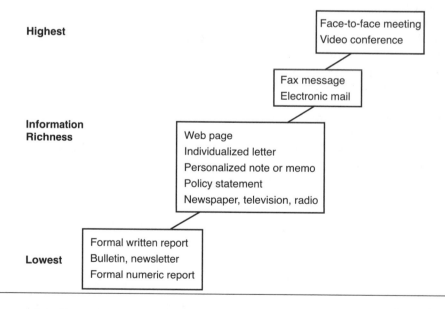

Figure 4–2 Communication Channels
SOURCE: Information richness: A new approach to managerial behavior and organizational design, by R. L. Daft and R. H. Lengel, 1984, in B. Staw and L. Cummings (Eds.), *Research in organizational behavior* (vol. 6, pp. 191–233, Greenwich, CT: JAI Press.

allow time to get to know one another—have dinner before, during, or after a meeting. Successful dialogue between group members in an organization enhances communication.

There are different forms of verbal communication, which should be used for different situations. Face-to-face meetings are information-rich, since they allow for emotions to be transmitted and immediate feedback to take place. Written communication is more appropriate for describing details, especially of a technical nature as in the example of monitoring a patient's complex medical condition. Although traditional written communication had been considered slow, now with the development of electronic mail and computer-aided communication, written communication through these channels has dramatically improved efficiency (See Case Study 4–1: Are We Getting the Message Across?).

Case Study 4–1 Are We Getting the Message Across?

James Warick, Director of Physical Plant at Southern Hospital, e-mailed Diane Curtis, Director of Nursing, informing her of a leak in Operating Room 1 that must be shut down for repairs early next morning. Curtis forwarded the message to Joanne Messing, the operating room nurse supervisor on duty for the night shift. Messing, tired from a long night's work, handwrote a message to the nurse supervisor in the day shift to switch the 8 am operation from Room 1 to Room 8 and taped it on the bulletin board. David Swanson, the day-shift nurse supervisor, arrived at 7:30 am and found Dr. Roberts shouting that his patient was ready for surgery, but no rooms were available because Dr. Jones had already taken Room 8.

Discussion Questions

1. What were the channels of communication used by each person?
2. Should a different channel of communication have been used instead?
3. What can be done to resolve the problem?
4. What future policies should be put in place to prevent this from occurring again?

Computer-aided Communication

The use of computers and information technology is dramatically affecting the way we communicate. The Internet is a global network of interconnected, yet independently operated computers. An intranet is an organization's private Internet. Especially in the case of healthcare organizations, the intranet helps to protect the privacy and confidentiality of company records, such as patient medical records. An extranet is an extended intranet that enables employees to stay connected with selected customers, clients, suppliers, and other partners, such as healthcare insurance companies and healthcare vendors. The Internet, intranets, and extranets enable employees to access, manage, and distribute information. These systems can enhance communication if properly set up and managed effectively. On the other hand, ineffective management can hinder communication and result in decreased productivity.

Electronic mail uses the Internet or intranet to send computer-generated text and documents. E-mail has revolutionized the communication process. E-mail allows messages to be rapidly created, changed, saved, and sent to many people at the same time. One can select any part of the message to read and skip to important parts of the message. E-mail is a preferred channel for coordinating work and schedules. Messages can be clearly defined through concrete and specific instructions rather than abstract words or generalization. For example, an e-mail can be sent to all physicians to inform them that a meeting starts promptly at 10 AM.

There are several problems and limitations to electronic mail. The most obvious is information overload. E-mail users are overwhelmed by the number of messages received on a daily basis, of which many are unnecessary to the receiver. Moreover, e-mail messages are frequently carrying computer viruses, which have caused major damage to computers and interruptions in work flow. Another problem with e-mail is its ineffectiveness to communicate emotion. Tones of messages are easily misinterpreted, causing misunderstandings between sender and receiver. Computer experts have even developed icons to represent emotions (emoticons) in e-mail messages. For instance, the symbol :-) or :) means happy (Peck, 1997). E-mail also reduces politeness and respect for others. Flaming is the act of sending an emotionally charged message to others, especially before emotions subside. This common problem occurs frequently over e-mail, whereas a traditional letter provides time to cool down and have second thoughts. To reduce these e-mail problems, some have recommended training for communication on the Internet, called netiquette (Extejt, 1998). Netiquette rules include keeping e-mail messages to fewer than 25 lines and not sending sensitive issues through e-mail. There are also key benefits to using e-mail. E-mail reduces time and cost of distributing information to employees. Furthermore, e-mail has increased the potential for more employee collaboration and teamwork. Rather than using the telephone, letters, or memos, employees can use e-mail to rapidly send and receive messages. For instance, if a hospital ethics committee comprises physicians, nurses, and administrators, staff responsible for setting up monthly meetings find that the fastest way to confirm a meeting date and time would be through e-mail. Another advantage of e-mail is its flexibility. This is especially so for those employees with portable computers, such as personal digital assistants (PDAs). PDAs are multifunctional, that is, they can accomplish many tasks, including managing appointments, sending and receiving e-mail, watching video clips, and completing a variety of tasks. These handheld devices have contributed to the increased demand for access to information.

Other Computer-aided Communication

In addition to e-mail technology, other forms of technology have entered healthcare organizations and directly enhanced and impacted the communication process. Coile (2002) describes several such technological advancements that can be used to bridge the communications gap between clinicians and administrators. Computer-aided drug discovery is expected to double the number of new medications. High-speed, high-definition images are created for rapid access via telemedicine. Wireless, handheld digital electronic medical records are capable of voice recognition. Telepresence surgery with minimally invasive, remotely guided instruments extends beyond the precision of humans. Medical applications of artificial intelligence are designed for diagnosis, treatment planning, and continuous monitoring of the chronically ill (Coile, 2002).

Nonverbal Communication

Nonverbal communication is sharing information without using words to encode messages. There are four basic forms of nonverbal communication: proxemics, kinesics, facial and eye behavior, and paralanguage (Nelson & Quick, 2003). Proxemics is the study of an individual's perception and use of space. Territorial space and seating arrangement are two examples. For instance, to encourage cooperation, coworkers working together on a quality-control report should sit next to each other. To facilitate communication, a manager should seat a subordinate at a 90 degree angle in order to discuss resolving staff complaints.

Kinesics refers to body language, which is used to convey meanings and messages. Pacing or drumming fingers are signs of nervousness. Wringing of the hands and rubbing temples signal stress. Facial and eye behavior is another example of nonverbal communication. For example, when a health-care manager interviews a candidate for a position as a clinical care coordinator, the manager attaches meanings to frowns and eye contact. Avoiding eye contact tends to close communication. However, cultural and individual differences influence appropriate eye contact. Moderate direct eye contact communicates openness, while too much direct eye contact can be intimidating.

Paralanguage consists of voice quality, volume, speech rate, and pitch. Rapid and loud speech may be taken as signs of anger or nervousness. The communication process is impeded by negative nonverbal cues. For example, arriving late for an interview with the vice president of finance, talking very fast, avoiding eye contact, getting very close during a conversation or in a seating arrangement for a committee meeting serve as negative factors in the communication process.

To determine the most appropriate channel of communication for sending messages, one needs to identify whether verbal or nonverbal communication should be used. At the same time, ideal channels of communications can be selected through an examination of the information richness and symbolic meaning of messages (Daft & Lengel, 1984). Information richness refers to the volume and variety of information that can be transmitted. As shown in Figure 4–2, face-to-face meetings have the highest information-carrying capability, because the sender can use verbal and nonverbal communication channels and the receiver can provide instant feedback. When a wrong channel of communication is used, this creates a waste of time and leads to more misunderstanding. When communication is nonroutine or unclear, information-rich channels are required. As an example, a gunshot victim is brought into the trauma center. Coordinating the care of this patient requires face-to-face instructions to quickly coordinate work flow and minimize the risk of confusion among various staff members. However, for routine communications, less information-rich channels can be used.

Choosing one communication channel over another lends meaning to the message. That is to say, there is symbolic meaning to the selection of a particular channel of communication beyond the message content. For example, when a manager tells an employee that they must have a face-to-face meeting, this symbolizes that the issue is important compared to a brief e-mail message with instructions.

In summary, one essential part of the communication process is selecting an ideal channel of communication. The use of different channels leads to differences in the amount and variety of information transmitted. Choosing an appropriate channel of communication involves understanding symbolic meanings and the information richness of messages.

BARRIERS TO COMMUNICATION

As illustrated in Table 4–1, several forms of barriers can impede the communication process. Longest et al. (2000) classify these barriers into two categories: environmental and personal. Environmental barriers are characteristic of the organization and its environmental setting. Personal barriers arise from the nature of individuals and their interaction with others. Both barriers can block, filter, or distort the message as it is encoded and sent, as well as when it is decoded and received.

Environmental Barriers

Examples of environmental barriers include competition for attention and time between senders and receivers. Multiple and simultaneous demands cause messages to be incorrectly decoded. The receiver hears the message, but does not understand it. As a result of inadequate attention paid to the message, the receiver is not really "listening." Listening is a process that integrates physical, emotional, and intellectual inputs into the quest for meaning and understanding. Listening is effective only when the receiver understands the sender's messages as intended. Thus, without engaging in active listening, the receiver fails to comprehend the message. Time is another barrier. Lack of time prevents the sender from carefully thinking through and thoroughly structuring the message accordingly, and limits the receiver's ability to decipher the message and determine its meaning.

Other environmental barriers include the organization's managerial philosophy, multiple levels of hierarchy, and power or status relationships between senders and receivers. Managerial philosophy can promote or inhibit effective communication. Managers who are not interested in promoting intraorganizational communication upward or disseminating information downward will establish procedural and organizational blockages. By requiring that all communication follow the chain of command, lack of attention and concern toward employees is a sign of a managerial philosophy that restricts communication flows. Furthermore, when subordinates encounter managers who fail to act, they are unwilling to communicate upward in the future, because communications are not taken seriously.

Managerial philosophy not only affects communication within the organization, but also impacts the organization's communications with external stakeholders. For instance, when the chief executive officer (CEO) of one hospital becomes aware that patients might have been exposed to a dangerous infection while hospitalized, he immediately decides to cover up the incident and communicates that message down to his managers. However, another hospital CEO deals with this incident in a very different manner. She uses the public media as a channel of communication to encourage patients to come forward and be tested. These reactions to similar events reflect different managerial philosophies about communication.

Multiple levels of hierarchy and complexities such as the size and degree of activity conducted in the organization tend to cause message distortion. As messages are transmitted up or down, they may be interpreted according to an individual's personal frame of reference. When multiple links exist in the communication chain, information could be misinterpreted. As a result, a message sent through many levels is likely to be distorted or even totally blocked. As an example, the CEO asked department administrators to relay his message of sincere congratulations and appreciation for their hard work to obtain their institutional Joint Commission on Accreditation of Healthcare Organizations accreditation status. The message went through several layers of the organization and was received in a more nonchalant manner than originally intended. In another scenario, a report generated by the management information system analyst was given to his supervisor, who went on vacation and left it on his desk without giving it to the vice president who had requested it a week ago. In this case, the message did not reach its destination.

Power or status relationships can also affect transmission of a message. An unharmonious supervisor–subordinate relationship can interfere with the flow and content of information. Moreover, a staff member's previous experiences in the workplace may prevent open communication because of fear of negative sanctions as a result. For instance, a poor supervisor–subordinate relationship inhibits the subordinate from reporting that the project is not working as planned. Fear of the power and status of the manager is a common barrier to communication. Another environmental barrier that may lead to miscommunication is the use of specific terminology unfamiliar to the receiver or when messages are especially complex. Managers and clinical staff in healthcare organizations use medical terminology, which may be unfamiliar to external stakeholders. Communication between people who use different terminology can be unproductive simply because people attach different meanings to the same words. Thus, misunderstanding can occur as a result of unfamiliar terminology.

Personal Barriers

Personal barriers arise because of an individual's frame of reference or beliefs and values. These barriers are based on one's socioeconomic background and prior experiences and shape how messages are encoded and decoded. One may also consciously or unconsciously engage in selective perception or be influenced by fear or jealously. For example, some cultures believe in "don't speak unless spoken to" or "never question elders" (Longest et al., 2000). These beliefs inhibit communication. Others accept all communication at face value without filtering out erroneous information. Still others provide self-promotion information, intentionally transmitting and distorting messages for personal gain. Unless one has had the same experiences as others, it is difficult to completely understand their message. In addition to frame of reference, one's beliefs, values, and prejudices also can alter and block messages. Preconceived opinions and prejudices are formed on the basis of varying personalities and backgrounds. As discussed in Chapter 3, selective perception is a tendency for retaining positive parts of the message and filtering out negative portions.

Two additional personal barriers are status quo and evaluating the sender to determine whether one should retain or filter out messages. For instance, a manager always ignores the complaints from Melissa, the medical receptionist, because Melissa tends to exaggerate issues and events. However, one must be careful to evaluate and distinguish exaggerations from legitimate messages. Status quo is when individuals prefer the present situation. They intentionally filter out information that is unpleasant. For example, a manager refuses to tell staff and patients that their favorite physician, Dr. Ames, has decided to leave the practice. To prevent patients from switching to another physician, the manager postpones the communication to retain status quo.

A final personal barrier is lack of empathy, in other words, insensitivity to the emotional states of senders and receivers. In the case where a physician demands that his assistants hurry and clean up the rooms because 50 patients are waiting, the assistants should empathize with the physician and understand that the physician is under stress and pressure to see his patients who are complaining that they have been waiting over three hours.

OVERCOMING BARRIERS TO IMPROVE COMMUNICATION

Recognizing that environment and personal barriers exist is the first step to effective communication. By becoming cognizant of their existence, one can consciously minimize their impact. However, positive actions are needed to overcome these barriers (see Table 4–1).

Longest and colleagues (2000) provide us with several guidelines for overcoming barriers:

1. Environmental barriers are reduced if receivers and senders ensure that attention is given to their messages and that adequate time is devoted to listening to what is being communicated.

2. A management philosophy that encourages the free flow of communication is constructive.

3. Reducing the number of links (levels in the organizational hierarchy or steps between the sender in the healthcare organization and the receiver who is an external stakeholder) reduces opportunities for distortion.

4. The power/status barrier can be removed by consciously tailoring words and symbols so that messages are understandable; reinforcing words with actions significantly improves communication among different power/status levels.

5. Using multiple channels to reinforce complex messages decreases the likelihood of misunderstanding.

Table 4–1 Overcoming Barriers to Communication

Barriers to Communication	Overcoming Barriers to Communication
Environmental Barriers	
1. Competition for time and attention	1. Devote adequate time and attention to listening
2. Multiple levels of hierarchy	2. Reduce the number of links or levels of hierarchy
3. Managerial philosophy	3. Change philosophy to encourage the free flow of communication
4. Power/status relationships	4. Consciously tailor words and symbols and reinforce words with actions so that messages are understandable
5. Organizational complexity	5. Use multiple channels of community to reinforce complex messages
6. Specific terminology	6. Consciously define and tailor words and symbols and reinforce words with actions so that messages are understandable
Personal Barriers	
1. Frame of reference	1. Consciously engage in efforts to be cognizant of other's frame of reference and beliefs
2. Beliefs	
3. Values	2. Recognize that others will engage in selective perception, jealousy, fear, and prejudices to help diminish the barriers
4. Prejudices	
5. Selective perception	
6. Jealousy	3. Engage in empathy
7. Fear	
8. Evaluate the source (sender)	
9. Status quo	
10. Lack of empathy	

Source: Based on *Managing health services organizations* (4th ed., pp. 808–810), by B.B. Longest, J.S. Rakich, and K. Darr, 2000, Baltimore, MD: Health Professions Press.

Personal barriers to effective communication are reduced by conscious efforts of senders and receivers to understand each other's values and beliefs. One must recognize that people engage in selective perception and are prone to jealously and fear. Sharing empathy with those to whom messages are directed is the best way to increase effective communication.

Communicating effectively among a complex, multisite healthcare system is challenging. Barriers may be difficult to overcome. Porter (1985) offers several approaches for achieving effective linkages among business units in a diversified corporation and suggests ways in which managers can overcome some of these barriers.

1. Use techniques that extend beyond traditional organizational lines to facilitate communication. For instance, the use of diagonal communication that

flows through task forces or committees enhances communication throughout the organization.

2. Use management processes that are cross-organizational rather than confined to functional or department procedures. Implementing management processes in the areas of planning, controlling, and managing information systems facilitates communication.

3. Use human resources policies and procedures (job training and job rotation) to enhance cooperation among members in organizations.

4. Use management processes to resolve conflicts in an equitable manner to produce effective communication.

EFFECTIVE COMMUNICATION FOR KNOWLEDGE MANAGEMENT

Communication plays an important role in knowledge management. Employees are the organization's brain cells, and communication represents the nervous system that carries information and shared meaning to vital parts of the organizational body. Effective communication brings knowledge into the organization and disseminates it to employees who require that information. Effective communication minimizes the "silos of knowledge" problem that undermines an organization's potential and, in turn, allows employees to make more informed decisions about corporate actions. Effective communication is one of the most critical goals of organizations (Spillan et al., 2002). Research suggests that an effective manager is one who spends considerable time on staffing, motivating, and reinforcing activities (Luthans et al., 1988).

Shortell (1991) identified multiple key elements to effective communication in a model developed for physicians and hospital administration to improve their communication abilities to disseminate knowledge within the organization. The following summarizes these key elements:

- An effective communicator must have a desire to communicate, which is influenced both by one's personal values and the expectation that the communication will be received in a meaningful way.

- An effective communicator must have an understanding of how others learn, which includes consideration of differences in how others perceive and process information (e.g., analytic versus intuitive, abstract versus concrete, verbal versus written).

- The receiver of the message should be cued as to the purpose of the message, that is, whether the message is to provide information, elicit a response or reaction, or arrive at a decision.

- The content, importance, and complexity of the message should be considered in determining the manner in which the message is communicated.

- The credibility of the sender affects how the message will be received.

- The time frame associated with the content of the message (long versus short) needs to be considered in choosing the manner in which the message is communicated. More precise cues are needed with shorter time frames (see Figure 4–3).

Effective Communication

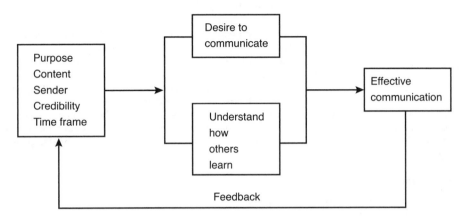

Figure 4–3 Interrelationships of Effective Knowledge-management Communication
SOURCE: Based on *Effective hospital-physician relationship* (p. 87), by S.M. Shortell, 1991, Ann Arbor, MI: Health Administration Press.

A formula to evaluate an individual's effectiveness in communicating to others can be calculated as shown in Exhibit 4–2.

The ICE is a percentage of the reaction to the intended message over the total number of messages sent. If managers find that their ICE is low over time, they should evaluate their communication processes to identify ways to make improvements (Certo, 1992). Research suggests that to improve healthcare organizational communication and cohesion, exchanges between employees and leaders should involve leaders' direct support and encouragement of employees' constructive expressions of dissatisfaction and innovative ideas (Sobo and Sadler, 2002) (see Case Study 4–2: What Should We Do Now?).

Exhibit 4–2 An Index of Communication Effectiveness

$$\text{Index of communication effectiveness (ICE)} = \frac{\text{RIM (reaction to intended message)}}{\text{TMS (total number of messages sent)}}$$

SOURCE: *Modern management: Quality, ethics, and the global environment* (5th ed.), by S. C. Certo, 1992, Boston, MA: Allyn and Bacon.

Case Study 4–2 What Should We Do Now?

Jenny Taylor, Receptionist at Caring Physicians Clinic, was responsible for calling patients to remind them of their appointments. Dr. Ann Ryan, Medical Director of the Clinic, found Jenny to be hardworking and pleasant to the patients. One morning, Dr. Ryan arrived and found Jenny crying in the supplies room, and when she questioned Jenny, Jenny sobbed that for the past three months she had forgotten to order supplies. Jenny had been borrowing supplies from the pediatrics office next door. Now, they were unwilling to lend her more. Jenny confessed that she had called once to the supply center and faxed a list of supplies over, but had not followed through. This morning, Jenny called the supply center again and found out that they were out of business. Jenny told her immediate supervisor, Barbara Lakes, Patient Care Coordinator for the Clinic. Lakes fired Jenny for incompetence. In the meantime, patients were waiting and there were no clean sheets, gloves, or gowns.

Discussion Questions

1. What was the beginning of the problem?
2. What should Jenny have done?
3. Using the elements of effective communication, discuss what should Dr. Ryan and Barbara Lakes do now?

STRATEGIC COMMUNICATION

Strategic communication is an intentional process of presenting ideas in a clear, concise, and persuasive way. A manager must make an intentional effort to master communication skills and use them strategically, that is, consistently with the organization's values, mission, and strategy. To plan strategic communication, managers must develop a methodology for thinking through and effectively communicating with superiors, staff, and peers. Sperry and Whiteman (2003) provide us with a strategic communication plan, which consists of five components.

1. *Outcome:* The specific result that an individual wants to achieve.
2. *Context:* The organizational importance of the communication.
3. *Messages:* The key information that staff need to know.
4. *Tactical Reinforcement:* Tactics or methods used to reinforce the message.
5. *Feedback:* The way the message is received and its impact on the individual, team, unit, or organization.

Strategic communication requires forethought about the purpose and outcome of the message. Managers must be able to link the needs of the staff to the organization's mission and deadlines.

FLOWS OF INTRAORGANIZATIONAL COMMUNICATION

Communication can flow upward, downward, horizontally, and diagonally within organizations. Upward communication occurs between supervisors and subordinates. Downward communication primarily involves passing on information from supervisors to subordinates. Horizontal flow is from manager to manager or from coworker to coworker. Diagonal flow occurs between different levels of different departments. Longest et al. (2000) provides us with several forms of intraorganizational communication for healthcare organizations, which are described in the following paragraphs.

Upward Flow

The purposes of upward communication flow are to provide managers with information to make decisions, identify problem areas, collect data for performance assessments, determine staff morale, and reveal employee thoughts and feelings about the organization. Upward flow becomes especially important with increased organizational complexity. Therefore, managers must rely on effective upward communication and encourage it as an integral part of the organizational culture. Upward communication flow helps employees meet their personal needs, by allowing those in positions of lesser authority to express opinions and perceptions to those with higher authority. As a result, they make contributions to the organization, and participate in the decision-making process. The hierarchical structure (chain of command) is the main channel for upward communications in healthcare organizations. To increase the effectiveness of upward communication, Luthans (1984) recommends the use of grievance procedures, open-door policies, counseling, employee questionnaires, exit interviews, and participative decision-making techniques and the use of an ombudsperson.

- *Grievance Procedure:* The grievance procedure allows employees to make an appeal upward beyond their immediate supervisor. It protects the individual from arbitrary action by their direct supervisor and encourages communication about complaints.
- *Open-door Policy:* The supervisor's door is always open to subordinates. It is an invitation for subordinates to come in and talk to the superior about things that trouble them.
- *Counseling, Questionnaires, and Exit Interviews:* The department of human resources in a healthcare organization can facilitate subordinate-initiated communication by conducting confidential counseling, administering attitude questionnaires, and holding exit interviews for those leaving the organization. Information gained from these forms of communication can be used to make improvements.
- *Participative Decision-making Techniques:* Through the use of informal involvement of subordinates or formal participation programs such as quality-improvement teams, union–management committees, and suggestion boxes, participative techniques can improve employee performance and satisfaction. Since employees can participate in the decision-making process, they feel that they can make valuable contributions to the organization.
- *Ombudsperson:* The use of an ombudsperson provides an outlet for persons who feel they have been treated unfairly.

In upward communication, subordinates can provide two types of information to supervisors: (1) personal information about ideas, attitudes, and performance and (2) technical information to provide feedback. Managers who encourage feedback enhance upward flow of communication.

Downward Flow

Downward communication involves passing information from supervisors to subordinates. This includes verbal and nonverbal communication, such as instructions for completing tasks, as well as communications on a one-to-one basis. Downward communications include meeting with employees, written memos, newsletters, bulletin boards, procedural manuals, and clinical and administration information systems.

Horizontal Flow

Upward and downward communications are inadequate for effective organizational performance. In complex healthcare organizations, horizontal flow or lateral communication must also occur. The purpose of lateral communication is the sharing of information among peers at similar levels to keep organizational staff informed of all current practices, policies, and procedures (Spillan et al., 2002). For example, coordinating the continuum of patient care requires communication among multiple units. Committees, task forces, and cross-functional project teams are all useful forms of horizontal communication.

Diagonal Flow

The least used channel of communication in healthcare organizations is diagonal flow although growing in importance. While diagonal flow does not follow the typical hierarchical chain of command, diagonal flow is especially useful in health care for efficient communication and coordination of patient care. For example, diagonal communication occurs when the director of nursing asks the data analyst in the medical records department to generate a report for the month on all patients in the intensive care unit (see Case Study 4–3: Communication Flows).

Case Study 4–3 Communication Flows

Sara Lang is a charge nurse at Sunny Nursing Home and has worked under the same president, Lisa Davis, for five years. In fact, the two have become good friends. They frequently socialize after hours. Rick Walters, Director of Nursing, is a capable person who has been working there for three years. Four nurses (Anna, Barbara, Charles, and Dan) report directly to Sara.

Anna, one of the nurses, was having personal difficulties. She asked Sara whether she could change her work schedule from the usual 8-hour shift of 4 days with 3 consecutive days off to 16-hour shifts for two days and 5 consecutive days off. Sara thought that was not a problem and told Anna that she would enter that information into the computerized scheduling system and that she would tell Lisa Davis of the change, since they were getting together for a drink after work.

Barbara overheard the conversation between Sara and Anna, and she immediately went to see Rick Walters and complained that Anna was getting preferential treatment and she wanted the same schedule. Rick, who always wanted to make sure that the nursing staff was happy and got along, approved Barbara's change in schedule. He made this change through the computerized schedule and did not tell anyone else. Barbara, who is good friends with Charles, told him of her new schedule. Charles, who works closely with Chief of

Staff, Dr. Goodman, told Dr. Goodman of the change in Barbara's schedule and asked Dr. Goodman to change his. Dr. Goodman thought it was a good idea and e-mailed Charles' new schedule to his assistant, Susan Stevens, to enter it into the scheduling system.

On the next Monday morning, changes were implemented to Anna's, Barbara's, and Charles' schedules. Yet, no one had discussed these changes with anyone else. When the schedule was printed out and posted, it showed that Anna, Barbara, and Charles were all off for 5 days that week from Monday to Friday and all three began work on Saturday. In the meantime, the only nurse left working was Dan.

Discussion Questions

1. What are the different forms of communication flow taking place?
2. What changes should have been implemented?
3. What should be done now?

COMMUNICATION NETWORKS

Flows of communication can be combined into patterns called communication networks. These networks are interconnected by communication channels. A communication network is the interaction pattern between and among group members. A network creates structure for the group because it controls who can and should talk to whom (Keyton, 2002). Groups generally develop two types of communication networks: centralized and decentralized (Figure 4–4).

Decentralized networks allow each group member to talk to every other group member without restrictions. An open, all-channel or decentralized network is best used for group discussions, decision making, and problem solving. The all-channel network tends to be fast and accurate compared with the centralized network such as the chain or Y-pattern networks (Longest et al., 2000). Nevertheless, a decentralized network can create communication overload, in which too much information or too complex communication may occur (Keyton, 2002). When a communication overload is produced, messages may conflict with one another and result in confusion or disagreement. To reduce communication overload, a facilitator should be used to monitor group discussions.

A centralized network restricts the number of people in the communication chain. In a group setting where a dominant leader takes over group discussions by controlling the number of messages and amount of information being passed, group members do not interact except through the leader. Such a network can create communication underload, in which too few or simple messages are transmitted. In this type of network, group members feel isolated from group discussions and generally feel dissatisfied. In the chain network, communication occurs upward and downward and follows line authority relationships. An example is a staff nurse who reports to the charge nurse, who reports to the director of nursing, who reports to the vice president for clinical services, who finally reports to the CEO of a large hospital. This network delineates the chain of command and shows clear lines of authority.

Other types of centralized networks include the Y-pattern, the wheel, and the circle network. The Y-pattern is similar to the chain network, with its hierarchical structure, except it shows two employees at the same level who then follow the chain. An example is of two medical assistants in the organ trans-

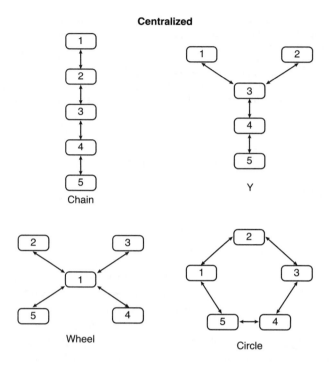

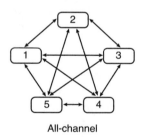

Figure 4–4 Two Types of Communication Networks: Centralized and Decentralized
SOURCE: *Managing health services organizations* (4th ed., p. 813), by B. B. Longest, J. S. Rackich, and K. Darr, 2000, Baltimore, MD: Health Professionals Press.

plant division who report to the clinical administrator for the division, who reports to the clinical administrator for the department of surgery, who reports to the vice president of clinical services, who finally reports to the CEO of the hospital.

The wheel pattern shows four subordinates reporting to one supervisor. Subordinates do not interact, and all communications are channeled through the manager at the center of the wheel. This pattern is rare in healthcare organizations and systems, although elements of it can be found in the example where four vice presidents report to a president if the vice presidents have little interaction. Even though this network pattern is not routinely used, it may be used when urgency or secrecy is required. For example, the president with an organizational emergency might communicate with the vice presidents in a wheel pattern because time does not permit using other modes. Similarly, if secrecy is important, such as when investigating possible embezzlement, then the president may require that all relevant communication with the vice presidents be confidential. The wheel pattern works well when there is pressure for time, secrecy, and accuracy.

The circle pattern allows communicators in the network to communicate directly only with two others. Since each communicates with another in the network, there is no central authority or leader. The circle network works well when there are open channels of communication among all parties; however, it can also slow down the communication process to enable everyone access to information.

Although there are different communication networks, there is not one that works for all situations. Different forms can be applied under varying circumstances. To be effective, healthcare managers must be able to select appropriate flows of communication for specific situations. Identifying an ideal communication network is critical to successful communication. Since health problems range from simple to complex, simple problems can be easily resolved using simple networks. As an example, scheduling patient appointments for Dr. Davis can be easily accomplished through the superior–subordinate chain network. However, complex problems require many levels of decision making. For instance, whether Horizons Hospital should merge with its major competitor to gain more market share at the risk of making a major capital investment can be accomplished through the all-channel network, which is more useful and effective for tackling complex problems. Hellriegel and Slocum (2004) compared the five communication networks using four assessment criteria. Figure 4–5 shows the specific criteria when making a selection among the different types of networks.

1. *Degree of Centralization:* Degree of centralization is the extent to which team members have access to more communication than others. In the case of the wheel network, because communication flows from and to only one member, this is the most centralized network. However, the all-channel network provides everyone in the network with the same opportunity for communication; thus, it is the least centralized network.

2. *Leadership Predictability:* Leadership predictability is the ability to anticipate which member of the communication network is likely to emerge as the leader. In the case of the Y and wheel, the most centrally positioned individual is the most likely person.

3. *Average Group Satisfaction:* Average group satisfaction reflects the level of satisfaction of members in the communication network. In the wheel network, average member satisfaction is the lowest compared to other networks, since the most centrally positioned person plays the most crucial roles and leaves small decision-making roles for those around the wheel.

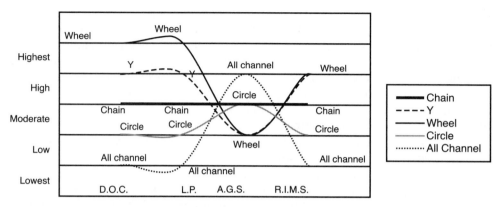

D.O.C. – Degree of Centralization
L.P. – Leadership Predictability
A.G.S. – Average Group Satisfaction
R.I.M.S. – Range in Individual Member Satisfaction

Figure 4–5 Effects of Five Communication Networks
SOURCE: *Organizational behavior* (10th ed., p. 301), by D. Hellriegel and J. W. Slocum, 2004, Mason, OH: South-Western.

4. *Range of Individual Member Satisfaction:* The range of an individual's satisfaction within the communication network shows an inverse relationship with the average group satisfaction. Again, in the wheel, although average member satisfaction is low, the range of individual member satisfaction is high, because they are highly dependent on the individual in the middle. In the case of the all-channel, average group satisfaction is high since there is greater participation by all members of the communication network; yet, individual satisfaction is very low.

INFORMAL COMMUNICATION

In addition to formal communication flows and networks within healthcare organizations, there are informal communication flows, which have their own networks. Employees have always relied on the oldest communication channel—the corporate grapevine. The grapevine is an unstructured and informal network founded on social relationships rather than organizational charts or job descriptions. According to some estimates, 75 percent of employees typically receive news from the grapevine before they hear about it through formal channels (McShane & Von Glinow, 2003).

Early research identified several unique features of the grapevine. It transmits information very rapidly in all directions (Newstrom & Davis, 1993). Figure 4–6 illustrates four common patterns that the grapevine can take.

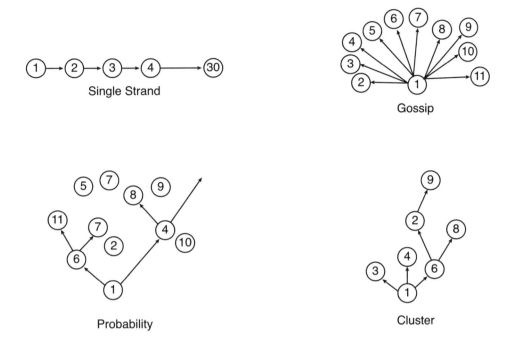

Figure 4–6 Grapevine Networks
SOURCE: *Organizational behavior: Human behavior at work* (9th ed., p. 445), by J. W. Newstrom and K. Davis, 1993, New York: McGraw-Hill Book Company.

The typical pattern is a cluster chain, whereby a few people actively transmit rumors to many others. The grapevine works through informal social networks, so it is more active where employees have similar backgrounds and are able to communicate easily. Many rumors seem to have at least a little bit of truth, possibly because rumors are transmitted through information-rich communication channels, and employees are motivated to communicate effectively. Nevertheless, the grapevine distorts information by deleting fine details and exaggerating key points of the message.

In this era of information technology, e-mail and instant messaging have replaced the traditional watercooler site of grapevine gossip. Instead, networks have expanded as employees communicate with one another inside and outside of the organization instantly through computer-aided communication. Furthermore, public Web sites have become virtual watercoolers for posting anonymous comments about specific companies for all to view. This technology extends gossip to anyone, not just employees connected to the social networks. A manager's responsibility is to utilize the informal network selectively to benefit the organization's goals (see Case Study 4–4: Did You Hear the Latest?).

Case Study 4–4 Did You Hear the Latest?

Sally Reeds, a medical secretary for the department of neurology at Western Heights Hospital in Colorado, turned on her computer and found an e-mail from her friend and coworker, Justin Zeels, a social worker in the same hospital. Justin wrote that Dr. Sites, Medical Director of Neurology, was found under a bench outside the ER. The hospital security allegedly reported that Dr. Sites was completely intoxicated, and he was rushed home. Sally spiced up the tale and immediately e-mailed 10 of her friends. This morning, Sally looked up and saw Dr. Sites seeing his patients as if nothing had happened. She confronted him and asked him how he could possibly face everyone after what happened last night. Dr. Sites looked confused until a copy of Zeels' e-mail was thrust into Dr. Sites' hands by another staff member. After reading it, Dr. Sites became livid and fired Justin for spreading such a malicious rumor. Meanwhile, Maria Hummingshire, another medical secretary, who saw the entire incident, ran to her computer to e-mail the latest to her friends.

Discussion Questions

1. What did Sally do wrong?
2. What should Justin have done?
3. What should the organization do to prevent the spread of gossip through the grapevine?

CROSS-CULTURAL COMMUNICATION

Increasing information technology, globalization, and cultural diversity present a number of communication opportunities and challenges for organizations. Organizational personnel must be sensitive and competent in cross-cultural communication. While ethnic and racial diversity enriches the environment, it can also cause communication barriers and impede efficient and effective service delivery. Communication difficulties arise from differences in cultural values, languages, and points of view. For instance, in the healthcare industry, one major barrier is language because as many as 20 languages may be encountered among staff and patients. In the United States, more than 25 percent of the population is foreign-born, and 15 percent speak a language at home other than English (Thiederman, 1996). Since language is the most obvious cross-cultural barrier, words can be easily misunderstood in verbal communication (Dutton, 1998). Although the English language is relied on as the common business language, English words may have different meanings in different cultures.

Voice intonation varies by country. For instance, in Japan, communicating softly is an expression of politeness, whereas in the Middle East, the opposite holds true, for the louder the voice, the more one is believed to be sincere (Mead, 1993). To achieve effective communication, healthcare professionals can apply several strategies to reduce communication barriers. Thiederman (1996) provides us with several verbal and nonverbal techniques to improve cross-cultural communication.

- Write down in simple English the issues that have been agreed upon in order to obtain feedback on accuracy.
- Repeat a message when there is doubt.
- Watch for nonverbal signs of a lack of understanding.

- Listen carefully to an entire message, especially when there is a foreign accent involved in the communication.
- Create a relaxed atmosphere so that tension is reduced to increase the flow of communication.
- Phrase questions in a different way to allow the sender the opportunity to respond, utilizing different words that may be easier for the receiver to understand.

COMMUNICATING WITH EXTERNAL STAKEHOLDERS

In healthcare organizations, managers must be competent communicators, because they spend most of their time and energy communicating with large numbers of external stakeholders, individuals, groups, and organizations that are interested in the healthcare organization's actions and decisions. A competent communicator is an individual who has the ability to identify appropriate communication patterns in a given situation and to achieve goals by applying that knowledge. Competent communicators quickly learn the meaning that listeners take from certain words and symbols, and they know which communication channel is preferred in a particular situation. Moreover, competent communicators use this knowledge to communicate in ways to achieve personal, team, and organizational objectives. A manager with high communication competence would be better than others at determining whether an e-mail, telephone call, or personal visit would be the best approach to convey a message to an employee.

To competently communicate with external stakeholders, organizations and their managers are responsible for assessing the environment to gain information in order to make strategic decisions. Managers must utilize their roles as liaisons and monitors to scan the environment for opportunities and minimize threats. Furthermore, managers must utilize their strategist role to formulate and implement policies that are consistent with their organization's strategic goals and plans (Guo, 2003). Exhibit 4–3 shows steps for analyzing stakeholders to increase the acquisition of useful information.

Exhibit 4–3 Stakeholder Analysis

1. Scan the environment of the organization (macroenvironment: economic, regulatory, social/cultural, political, demographics, competitive, technology) (microenvironment: healthcare industry)
2. Identify strategically important issues (i.e., identify important stakeholders)
3. Monitor these issues (track stakeholders' views and positions)
4. Forecast trends (project trends in stakeholders' views and positions)
5. Assess their importance (assess the implications of stakeholders' views and positions)
6. Diffuse information (diffuse stakeholder information to those who need it)

SOURCE: Based on *Managing health services organizations* (4th ed., p. 820), B. B., Rakich, J. S. Longest and K. Darr, 2000, Baltimore, MD: Health Professions Press.

First, scanning the macro- and microenvironments results in information about stakeholders. In the case of one state's department of health, shown in Figure 4–7, the diversity of stakeholders is illustrated (Ginter et al., 1998).

The relationships and communications between the organization and its external stakeholders are complex since the organization is a dynamic, open system operating in a complex and turbulent external environment. The size and variety of external stakeholders make communication complex, especially since stakeholders attempt to influence the decision making of organizations. Fottler et al. (1989) examined communication between a large hospital and its stakeholders and found different relationships. While some relationships are positive, others are neutral or negative. Positive relationships with external stakeholders are easier to manage, and communication tends to be more effective than negative relationships.

In the stakeholder analysis, important issues and stakeholders are identified through the environmental scan. Next, monitoring the activities of stakeholders is crucial. Managers must be able to take the views of stakeholders and use that information to incorporate trends into their decision-making process. Finally, managers must evaluate the value of the information, and take the information gathered and transmit it to those who need the information.

Another way to describe communication with external stakeholders is called boundary spanning. Boundary spanning, or external communication links, provides opportunities for organizational learning in areas such as strategic plan-

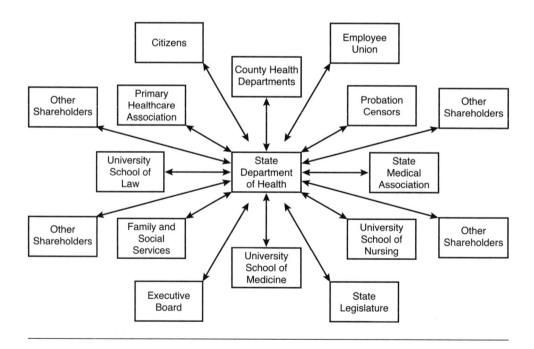

Figure 4–7 Grapevine Networks
SOURCE: *Organizational behavior: Human behavior at work* (9th ed., p. 445), J. W. Newstrom and K. Davis, 1983). New York: McGraw-Hill Book Company.

ning or marketing (Johnson & Chang, 2000). Communicating with all external stakeholders is essential; however, each may be viewed for its unique position and benefits to the organization. For instance, in interactions with the public sector, healthcare organizations are affected by public policies. Government is a major stakeholder because of its legislative and regulatory powers and as one of the largest purchasers of health services. For example, issues such as access to care, cost containment, and quality concerns have driven federal government debate and involvement in health care. Thus, healthcare organizations cannot be insulated from public policies and must make strategic responses to reflect the needs of the public sector. A healthcare organization holds a special relationship with the geographical community where the organization is located. Meeting the particular needs of the community is a primary goal of healthcare organizations. For effective communication to take place, realistic expectations must be formed by both parties. There are six areas of responsibility toward their communities for healthcare organizations (Longest et al., 2000). They include:

1. Engaging in the core, health-enhancing activities in the community.
2. Providing economic benefits to the community.
3. Offering unique benefits or a niche to the community.
4. Pursuing philanthropic activities in a broad and generous manner.
5. Being in full compliance with legal requirements.
6. Meeting ethical and fiduciary obligations.

SUMMARY

Communication in the workplace is critical to establishing and maintaining quality working relationships in organizations. Communication is the creation or exchange of thoughts, ideas, emotions, and understanding between sender(s) and receiver(s). Feedback is information that individuals receive about their behavior. Feedback can be used to promote more effective communication. The Johari Window is a model to improve an individual's communication skills through identifying one's capabilities and limitations. The channels of communication are the means by which messages are transmitted. Verbal communication relies on spoken or written words to share information with others. Computer-aided communication, such as electronic mail, has greatly enhanced the communication process. Especially in health care, other forms of technology, such as high-speed, high-definition images, telemedicine, and wireless, hand-held digital electronic medical records can be used to bridge communications gaps between clinicians and administrators. Nonverbal communication is the sharing of information without using words to encode messages. This includes proxemics, kinesics, facial and eye behavior, and paralanguage.

There are two types of barriers to communication: environmental and personal. Barriers can be overcome by conscious efforts to devote time and attention to communication, reduce hierarchical levels, tailor words and symbols, reinforce words with action, use multiple channels of communication, and understand one another's frame of reference and beliefs.

Key elements of effective communication include the desire to communicate; understanding how others learn; the intent; the content; the sender's credibility; and the time frame. Strategic communication is an intentional process of presenting ideas in a clear, concise, and persuasive way. Five components of strategic communication are outcome, context, messages, tactical reinforcement, and feedback.

Intraorganizational communication flows upward, downward, horizontally, and diagonally. The various flows can be combined to form communication networks, such as the chain, Y, wheel, circle, and all-channel. Certain networks work better than others in varying situations. A manager's role is to determine the best network to use for simple or complex communications. Informal communication results from interpersonal relationships developed in the workplace. Although informal networks can be useful, they can also be misused.

Cross-cultural communication can be challenging. Communication difficulties arise from differences in cultural values, languages, and points of view. Organizational personnel must be sensitive and competent in cross-cultural communication. Several techniques for improving cross-cultural communication include writing down the message, repeating it, listening to the entire message, asking questions using different words, and creating a relaxed atmosphere for communications.

Healthcare organizations must manage relationships with large numbers of external stakeholders, individuals, groups, and organizations that are interested in the organization's actions and decisions. Effective communication with external stakeholders involves environmental assessments to enable managers to identify and make strategic decisions for their organizations.

END-OF-CHAPTER DISCUSSION QUESTIONS

1. What are the various components of the communication process?
2. What are the three forms and four levels of feedback?
3. What is the Johari Window? How is it used in communication?
4. What is verbal communication? Give an example.
5. What are the different types of nonverbal communication?
6. What are the appropriate uses of verbal and nonverbal communication channels?
7. What are the two types of barriers to effective communication?
8. What methods are available to overcome these barriers?
9. What are the elements of effective communication?
10. What are the five components of a strategic communication plan?
11. What are the different forms of intraorganizational flows of communication?
12. What are the various networks available for formal and informal communication?

13. Why is cross-cultural communication important to today's health services organizations?

14. What competencies are needed by managers for communicating with external stakeholders?

END-OF-CHAPTER CASE STUDIES

Case Study 1 Tri-Star Health Insurance Company

At Tri-Star Health, Paul Fisher, Director of Medical Cost Management, recently reconstructed the company's internal codes used to process medical claims. This action not only changed the monetary value of certain codes, but it also altered the numeration assigned to a particular treatment drug. Fisher submitted all the documentation to alter these codes, but failed to submit an update to the physician representatives.

Fisher's busy schedule hindered him from requesting a newsletter explaining how to use the new codes as well as their payment schedule. Shortly after the new codes were implemented, various physicians had their claims denied and subsequently were left unpaid. The contracted physicians were reasonably upset and sought financial settlement with interest for the company's failure to update their provider network.

Discussion Questions

1. What should Fisher have done when he first decided to tackle this project?
2. What protocols should have been in place to avoid the present situation?
3. What positive resolution can be implemented in order to keep these contracted physicians with the plan?

Case Study 2 Good Work Goes Unrewarded

Iris Jones is the Associate Vice President of a large chain pharmaceutical company based in the northeastern part of the country. Recently her chief operating officer, Philip Walker, asked her to complete five high revenue–generating projects for the company. Her expeditious completion of these projects would enable her to advance into a senior-level management position.

Determined to get a promotion, Jones handed these projects over to her very competent network team. The team was hesitant to work hard, for in the past Jones took all the credit and bonuses for herself, when they were the ones who accomplished all the tasks. Nonetheless, the team took on these new high-profile projects and completed them with a very high success rate.

Months later as the profits began to rise, Jones was summoned into Walker's office. When asked if her team contributed in any way to her successful projects, Jones simply answered "No" and took all the credit. Walker was planning to increase her team's salary, but felt no reason for it after Jones' response.

Discussion Questions

1. What should the team have done before accepting Jones' new projects?
2. Did the team have motive to jeopardize these high-profile projects?
3. What do you think of Jones's inability to highlight her employees' meritorious work?

Case Study 3 Sunrise Hospital

Sunrise Hospital is a 300-bed general hospital located in northeastern New York. The last couple of months have been very stressful for its nursing personnel because of an increased volume of patients after the closing of its nearby competitor. The hospital acquired all its competitor's workload and saw a significant rise in profit.

The associate managers were inundated with complaints from the nurses and requests to seek assistance from upper management. The managers resisted informing upper management of this dilemma to prevent showing that they were unable to handle the new workload. Additionally, they did not know how to address the nurses' concerns with upper management. After a couple of weeks of heavy work flow, the nurses decided unanimously to go on strike on a very busy day in the hospital.

Upper management was stunned when they arrived at the hospital and saw all the nurses picketing outside their building.

Discussion Questions

1. What should the managers have done upon initially hearing of the nurses' complaints?
2. What would you have done if placed in the positions of the associate managers?
3. What remedy can upper management have to facilitate fair hospital working conditions?

REFERENCES

Certo, S. C. (1992). *Modern management: Quality, ethics, and the global environment* (5th ed.). Boston, MA: Allyn and Bacon.

Coile, R. C., Jr. (2002). Physician executives explore "New Science" frontier: Bridging the communications gap between medical staff and administration. *Physician Executive, 28*(1), 81–83.

Daft, R. L., & Lengel, R. H. (1984). Information richness: A new approach to managerial behavior and organizational design. In B. Staw & L. Cummings (Eds.), *Research in organizational behavior* (pp. 191–233). Greenwich, CT: JAI Press.

Dunn, R. (2002). *Haimann's healthcare management* (7th ed.). Chicago: Health Administration Press.

Dutton, G. (1998). One workforce, many languages. *Management Review, 87,* 42–47.

Edgley, G., & Robinson, J. (1991). The dialogue process. *Association Management, 43*(10), 37–40.

Extejt, M. M. (1998). Teaching students to correspond effectively electronically: Tips for using electronic mail properly. *Business Communication Quarterly, 61,* 57.

Fottler, M. D., Blair, J. D., Whitehead, C. J., Laus, M. D., & Savage, G. T. (1989). Assessing key stakeholders: Who matters to hospitals and why? *Hospital & Health Services Administration, 34,* 530.

Ginter, P. M., Swayne, L. M., & Duncan, W. J. (1998). *Strategic management of healthcare organizations* (3rd ed.). Malden, MA: Blackwell.

Guo, K. L. (2003). A study of the skills and roles of senior level healthcare managers. *The Healthcare Manager, 22*(2), 152–158.

Hellriegel, D., & Slocum, J. W. (2004). *Organizational behavior* (10th ed.). Mason, OH: South-western.

Johnson, J. D., & Chang, H. J. (2000). Internal and external communication, boundary spanning and innovation adoption: An over-time comparison of three explanations of internal and external innovation communication in a new organizational form. *The Journal of Business Communication, 37*(3), 238.

Keyton, J. (2002). *Communicating in groups: Building relationships for effective decision making* (2nd ed.). Boston: McGraw-Hill Book Company.

Liebler, J. G., & McConnell, C. R. (2004). *Management principles for health professionals* (4th ed.). Sudbury, MA: Jones and Bartlett.

Longest, B. B., Rakich, J. S., & Darr, K. (2000). *Managing health services organizations* (4th ed.). Baltimore, MD: Health Professions Press.

Luft, J. (1984). *Group processes: An introduction to group dynamics* (3rd ed.). Palo Alto, CA: Mayfield.

Luthans, F. (1984). *Organizational behavior* (5th ed.). New York: McGraw-Hill Book Company.

Luthans, F., Welsh, D. H. B., & Taylor, L. A., III (1988). A descriptive model of management effectiveness. *Group & Organization Studies, 13*(2). ABI/INFORM Global 148.

McShane, S. L., & Von Glinow, M. A. (2003). *Organizational behavior: Emerging realities for the workplace revolution* (2nd ed.). Boston, MA: McGraw-Hill Book Company.

Mead, R. (1993). Cross-cultural management communication. In J. V. Thill & C. L. Bovee (Eds.), *Excellence in business communication* (2nd ed., pp. 161–162). New York: McGraw-Hill Book Company.

Nelson, D. L., & Quick, J. C. (2003). *Organizational behavior: Foundations, realities and challenges* (4th ed.). Mason, OH: South-Western.

Newstrom, J. W., & Davis, K. (1993). *Organizational behavior: Human behavior at work* (9th ed.). New York: McGraw-Hill Book Company.

Peck, R. (1997, June 5). Learning to speak computer lingo. (New Orleans) *Times-Picayune*, p. E1.

Porter, M. (1985). *Competitive advantage: Creating and sustaining superior performance*. New York: The Free Press.

Shortell, S. M. (1991). *Effective hospital-physician relationship* (p. 87). Ann Arbor, MI: Health Administration Press.

Sobo, E. J., & Sadler, B. L. (2002). Improving organizational communication and cohesion in a healthcare setting through employee-leadership exchange. *Human Organization, 61*(3), 277–287.

Sperry, L. with Whiteman, A. (2003). Communicating effectively and strategically. In L. Sperry (Ed.), *Becoming an effective healthcare manager: The essential skills of leadership* (pp. 75–98). Baltimore, MD: Health Professions Press.

Spillan, J. E., Mino, M., & Rowles, M. S. (2002). Sharing organizational messages through effective lateral communication. *Communication Quarterly, 50*(2): Research Library Core, Q96.

Thiederman, S. (1996). Improving communication in a diverse healthcare environment. *Healthcare Financial Management, 50*(11), 72–74.

Tubbs, S. L. (2001). *A systems approach to small group interaction* (7th ed.). Boston, MA: McGraw-Hill Book Company.

Understanding Individual Behaviors

"What conditions of work, what kinds of work, what kinds of management, and what kinds of reward or pay will help motivate humans?" (Maslow, in Motivation and Personality, 1954)

In Part II, we try to answer the questions posed by Maslow with three chapters on motivation.

In Chapter 5, we describe and explain four content theories of motivation: (1) Maslow's Hierarchy of Needs, (2) Alderfer's ERG Theory, (3) Herzberg's Two-Factor Theory, and (4) McClelland's 3-Needs Theory. Each of these theories contains some parts of the others, as they attempt to explain what motivates employees.

In Chapter 6, we will examine five process theories of motivation: (1) Expectancy Theory, (2) Equity Theory, (3) Satisfaction-Performance Theory, (4) Goal Setting Theory, and (5) Reinforcement Theory. Although Reinforcement Theory is not usually included with process theories of motivation, it does assist managers with understanding what reinforcements control an individual's behavior. Process theories contain some components of the content theories and vice versa.

In Chapter 7, we examine attribution theory, which was introduced to the reader in Chapter 3. The discussion of attribution theory and its relevancy in the workplace provides managers with a better understanding of the highly cognitive and psychological mechanisms that influence individuals' motivation levels.

CHAPTER 5

Content Theories of Motivation

Nancy Borkowski, DBA, CPA, FACHE

LEARNING OUTCOMES

After completing this chapter, the student should be able to understand:

- ☛ The definition of motivation.
- ☛ The difference between content theories and process theories of motivation.
- ☛ Maslow's Hierarchy of Needs and its criticisms.
- ☛ Alderfer's ERG Theory.
- ☛ Herzberg's Two-Factor Theory and how it relates to job design.
- ☛ Hackman and Oldham's Job Characteristic Model.
- ☛ McClelland's 3-Needs Theory.

OVERVIEW

We will begin by defining motivation before we explore two groups of motivation theories—content and process. Motivation is described as the conscious or unconscious stimulus, incentive, or motives for action toward a goal resulting from psychological or social factors, the factors giving the purpose or direction to behavior (see Figure 5–1). In other words, motivation is the psychological process through which unsatisfied needs or wants lead to drives that are aimed at goals or incentives. The purpose of an individual's behavior is to satisfy needs or wants. A need is anything a person requires or desires. A want is the conscious recognition of a need. The presence of an unsatisfied need or want creates an internal tension, from which an individual seeks relief.

In organizational behavior the concept of motivation has been researched over many years. Through this research, we have identified and grouped motivation into two theories of motivation: (1) content and (2) process.

Content theories of motivation (also referred to as needs theories) explain the specific factors that motivate people. The content approach focuses on the assumption that individuals are motivated by the desire to satisfy their inner

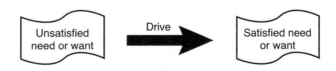

Figure 5–1 Process of Motivation

needs. Content theories answer the question "what drives behavior?" Content theories help managers understand what arouses, energizes, or initiates employee behavior.

Process theories of motivation (also referred to as cognitive theories) focus on the cognitive processes underlying an individual's level of motivation. This approach provides a description and analysis of how behavior is energized, directed, sustained, and stopped. Process theories help explain how an employee's behavior is initiated, redirected, and halted.

Employee motivation has a direct impact on a health service organization's performance; therefore, managers need to understand what motivates employees. By understanding what motivates employees, managers can assist them in reaching their fullest potential. There are some factors the manager can control (e.g., extrinsic factors such as salary, working conditions, interpersonal relationships). For the motivating factors that are intrinsic to the employee (e.g., need for recognition, achievement), managers can be influential by providing a work environment that allows employees the opportunity to satisfy their personal needs and, simultaneously, the organization's goals.

Motivating staff is not about hanging posters with cute sayings in the office. Motivating is something managers do by establishing an organizational structure and environment that provide the opportunity for employees to satisfy both their intrinsic and extrinsic needs (see Section II of this textbook for a full discussion on organizational structure). Remember, motivation is an individual's voluntary drive to satisfy a need or want!

MASLOW'S HIERARCHY OF NEEDS

The most popular and widely cited human motivation theorist is Abraham Maslow. Maslow (1954) is considered the father of humanistic psychology. As a brief background, humanistic psychology incorporates aspects of both behavioral and psychoanalytic psychology. Behaviorists believe that human behavior is controlled by external environmental factors, whereas psychoanalytic psychology is based on the idea that human behavior is controlled by internal unconscious forces. Early in his career, Maslow concluded that human behavior is not controlled only by internal or external factors (e.g., needs), but by both and that some factors have precedence over others. From this concept, Maslow created his five-tier hierarchy of needs (see Figure 5–2).

According to Maslow, humans have five levels of needs and are driven to fulfill these needs. The most basic needs are physiological, such as the need for air, water, and food. After the basic physiological needs are achieved, an individual moves toward satisfying safety and security needs. At this lower level of the hierarchy, individuals are interested in having a home in a safe neighborhood, job security, a retirement plan, and health/medical insurance. Because employees are concerned about satisfying these external or "extrinsic" needs, these motivators need to be addressed by employers, such as by providing employees with an adequate benefits package.

The next three levels in Maslow's Hierarchy of Needs are somewhat less tangible and more psychological. The third level in the hierarchy is a desire to be loved, to belong, and to be approved of by others. Humans have a drive to

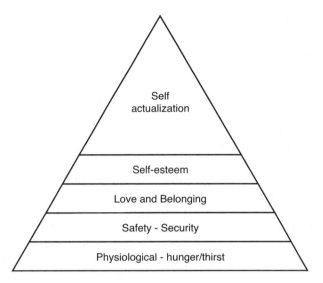

Figure 5-2 Maslow's Hierarchy of Needs
Source: *Motivation and personality*, by A. H. Maslow, 1954, New York: Harper & Row.

feel needed and loved. Within the workplace, employees seek a sense of community and belonging. As such, they seek the approval and acceptance of their peers and supervisors. Managers, by helping staff feel connected to the organization and its mission, can provide this sense of belonging and community.

After an individual's physiological, safety, and belonging needs are satisfied, the next tier in the hierarchy is self-esteem. Maslow noted two versions of esteem needs—a lower one (external) and a higher one (internal). External esteem is satisfied by achieving the respect of others, social and professional status, recognition, and appreciation. The higher form of esteem, internal esteem, involves the need for self-respect, a feeling of confidence, achievement, and autonomy. Individuals want to be competent in what they do, and self-esteem grows when one receives attention and recognition from others for one's accomplishments. Therefore, careful use of praise and of positive feedback to staff is an important means of motivating employees. A pat on the back or other forms of positive feedback goes a long way toward motivating staff to perform. Managers should also provide employees with opportunities to demonstrate their competence. Staff participation in continuing education and other professional development activities and providing opportunities for challenging and meaningful work are effective motivators. These opportunities allow employees to achieve feelings of self-esteem and accomplishment.

Maslow described the preceding four levels (physiological, safety, belonging, and self-esteem) as deficit needs because if any of these motivators are not satisfied, they create an inner tension within the individual that must be relieved. However, if an individual has satisfied his or her needs, those needs cease to motivate the individual and the person moves to the next level in the hierarchy. Individuals must satisfy their lower-level needs, *at least to an acceptable state*, before they can be motivated to achieve the higher levels in the hierarchy.

The highest level of need is an individual's desire to become all that he or she can be. Although Maslow used a variety of terms to refer to this level, it is most commonly referred to as self-actualization. Self-actualization is the desire to become more of what we are, and to become everything that one is capable of becoming. In Maslow's view, self-actualization is not an end point, but rather an ongoing process that involves many growth choices that entail risk and require courage (O'Connor & Yballe, 2007). Maslow noted that self-actualizing people were deeply committed in action to core values (i.e., truth, justice, goodness, purposefulness) and were attuned to their own uniqueness (i.e., talents, likes). In general, self-actualizing individuals seek to put things right and to do it the right way (O'Connor & Yballe, 2007). Although progress to self-actualization is often interrupted by failure to meet lower-level needs due to illness (lack of physiological well-being), loss of job (lack of security), or divorce (lack of sense of being loved), individuals can learn that satisfying basic needs becomes an integrated, consciously managed aspect of a whole life and is not compulsive or dominating of all other concerns. As O'Connor and Yballe (2007, p. 749) point out, "a paradigm shift takes place. An individual becomes a person who has needs, not a needy person."

Managers need to ask themselves, "How can I motivate my employees?" When answering this question, managers need to be conscious of the fact that all employees are not driven by the same needs, nor is any employee driven by the same need at the same time. For example, right now as you read this book, you may have several needs operating simultaneously—curiosity, need for new knowledge, thirst, and so forth. Managers need to recognize the needs of each employee, individually. Managers who simultaneously address each employee's lower level of needs will benefit from workers who are motivated to achieve the highest level in Maslow's Hierarchy of Needs—self-actualization (see Figure 5–3).

Although Maslow introduced his Hierarchy of Needs theory over 60 years ago, there has been only a limited number of studies that support his needs theory, and those published have reported mixed findings (Alderfer, 1972). In fact, some research contradicts Maslow's specific "ordering" of needs. For example, Huizinga, as cited in Griffin (1991), attempted to validate the theory in the workplace.

Because of its scope and different cultural setting, Huizinga's study is one of the more ambitious attempts to verify the principles of the hierarchy. He surveyed over 600 managers drawn from five industries in the Netherlands. His sample included people from production, personnel, research and development, finance, and top management. They ranged in age from 20 to 65, and their educational backgrounds extended from the Dutch equivalent of grade school to university graduates. Huizinga found that no matter how many ways he analyzed the data, there was simply no evidence that workers had a single dominant need, much less that the need diminished in strength when gratified (p. 131).

In addition, Maslow's needs theory also had difficulty explaining individuals such as Mother Theresa, who neglected her lower-level needs in pursuit of her spiritual calling to serve the poor in India. Maslow himself used the example

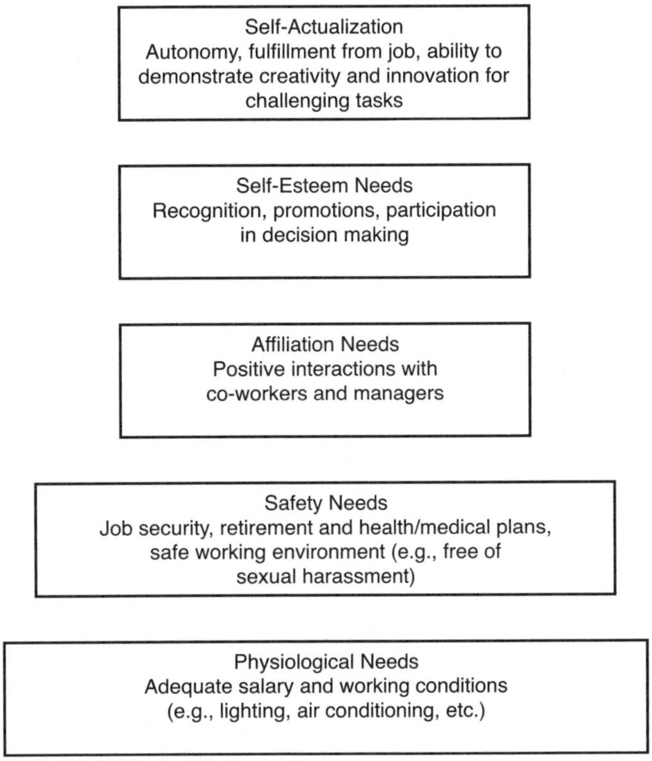

Figure 5–3 How Managers Can Satisfy Employees' Needs at Different Levels of Maslow's Hierarchy of Needs

of a starving artist pursuing his creativity needs (e.g., self-actualization) while ignoring physiological needs.

ALDERFER'S ERG THEORY

To address the criticisms of Maslow's Hierarchy of Needs, in the late 1960s, Clayton Alderfer (1972) introduced an alternative needs hierarchy, referred to as the ERG Theory. Alderfer's hierarchy relates to three identified categories of needs: existence, relatedness, and growth (see Table 5–1).

- Existence refers to an individual's concern with basic material and physiological existence requirements, such as food, water, pay, fringe benefits, and working conditions.
- Relatedness refers to the need for developing and sustaining interpersonal relationships such as relations with family, friends, supervisors, coworkers, subordinates, and other significant groups.
- Growth refers to an individual's intrinsic need to be creative, and to make useful and productive contributions, including personal development with opportunities for personal growth.

Table 5-1 Alderfer's ERG Theory

Level of Need	Definition	Properties
Growth	Impel a person to make creative or productive effects on himself or herself and the environment.	Satisfied through a person using his or her capabilities fully (and developing additional ones) in problem solving; creates a greater sense of wholeness and fullness as a human being.
Relatedness	Involves relationships with significant other people.	Satisfied by mutually sharing their thoughts and feelings; acceptance, confirmation, understanding, and influence are elements of the relatedness process.
Existence	Includes all of the various forms of psychological and material desires.	When divided among people, one person's gain is another's loss when resources are limited.

When compared to Maslow's Hierarchy of Needs, Alderfer's ERG Theory differs on three points. First, the ERG theory allows for an individual to seek satisfaction of higher-level needs before lower-level needs are satisfied. In other words, the ERG Theory does not require an individual to satisfy a lower-level need for a higher-level need to become the driver of the person's behavior. Although the ERG Theory retains the concept of a need hierarchy, it does not require a strict ordering, as compared to Maslow.

Second, the ERG theory accounts for differences in need preferences between cultures; therefore, the order of needs can be different for different people. This flexibility allows the ERG theory to account for a wider range of observed behaviors. For example, it can explain Mother Theresa's behavior of placing spiritual needs above existence needs.

Third, which may be the most important aspect of the ERG theory, is the frustration–regression principle. The frustration–regression principle explains that when a barrier prevents an individual from obtaining a higher-level need, a person may "regress" to a lower-level need (or vice versa) to achieve satisfaction. For example, a person wants existence-related objects when his or her relatedness needs are not satisfied; a person wants relationships with significant others when growth needs are not being met.

Managers must recognize that an employee may have multiple needs to satisfy simultaneously; focusing exclusively on one need at a time will not effectively motivate an employee. In addition, the frustration–regression principle impacts workplace motivation. For example, if growth opportunities are not provided to employees, they may regress to relatedness needs and socialize more with coworkers, or even look to other types of organizations for satisfaction of this need, for example, a union. If the work environment does not satisfy an employee's need for social interaction, an increased desire for more money or better working conditions may occur. If a manager is able to recognize these conditions, steps can be taken to satisfy the employee's frustrated needs until the employee is able to pursue growth again. (See Case Study 5–1: I Get by with a Little Help from My Friends.)

Case Study 5–1 I Get by with a Little Help from My Friends

Jennifer Smith, RN, has worked at St. Joe's Medical Center for the past five years as an operating room nurse. She enjoys her work and the interaction it provides with patients, physicians, and especially her coworkers. In fact, she has developed strong friendships with her coworkers. Almost every day, they eat lunch together. They have monthly dinner parties at each other's homes and frequently go on vacations together. Helen Jones, the Director of Surgical Services, has remarked about the cohesiveness of the group and how well they work together, creating a well-functioning team. However, during the past year, Jennifer has made frequent remarks to her coworkers that she felt her nursing career was at a stalemate and that she was getting bored with "doing the same thing every day." Jennifer questioned why she went back to school to earn her MSN degree, when Helen never gave her an opportunity to apply what she learned! Jennifer started to think about looking for a new position at a different hospital that would give her the opportunity to grow professionally. Jennifer's coworkers empathized with her, and when a vacancy was posted on the hospital's job bulletin board for an assistant clinical manager position in her department, they encouraged her to apply. After reviewing the job description, Jennifer agreed that with her clinical experience and graduate degree, she was the perfect candidate for the job! She submitted her application, fully confident that Helen would offer her the position. Jennifer was very excited and looked forward to the challenges she would face when promoted.

However, when Jennifer was informed by Helen that another staff member with more "management" experience was offered the position, Jennifer could not disguise her disappointment. She wondered what she would do now. Should she quit and seek a new position at a different hospital? But what about her friends at St. Joe's?

Jennifer's coworkers knew how upset she was and made special efforts to ease her disappointment by scheduling more outings together. They told her that other opportunities would come and that, with a little more experience, she would be promoted. Being with her coworkers was like group therapy for Jennifer.

After a few weeks, Jennifer returned to the level of enjoyment she obtained from her work before this episode. In addition, Helen approached Jennifer to discuss her enrolling in a mentorship program that the hospital had recently established. The mentorship program, similar to an internship, would provide clinical staff with hands-on management experience. Jennifer did not hesitate; she enrolled in the program the following week. Jennifer was confident that she would be ready when the next opportunity presented itself.

Discuss how Jennifer displayed the frustration–regression principle of Alderfer's ERG theory.

HERZBERG'S TWO-FACTOR THEORY

Frederick Herzberg developed his Two-Factor Theory, also known as the Motivation–Hygiene Theory, from a study designed to test the concept that people have two sets of needs: (1) avoidance of unpleasantness and (2) a personal growth. In Herzberg's original study (1959, 1966), 200 engineers and accountants were asked about events they had experienced at work, which had resulted in either a marked improvement in their job satisfaction or had led to a marked reduction in job dissatisfaction. From Herzberg's research

(1966), five factors stood out as strong determiners of job satisfaction (i.e., motivator factors) and are related to job content: (1) achievement, (2) recognition, (3) work itself, (4) responsibility, and (5) advancement. The determinants of job dissatisfaction (i.e., hygiene factors) that are related to job context were found to be: (1) company policies, (2) administrative policies, (3) supervision, (4) salary, (5) interpersonal relations, and (6) working conditions. It is important to note that Herzberg used the term "hygiene" to describe factors that are necessary to avoid dissatisfaction, but that by themselves do not provide satisfaction or motivation (see Exhibit 5–1).

Herzberg's research findings are significant to managers because the factors involved in producing job satisfaction are separate and distinct from the factors that lead to job dissatisfaction. As illustrated in Exhibit 5–1 these two factors are not opposites of each other. As Herzberg pointed out, the opposite of job satisfaction is not job dissatisfaction, but rather no job satisfaction; similarly, the opposite of job dissatisfaction is no job dissatisfaction, not satisfaction with one's job.

In a practical sense, this means that dissatisfiers, referred to as hygiene factors, support and maintain the structure of the job (job context), while the satisfiers, referred to as motivators, assist employees to reach self-actualization and increase their motivation to do their work (job content). Unfortunately, Timmreck's (2001) study of 99 health service midmanagers found

---

Exhibit 5–1 Job Satisfaction

Job Satisfaction ◄─────────────────────────► No Job Satisfaction

Motivators/Satisfiers

(Intrinsic—Job Content)

Achievement
Recognition
Work Itself
Responsibility
Advancement

No Job Dissatisfaction ◄─────────────────────────► Job Dissatisfaction

Hygiene Factors/Dissatisfiers

(Extrinsic—Job Context)

Company Policies
Administrative Policies
Supervision
Salary
Interpersonal Relations
Working Conditions

that only a minority actually believed in and used motivators to stimulate subordinates' behavior.

One of the criticisms of Herzberg's Two-Factor Theory is that a single factor may be a motivator for one person, but cause job dissatisfaction for another. As an example, increased responsibility may be welcomed by one employee, but avoided by another. Another criticism has been Herzberg's placement of salary/pay in the dissatisfier category, which has caused some to believe that Herzberg did not value money as a motivator. However, what Herzberg meant was that if pay did not meet expectations, employees were dissatisfied, but if pay met employees' expectations, salary was not a need to achieve satisfaction. Herzberg believed that the absence of good hygiene factors, including money, would lead to dissatisfaction and thus potentially block any attempt to motivate the worker.

Dent (2002) relates that when Herzberg first presented his work it was very controversial in the academic community, but very popular in industry because it helped to answer employers' questions as to "why the level of an employee's productivity did not equate to the compensation received by their workers?"

In the late 1950s, the US economy was in a tremendous economic upswing. The issue of motivation was critical for retaining good people, who often had several other opportunities. The primary advice coming from industrial psychologists was to motivate through compensation packages. As a result, employers were paying higher and higher salaries, but felt that they were not getting higher amounts of performance. Herzberg's work validated what the employers were feeling. Herzberg suggested that higher performance levels would come not from higher salaries but by giving employees the opportunity to create and impact their environments (Dent, 2002, p. 276).

Although managers need to provide employees with a reasonable salary, a degree of job security, and safe and comfortable working conditions (hygiene factors), focusing on these matters will not contribute to an employee's motivation or performance improvement (Sashkin, 1996). Herzberg promoted the concept that if the work one does is significant, it will ultimately lead to satisfaction with the work itself. In other words, employees will be motivated to do work that they perceive to be significant (see Case Study 5–2: Why Don't I Just Quit!).

Case Study 5–2 Why Don't I Just Quit!

Robin Williams sat at her desk going through her mail and asked herself the same question she had asked herself 100 times before, "Why don't I just quit!" Robin thought to herself, "I don't need this job; I have enough money in my savings account to last a year, and with my degree and experience, I could go anywhere." Robin graduated from one of the top schools in the country with an MSW and has been a social worker for the Alpine Medical Center for the past four years. Although she loves her interaction with her clients, with the ability and freedom to help them through the "system" satisfying all their social and medical needs, she is unhappy with the required 60 hours work week, for a salary far less than what her friends who graduate with an AS/Nursing are earning. In addition, Robin believes her boss is trying to set her up to be fired just because she told him that he was an incompetent administrator.

"Well, he is," thought Robin. He hasn't been able to find the money in the department budget to purchase a new computer that she desperately needs to help her clients. To make matters worse, her coworkers, who "live in their own worlds," never extend the courtesy of asking her to join them for lunch. "Not that I would go with them," Robin thought. "They are just as useless as the Director; and didn't they forget yesterday was my birthday!"

As she thought the issues over in her mind, she opened a thank-you letter from a client she helped last month. He just wanted to tell her how much he appreciated her help through his illness and tell her that without her assistance, he would not have known all the community services available to him so he could remain at home versus being admitted into a nursing home.

Robin smiled and put the card aside; she was still trying to figure out why she didn't quit her job. She wished she knew the answer.

Using Herzberg's Two-Factor Theory, discuss why Robin has not resigned from her position.

Building on this concept, jobs should be designed with special attention for opportunities relating to achievement, responsibility, meaningfulness, and recognition (see Table 5–2).

According to Herzberg, motivation comes from job content. Therefore, it is important for managers to consider the nature of the jobs they ask their employees to do. Herzberg's approach can be summarized by "if you want people to do a good job for you, then you must give them a good job to do." Managers need to be concerned with job-design characteristics, including job enrichment. Job enrichment is the vertical expansion of the job as opposed to a horizontal expansion (job enlargement) (see Table 5–3).

JOB DESIGN

Job-design research in the past three decades has generated many insights into the relationship between job characteristics and job satisfaction. The well-known and widely researched job characteristics model was developed by Hackman and Oldham (1976, 1980) (see Figure 5–4).

Hackman and Oldham (1980) listed five core motivational job characteristics:

- *Skill Variety:* The degree to which a job requires a variety of different activities in carrying out the work, involving the use of a number of different skills and talents of the person.
- *Task Identity:* The degree to which a job requires completion of a "whole" and identifiable piece of work, that is, doing a job from beginning to end with a visible outcome.
- *Task Significance:* The degree to which the job has a substantial impact on the lives of other people, whether those people are in the immediate organization or in the world at large.
- *Autonomy:* The degree to which the job provides substantial freedom, independence, and discretion to the individual in scheduling the work and in determining the procedures to be used in carrying it out.
- *Feedback:* The degree to which the work activities required by the job provide the individual with direct and clear information about the effectiveness of his or her performance (pp. 78–80).

Table 5–2 Relationship of Herzberg's Two-Factor Theory and Motivators to Job Design

Motivator	Growth Principle	Description
Achievement and recognition for achievement	Opportunity to increase knowledge	The job must allow for achievement opportunities, and these achievements must result in the employee's knowing more about his/her job than he/she did previously. The recognition for achievement is the reinforcement that is necessary at the early stages of all learning. Eventually, the employee will develop his own "generator" and will rely less on outside recognition of his growth and more on his own evaluation.
Responsibility	Opportunity to increase understanding	Increased responsibility relates to a more complex task. Increasing the complexity of the job can provide the opportunity for understanding the relationships among the various components of the assignment and thereby provide for the next level of growth.
Possibility of growth	Opportunity for creativity	The task must contain an open end in its description to allow for possible growth. If the job allows for possible growth, it may then provide the opportunity for the employee to be creative.
Advancement	Opportunity to experience ambiguity in decision making	Advancement, whether including job promotion or not, requires that a higher-order of task be presented to the employee. The higher-order task gives the opportunity to the employee to be successful with "uncertainty," and thus leads to a higher level of growth.
Interest	Opportunity to individuate and seek real growth	If the employee finds that the actual task she has to do is of direct interest to him or her, then his or her job can provide a sense of personal worth and individuality. If the job has "intrinsic attractive powers," the employee is less likely to be concerned with other people's hygiene and less tempted to seek substitute growth from her own hygiene need. This enables an individual to experience the highest level of growth.

SOURCE: *Work and the nature of man* (pp. 177–178), by F. Herzberg, 1966, New York: The World Publishing Company.

Table 5–3 Herzberg's Principles of Vertical Job Loading

Principle	Motivators Involved
Removing some controls while retaining accountability	Responsibility and personal achievement
Increasing the accountability of individuals for own work	Responsibility and recognition
Giving a person a complete natural unit of work (module, division, area, and so on)	Responsibility, achievement, and recognition
Granting additional authority to an employee in his or her activity; job freedom	Responsibility, achievement, and recognition
Making periodic reports directly available to the worker himself or herself rather than to the supervisor	Internal recognition
Introducing new and more difficult tasks not previously handled	Growth and learning
Assigning individuals specific or specialized tasks, enabling them to become experts	Responsibility, growth, and achievement

SOURCE: "One more time: How do you motivate employees?" by F. Herzberg, 1983. *Harvard Business Review, 81*(1), p. 93.

As reflected in Figure 5–4, each core job characteristic, or combination of factors, leads to critical psychological states for an employee. Hackman and Oldham (1980) relate that the combination of skill variety, task identity, and task significance leads to the psychological state of experienced meaningfulness, where the worker perceives that the job is significant. Autonomy leads to the psychological state of experienced responsibility for outcomes (i.e., the employee feels individual responsibility for the work), and feedback leads to the psychological state of knowledge of the actual results of work activities. These critical psychological states lead to an employee's high levels of internal motivation, growth and job satisfaction, and work effectiveness (quality and quantity).

Using the moderators in the Job Characteristics Model, Hackman and Oldham (1980, pp. 82–88) attempted to explain why some employees "take off" on jobs that are high in motivating potential and others are "turned off." The first moderator is knowledge and skills. If people have sufficient knowledge and skills to perform their job well, they will experience positive feelings as a result of their work activities. However, people who are not competent to perform their tasks well will experience unhappiness and frustration at work.

The second moderator is growth-need strength. Some people have strong needs for personal accomplishment, for learning, and for developing themselves beyond where they currently are. These people are said to have strong

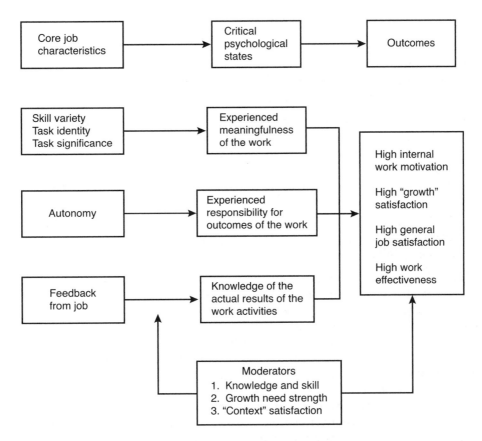

Figure 5–4 The Job Characteristics Model of Work Motivation
Source: *Work redesign* (p. 90), by J. R. Hackman and G. R. Oldham, 1980, Reading, MA: Addison-Wesley.

"growth needs." Others have less strong needs for growth or personal accomplishment. Therefore, individuals with strong growth needs respond positively to the opportunities provided by enriched work. However, individuals with low growth needs may not recognize the existence of enriching opportunities, or may not value them, or may find them threatening and complain at being pushed or stretched too far at work.

The third moderator is satisfaction with the work context. Employees who are relatively satisfied with their job context (pay, job security, coworkers, etc.) will respond more positively to enriched and challenging jobs than employees who are dissatisfied with their job context.

Managers need to pay close attention to the moderators. If an employee is fully competent to carry out the work required by a complex, challenging task, and has strong needs for personal growth and is well satisfied with the work context, then the manager should expect the employee to exhibit high personal satisfaction and high work motivation and performance. If an employee lacks any of these moderators, the opposite results would occur.

McCLELLAND'S 3-NEEDS THEORY

David McClelland (1985) experimented with individuals' responses to pictures of various groups of persons gathered together. On the basis of the participants' responses, McClelland identified three types of motivational needs: achievement, power, and affiliation.

- Achievement (n-Ach) is described as the need to excel or succeed. In general, high achievers tend to seek moderately challenging tasks, take personal responsibility for their performance, and require feedback to confirm their successes.
- Power (n-Pow) is described as an individual's need to influence others. This can be positive or negative, as we will discuss later.
- Affiliation (n-Aff) is described as an individual's need to be liked and approved of by others. As such, n-Aff people have a strong need for interpersonal relationships.

McClelland (1985) believed that most persons have a combination of these motivational needs, with some exhibiting a stronger tendency to one particular motivational need (e.g., a high power need versus a high achievement need). This tendency affects a person's behavior and management style. For example, McClelland suggested that a high affiliation need weakens a manager's objectivity and decision-making capability, because of the need to be liked by his or her subordinates, colleagues, and supervisors. Although persons with high power needs are attracted to leadership roles, they may not have the required flexibility and human relations skills necessary to be effective. McClelland argues that persons with strong achievement needs make the best leaders, although they can have a tendency to demand too much of their staff in the belief that they are all similarly and highly focused on achievement (i.e., results driven). One interesting aspect of McClelland's theory is that individuals can learn or acquire a need for achievement by being associated with success and failure in the past (and the effect that accompanies success and failure).

Achievement

A significant part of McClelland's research focused on the achievement motivational need (n-Ach). Through his research, McClelland concluded that while most persons do not possess a strong n-Ach motivation, those who do display a consistent behavior of moderate risk-taking. To support his theory, McClelland (1985) performed the now famous ring-toss experiment.

Participants played a ring-toss game where the subjects determined how close or far away they would stand from the peg. One group of participants stood very close to the peg to ensure they would never miss. Another group stood so far away that if they actually did place the ring on the peg, it was due to chance, not ability. The third group calculated their distance from the peg. They didn't stand too far away to make the task impossible, nor did they stand too close to make it too easy. If they missed the first toss, they would move closer; if they made the toss, they would take a step back for the next toss.

McClelland referred to the third group as moderate risk-takers—individuals who desired a challenge, but whose success was based on their abilities, not chance, as with the second group.

McClelland (1961) relates that n-Ach persons have various attributes. First, n-Ach persons are not high risk-takers as compared to a gambler who has no control over the outcomes. High achievers are moderate risk-takers. Achievement-motivated individuals set difficult goals, but goals they believe to be achievable through their efforts and abilities. High achievers work harder and more efficiently when the task is challenging and requires creativity, such as designing new systems or just a better way of doing things. Second, n-Ach persons view goal achievement as their reward and require feedback that is quantifiable and factual. As such, they equate more money and/or higher profits as the measurement or feedback of their success. Job security is not an important issue for n-Ach people. They prefer occupations that allow them the flexibility and the opportunity to set their own goals, such as in sales, business, or entrepreneurial roles. Although high achievers can work in groups, they receive their satisfaction by knowing that they initiated an action that contributed to the group's success.

McClelland (1961) believed that n-Ach persons are the ones who make things happen and get results in an organization. They are successful in obtaining the resources, including employee "buy-in" to achieve organizational goals. However, high achievers may be viewed as demanding of staff and insensitive to the needs of others, because of their results-driven attitude.

Power

McClelland (1985) relates that a high need for power may be expressed as personalized power or socialized power. Those with a high need for personalized power have tendencies to display impulsive aggressive actions, abuse alcohol, and collect prestige "toys" such as fancy cars. They seek to control others for their own benefit. Their attitude is "I win, you lose." Individuals with a high need for personalized power demand personal loyalty from staff versus loyalty to the organization. Yukl (2001) points out that when a high personalized power leader leaves an organization, it usually results in chaos, loss of direction, and low morale.

Socialized power need is associated with effective leadership. These leaders direct their power in ways that benefit others and the organization versus their own personal gain. As McClelland (1985) and Yukl (2001) relate, they are more interested in seeking power because it is through power that they can influence others to accomplish tasks. They empower others who use that power to enact and further the leader's vision for the organization.

Affiliation

Individuals with a high need for affiliation seek to be with and interact with others. McClelland (1985) relates that they are concerned with establishing, maintaining, or restoring positive relationships with others. High affiliation individuals want to please others and engage in more dialogue with others.

Individuals are very important to persons in n-Aff. They prefer friends over experts when working in groups (n-Ach prefer experts over friends as working partners), and prefer feedback on how well the group is getting along rather than how well they are performing on the task. They avoid conflict and criticism, and have a fear of rejection by others. As such, individuals with a high need for affiliation do not make good managers (see Case Study 5–3: The Office Manager's Dilemma).

Case Study 5–3 The Office Manager's Dilemma

When Karen Lewis was promoted to office manager for Dr. Green's orthopedic practice, she was thrilled. She had worked for Dr. Green for almost six years and considered it her home away from home and her coworkers as her extended family. Karen was the office organizer for picnics, Friday night get-togethers, and holiday parties. She always made sure that staff's birthdays and anniversaries were recognized and celebrated. She was very concerned that everyone was happy and was always available to help other coworkers with any problems.

In addition, Karen was competent in all areas of the office operations. Although originally hired as an X-ray technician, she had performed, at one time or another, the duties of all the positions within the practice. She had covered the receptionist, medical records, and billing staff's positions when they were on vacation or ill, or when there was an unfilled vacancy. Not only was she responsible for running the X-ray area of the practice, but also over the years she had assumed the responsibilities for ordering supplies and scheduling surgeries.

Karen thought making the transition to office manager would be easy. The first few months went well. But in her fourth month, other staff members came to her complaining about Suzie, the new appointment-scheduling clerk. Karen was surprised to hear that Suzie was not doing her job well and that her errors were affecting the entire office operations. Suzie was scheduling patients to come to the office when Dr. Green was at the hospital performing surgery, and during the staff's lunch periods. In addition, she was overscheduling, causing patients to wait hours. Karen told the office staff that she would discuss the matter with Suzie as soon as possible.

However, Karen found it very difficult to schedule a meeting with Suzie to discuss her problems. Every time Karen approached Suzie about the subject, she found that her stomach tightened and she began to sweat. The best she could do was to ask Suzie, "How is everything going?" Suzie replied, "Everything is great and I love working in such a warm and friendly office."

A week later, the staff approached Karen again and asked if she had spoken with Suzie because the problems were getting worse. Karen lied and said that last week was so busy, she did not get an opportunity but that she would talk with Suzie this week. Again, Karen found it difficult to discuss the matter with Suzie. She didn't want to hurt Suzie's feelings because Suzie thought she was doing a good job. However, if she didn't speak with Suzie soon, Karen knew Dr. Green would start to question whether she was capable of handling the duties of the office manager position. She couldn't bear to think that she let Dr. Green down and that he might be displeased with her work. In addition, there were rumors circulating through the office grapevine that if the "appointment-scheduling" problem was not fixed soon, a few staff members were thinking about quitting because the mistakes caused their workload to increase 20 percent.

Karen decided that she would discuss the matter with Suzie the following day. Karen asked Suzie to come in 10 minutes before office hours started so they could have a chat. Karen had a restless night's sleep. When she awoke, she noticed that she had developed a rash over her entire body! She had no choice; she called the answering service to tell Dr. Green and the staff that she was too ill to come to work.

Using McClelland's 3-Needs Theory, discuss if Dr. Green made the right decision promoting Karen Lewis to office manager. Why?

Table 5–4 Comparisons of Content Theories of Motivation

Herzberg's Two-Factor Theory	Maslow's Hierarchy of Needs	Alderfer's 3-Need Theory	McClelland's 3-Need Theory
Motivators	Self-actualization	Growth	Achievement
	Self-esteem		
Hygiene factors	Love	Relatedness	Power (influencing others)
			Affiliation (exchange of warm feelings)
	Safety	Existence	
	Physiological		

SUMMARY

When a comparison is made of the content theories of motivation, there are noted similarities (see Table 5–4). Each theory describes an individual's various needs in similar terms. Herzberg's hygiene factors parallel Maslow's physiological, security, and belongingness needs, and Alderfer's existence and relatedness needs. Maslow's self-esteem and self-actualization needs are similar to Herzberg's motivators and Alderfer's growth requirement. McClelland's achievement is closely related to Herzberg's motivators, and his power and affiliation can be related to Alderfer's relatedness needs because of an individual's need to influence (power) or satisfy a need for warm feelings (affiliation) (Alderfer, 1972). It is clear that Maslow's Hierarchy of Needs theory has had a great influence on the study of organizational behavior and continues to do so after 60 years (Latham & Pinder, 2005).

END-OF-CHAPTER DISCUSSION QUESTIONS

1. Define motivation.
2. Explain the connection of the five tiers of Maslow's Hierarchy of Needs to the workplace.
3. Discuss how Alderfer's ERG Theory satisfied the criticisms of Maslow's Hierarchy of Needs.
4. Explain Herzberg's Two-Factor Theory as it relates to job design.
5. Explain the various components of Hackman and Oldham's Job Characteristics Model.
6. Discuss McClelland's 3-Needs Theory as it relates to a manager's success in the workplace.
7. Discuss the relationship between the various content theories of motivation.

END-OF-CHAPTER CASE STUDIES

Case Study 1 All in a Day's Work (Part One)[a]

Sarah Goodman, Senior Manager of Network Development for Holy Managed Care Company, looked over her calendar for the day and sighed deeply. It seemed as if there would be no time at all to work on the project she'd been putting off for most of the week. Circumstances seemed to be such that she simply didn't have any control over her own time anymore.

Well, first things first, she determined. At 9 o'clock she was due at a meeting of senior managers who were involved in trying to devise a strategy for counteracting a threatened unionization drive by the company's nonexempt employees. As Sarah thought about the people working for her, she began to wonder exactly what they wanted. They had a pleasant working space, good benefits package, and secure employment. She heard the laughter and chatter drifting into her office as people came into work and thought what a pleasant and congenial group they were. What more could they want?

Then at 10:30 there was another meeting. This one could be very exciting! In six months Sarah's office was scheduled to be moved to a new industrial park on the west side of town. The plans she'd seen so far had all kinds of great perks for employees: on-site day-care center, fitness center, ample parking, great facilities for training. The company was certainly spending a lot of money on this new site. Sarah certainly hoped it would help increase productivity; it certainly would make the employees happier and make recruitment easier.

She'd have to hurry to her lunch meeting with the advisor for the MHA program at Saint Thomas University. Sarah had decided as a part of her New Year's resolution that she was finally going to begin her graduate degree. She felt she was simply stagnating in her job and, after looking around at positions in her company that looked interesting, she realized she needed a graduate degree if she were going to progress. The only problem was that she wasn't sure how enthusiastic Richard, her husband, would be about the whole idea. And her mother certainly wouldn't be happy! The hints about grandchildren had become an outright discussion over the holidays.

Discuss the various motivation theories reflected in this case study.

AUTHOR: Pidge Diehl, EdD. Reprinted with permission.
[a]Part Two is presented at the end of Chapter 6.

Case Study 2 Develop a Motivation Plan

You are the Director of Nursing for a 400-bed nonprofit hospital in the Southwest. Susan Smith joined your hospital as a staff nurse three years ago after relocating from the northeast. She is 30 years old and has been a staff nurse since graduating from a two-year college nursing program 10 years ago. She is married to a lawyer and they have two children ages six and eight.

Your hospital's inpatient census has been extremely high because of another hospital's closing. The tension on the nursing floors has been running pretty high because of time pressures to discharge patients early, lack of professional staff, and an upcoming accreditation visit from the Joint Commission. Because of time restraints, you were unable to complete the annual performance evaluations. However, all nurses received a 5 percent pay increase. With this increase, your hospital staff is now the highest paid as compared to other hospitals within your region. You believe the higher pay compensates your nursing staff for their increased workload and related stress levels.

Until recently, you have been pleased with Susan's performance. She had demonstrated, in the past, her willingness to work hard and has made very few, if any, patient-care errors. However, over the last three months, you have noticed that Susan is not performing at her

Exhibit 5–2 123

same level of productivity and appears to argue frequently with the treating physicians and other staff nurses about the patients' treatment plans. You frequently hear Susan complaining that "no one listens to me," "no one wants to hear my opinion," and "they don't pay me enough to do this job."

Susan was once a highly motivated, productive member of your nursing staff. You understand that everyone is experiencing more stress than usual because of the increased workload, but what can be done to motivate Susan to her prior "self"?

Within the principles of the content theories of Maslow, Herzberg, and Alderfer, develop a motivation plan.

EXHIBIT 5–2 Job Survey

Introduction

Objective: To learn how job design affects performance.

Time: About 25 minutes.

Instructions: Take the survey below. Once you have completed it, total your scores. Compare your score with others in the class and discuss the following questions:

- Normally, persons who are in a position of leadership will have scores that are higher than their workers. Why is this?
- If your employees were to take this survey today, what do you think their average scores would be?
- Discuss Hackman and Oldham's Five Dimensions and how they help to motivate a jobholder. Ask for a few examples of how a job could be redesigned under each of the five dimensions.

Job Design Questionnaire

Directions: Listed below are some statements about your job. For each statement, write in your response based on how much you agree or disagree with it.

Strongly Disagree (1)	Slightly Disagree (2)	Disagree (3)	Undecided (4)	Slightly Agree (5)	Strongly Agree (6)	Agree (7)

My job:

1. Provides much variety. _____
2. Allows me the opportunity to complete the work I start. _____
3. Is one that may affect a lot of other people by how well the work is performed. _____
4. Lets me be left on my own to do my own work. _____
5. Provides feedback on how well I am performing as I am working. _____
6. Provides me with a variety of work. _____
7. Is arranged so that I have a chance to do the job from beginning to end. _____
8. Is relatively significant in the organization. _____
9. Provides the opportunity for independent thought and action. _____
10. Provides me with the opportunity to find out how well I am doing. _____
11. Gives me the opportunity to do a number of different things. _____

(Continued)

12. Is arranged so that I may see projects through to their final completion.   _____

13. Is very significant in the broader scheme of things.   _____

14. Gives me considerable opportunity for independence and freedom in how I do my work.   _____

15. Provides me with the feeling that I know whether I am performing well or poorly.   _____

SUMMARY

Scoring for Job Design Questionnaire

The survey is designed to analyze five dimensions of the job:

- Skill Variety—Total the scores for questions 1, 6, 11 _____
- Task Identity—Total the scores for questions 2, 7, 12 _____
- Task Significant—Total the scores for questions 3, 8, 13 _____
- Autonomy—Total the scores for questions 4, 9, 14 _____
- Feedback about Results—Total the scores for questions 5, 10, 15 _____

The lower scoring dimensions (normally, anything below 15) should be investigated to see whether the job environment can be improved.

About the Survey

Hackman and Oldham's Five Dimensions of Motivating Potential

- Skill variety—the degree to which a job requires a variety of challenging skills and abilities.
- Task identity—the degree to which a job requires completion of a whole and identifiable piece of work.
- Task significance—the degree to which the job has a perceivable impact on the lives of others, either within the organization or the world at large.
- Autonomy—the degree to which the job gives the worker freedom and independence in scheduling work and determining how the work will be carried out.
- Feedback—the degree to which the worker gets information about the effectiveness of his or her efforts, either directly from the work itself or from others.

SOURCE: © Donald Clark, created March 18, 2000, last update March 26, 2000. Available at: http://www.nwlink.com/~donclark/leader/jobsurvey.html.

REFERENCES

Alderfer, C. (1972). *Existence, relatedness, & growth*. New York: Free Press.

Dent, E. B. (2002). The messy history of OB&D: How three strands came to be seen as one rope. *Management Decision, 40*(3), 266–280.

Griffin, E. (1991). *A first look at communication theory* (1st ed.). New York: McGraw-Hill Book Company.

Hackman, J. R., & Oldham, G. R. (1976). Motivation through the design of work: Test of a theory. *Organizational Behavior and Human Performance, 16,* 250–279.

Hackman, J. R., & Oldham, G. R. (1980). *Work redesign*. Reading, MA: Addison-Wesley.

Herzberg, F. (1966). *Work and the nature of man.* New York: The World Publishing Company.

Herzberg, F., Mausner, B., & Snyderman, B. (1959). *The motivation to work.* New York: John Wiley & Sons.

Maslow, A. H. (1954). *Motivation and personality.* New York: Harper & Row.

Latham, G.P., & Pinder, C.C. (2005). Work motivation theory and research at the dawn of the twenty-first century. *Annual Review of Psychology, 56*(4), 85–516.

McClelland, D. C. (1961). *The achieving society.* New York: The Free Press.

McClelland, D. C. (1985). *Human motivation.* Glenwood, IL: Scott-Foresman.

O'Connor, D., & Yballe, L. (2007). Maslow revisited: constructing a road map of human nature. *Journal of Management Education, 31*(6), 738–756.

Sashkin, M. (1996). The MbM questionnaire: Managing by motivation (3rd ed.). Amherst, MA: Human Resource Development Press.

Timmreck, T. C. (2001). Managing motivation and developing job satisfaction in the health care work environment. *The Health Care Manager, 20*(1), 42–58.

Yukl, G. A. (2001). *Leadership in organizations* (5th ed.). Upper Saddle River, NJ: Pearson Education.

OTHER SUGGESTED READING

Campbell, J. P., Dunnette, M. D., Lawler, E. E., & Weick, K. E. (1970). *Managerial behavior, performance and effectiveness.* New York: McGraw-Hill Book Company.

Maslow, A. H. (1943). A theory of human motivation. *Psychological Review, 50,* 370–396.

CHAPTER 6

Process Theories of Motivation

Nancy Borkowski, DBA, CPA, FACHE

LEARNING OUTCOMES

After completing this chapter, the student should be able to understand:

- ☛ The various components of Expectancy Theory and how they impact an individual's level of motivation.
- ☛ Equity Theory and the methods to resolve inequity tension.
- ☛ The significance of the Satisfaction–Performance Theory.
- ☛ Goal-setting Theory and the steps necessary for successful implementation.
- ☛ Reinforcement Theory and the four types of reinforcement.

OVERVIEW

Understanding individuals and what motivates them is a conundrum for healthcare managers, especially since we need to manage such diverse groups of employees. These employees are diverse not only in culture, race, and gender, but also in varying levels of education. On a daily basis, we need to manage not only secretarial staff with minimal educational requirements, but also highly skilled individuals such as nurses, physicians, and other licensed healthcare professionals. As such, process theories assist us in predicting employees' behavior so we may influence the behavior, if necessary.

In this chapter, we will examine five theories of motivation: (1) Expectancy Theory, (2) Equity Theory, (3) Satisfaction–Performance Theory, (4) Goal-setting Theory, and (5) Reinforcement Theory.

EXPECTANCY THEORY

One widely cited theory of motivation is Victor Vroom's (1964) Expectancy Theory (also referred to as the VIE Theory). Expectancy Theory suggests that for any given situation, the level of a person's motivation (force in Vroom's conceptualization) with respect to performance is dependent upon (1) his or her desire for an outcome; (2) the perception that individual's job performance is related to obtaining other desired outcomes; and (3) the perceived probability that his or her effort will lead to the required performance. The theory may be expressed as $M = V \times I \times E$ (see Figure 6–1).

Vroom (1964) explains that the force that drives a person to perform is dependent upon three factors: valence, instrumentality, and expectancy (pp. 15–19).

Valence is the strength of an individual's want or need, or dislike, for a particular outcome. An outcome has a positive valence when the person prefers attaining it to not attaining it, a valence of zero when the person is indifferent

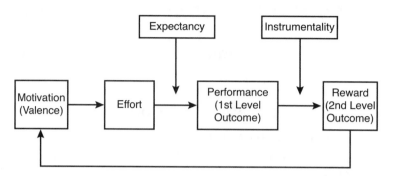

Figure 6–1 Vroom's Expectancy Theory (VIE)

to attaining or not attaining it, and a negative valence when the person prefers not attaining it to attaining it. As such, valence can have a wide range of both positive and negative values. The strength of a person's desire for, or aversion to, an outcome is based on the intrinsic properties of an outcome that are valued or not (a second-level outcome in Vroom's conceptualization), and/or on the anticipated satisfaction or dissatisfaction associated with other outcomes that are related to any given outcome (a first-level outcome in Vroom's conceptualization). For example, some workers may value an opportunity for promotion or advancement because of their need for achievement. (One outcome, advancement, is positively related to or instrumental with respect to achieving another outcome—achievement.) Others may not want the promotion because it would require additional time commitment and, therefore, less time for family or friends. (One outcome, advancement, is negatively related to or instrumental with respect to another outcome—need for affiliation.)

Instrumentality is an individual's perception that his or her performance is related to other outcomes, either positively or negatively. It is an outcome–outcome association. In other words, an individual will perform in a certain manner because he or she believes that behavior will be rewarded with something that has value to the individual. For example, a person believes that by producing both high-quality and -quantity of work, it will result in recognition (e.g., praise or bonus) or a promotion from his or her supervisor.

Expectancy is an individual's perception that his or her effort will positively influence his or her performance. It is an action–outcome association. It can be defined as a momentary belief concerning the likelihood that a particular act (effort) will be followed by a particular outcome (performance). Expectancies can be described in terms of their strength. Maximal strength is indicated by subjective certainty that the act will be followed by the outcome, while minimal (or zero) strength is indicated by subjective certainty that the act will not be followed by the outcome. For example, an individual perceives that if he or she works overtime, the management report will be completed by the deadline (maximal strength). However, if the employee perceives the deadline to be unrealistic and not obtainable because of the time required to complete the report, the expectancy strength is minimal.

Newsom (1990) summarized Expectancy Theory with what he termed the "Nine Cs":

1. *Challenge:* Does the individual have to work hard to perform the job well? Managers need to review an employee's job design. Is it routine and unchallenging? Does the job incorporate Herzberg's motivators (see Chapter 5)?

2. *Criteria:* Does he or she know the difference between good and poor performance? Managers need to effectively communicate to an employee the responsibilities and or requirements of the task and how the employee will be measured as to its successful completion. A manager should not assume that an employee knows the criteria for performing satisfactorily. In addition, managers need to provide feedback so an employee is aware of what he or she is doing right and what needs to be improved.

3. *Compensation:* Do the outcomes associated with good performance reward the individual? Nadler and Lawler (1983) discussed the mixed message an organization sends to employees when employees are rewarded for seniority rather than performance. What the organization gets is behavior oriented toward safe, secure employment rather than efforts directed at performing well.

4. *Capability:* Does the individual have the ability to perform the job well? Employees who lack the necessary skills, knowledge, and experience to perform a task well will become frustrated and avoid future growth opportunities.

5. *Confidence:* Does the individual believe he or she can perform the job well? Employees need to perceive that they can perform a task well. Although an employee may have the knowledge and skill, he or she may not see himself or herself with the ability to perform the task well. This may be based on past experiences of failure.

6. *Credibility:* Does the individual believe that management will deliver on promises? Managers must deliver what they promised.

7. *Consistency:* Does the individual believe that all workers receive similar preferred outcomes for good performance and similar less preferred outcomes for poor performance? Managers need to treat all employees equally, on the basis of objective criteria.

8. *Cost:* What does it cost an individual in time and effort to perform well?

9. *Communication:* Does management communicate well and consistently with the individual in order to affect the other eight Cs? Managers need to set clear goals and provide the right rewards for different people. (See Figure 6–2.)

For managers, Expectancy Theory is very useful because it helps to understand a worker's behavior. If employees lack motivation, it may be caused by their indifference toward, or desire to avoid, the existing outcomes. Expectancy Theory is based on the assumption that individuals calculate the "costs and benefits" in choosing among alternative behavioral actions. So the important question for managers to ask is, "What rewards (outcomes) do my employees value?" (See Case Study 6–1: Why Aren't My Employees Motivated?)

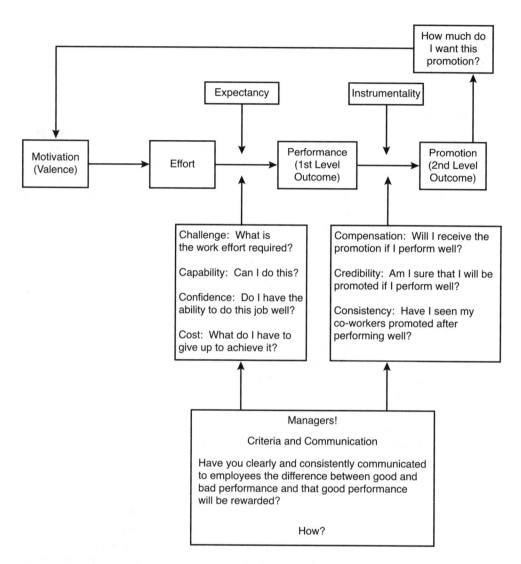

Figure 6–2 Application of Expectancy Theory Using Newsom's Nine Cs

Case Study 6–1 Why Aren't My Employees Motivated?

Roger Harris is the founder and managing partner of a large health management consulting firm that specializes in strategic planning for hospitals. The firm has six partners, including Roger, and 20 professional staff (all with graduate degrees in health administration). The staff is evenly divided between males and females, single and married individuals between 25 to 35 years old. Of the 10 married, two spouses work outside the home. All the married individuals have families of at least two children and all children are under 10 years old.

The philosophy of the firm is to serve the needs of the client and have fun serving those needs while making a profit. Because of the tight labor market, the firm's salaries for its professional staff are well above the market in order to attract and retain the best talent. In addition, each employee has a private office, breakfast served daily, free weekly car washes, and his or her dry cleaning delivered to the office. The firm also offers the staff home computers if they prefer to work at home on weekends during the firm's busy time, which usually runs from October to May.

During this period, staff are required to work approximately 55 to 60 hours per week. Staff receive two weeks vacation annually, in addition to one week for continuing professional education and one week personal time, which is utilized by 100 percent of the staff.

Roger Harris is concerned because, although partners' billable hours (i.e., hourly rates charged to clients for services rendered) have increased 12 percent over the last two years, the staff's billable hours have decreased by 14 percent. In addition, Roger Harris noted that the turnover rate (i.e., percentage of the newly hired graduates that stay with the firm for approximately three to four years before taking a position in one of their client's hospitals) has increased to 50 percent (from 10 percent five years earlier).

In order to increase the firm's productivity and retention rate, Roger Harris initiated a bonus program as follows:

If a staff member bills out 2,000 hours annually, he or she receives a bonus equal to 5 percent of his or her annual salary. For every hour billed over the minimum 2,000 hours, the employee is paid twice the hourly rate.

All employees earned their 5 percent bonus, but no one's productivity increased over the minimum 2,000 hours base.

Roger Harris is quite concerned by this lowering productivity and increasing turnover rate. Thinking that the staff needed outside professional recognition, he encouraged everyone to publish articles for the various health management journals discussing aspects of their most interesting cases. All the staff displayed their willingness to do so, as long as the time required to develop the articles would be applied toward their minimum 2,000 hours bonus calculation.

Roger Harris related to staff that anyone who demonstrated technical competence and the ability to attract and retain clients to the firm has the opportunity to become a partner. Even though individuals from the outside filled the last two senior management-level positions, four of the six partners were promoted from within (after 8 to 10 years of continuous employment with the firm). However, the most recent promotion to partner was made to an individual hired from the outside after only three years of employment with the firm.

Roger Harris thinks that the consulting firm is a great place to work with interesting and challenging cases, an excellent compensation package, and growth opportunity. Therefore, he cannot understand why staff's productivity continues to decline and the turnover rate continues to increase.

Using Expectancy Theory, explain to Roger Harris why nonpartner productivity level is low and why the firm is experiencing a high turnover rate with its professional staff.

EQUITY THEORY

J. Stacy Adams (1963, 1965) proposed his Equity Theory, stating that a person evaluates his or her outcomes and inputs by comparing them with those of others. Adams' theory is based in the social-exchange theories that center on two assumptions. First, that there is a similarity between the process through which individuals evaluate their social relationships and economic transactions in the market. Social relationships can be viewed as exchange processes in which individuals make contributions (investments) for which they expect certain outcomes (Mowday, 1983). The second assumption concerns the process through which individuals decide whether a particular exchange is satisfactory. If there is relative equality between the outcomes and contributions of both parties to an exchange, satisfaction is likely to result from the interaction (Mowday, 1983). If an inequality is perceived, then dissatisfaction occurs, which triggers an internal tension within one or more of the individuals.

The two major components in Equity Theory are inputs and outcomes. Inputs are defined as those things a person contributes to an exchange. In the workplace, an employee's inputs would be experience, education, efforts, skills, and abilities. Outcomes are those things that result from the exchange, such as salary, bonuses, promotions, and recognition. Adams states that equity exists when the ratio of a person's outcomes to inputs is equal to the ratio of others' outcomes and inputs (see Figure 6–3).

Several important aspects of Adams' theory are noted. First, the determination of whether inequity exists is based on the individual's perceptions of input and outcomes, which may or may not be reality. Second, inequity will not exist if the person has high inputs and low outputs, as long as the other person has the similar ratio. Third, inequity exists when a person is either underpaid or overpaid. For example, if employees perceive they are overcompensated, they may increase their level of productivity. If employees perceive they are undercompensated, they may either decrease their level of productivity or attempt to obtain additional compensation.

Adams (1965) proposed that when an inequity is perceived by an individual, (1) it creates tension within the person, (2) the tension is proportional to the degree of inequity, (3) the tension created within the individual motivates him or her to relieve it, and (4) the strength of the motivation to reduce the tension is proportional to the perceived inequity. Adams states that there are several cognitive and behavioral mechanisms available to individuals to reduce the psychological discomfort (i.e., inequity tension) associated with the perceived inequity. He refers to these cognitive and behavioral mechanisms as methods of inequity resolution. The six methods described by Adams are:

1. *Altering Inputs:* Reduce productivity, take longer break times, and use sick days for personal activities.
2. *Altering Outcomes:* Try to obtain an increase in pay, a bonus, or a new job title or resort to taking supplies from the company for personal use (i.e., stealing).
3. *Cognitively Distorting Inputs or Outcomes (self):* Describe how much harder he or she is working.

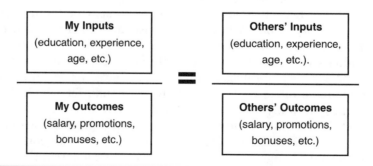

Figure 6–3 Adams' Equity Theory

4. *Leaving the Field:* Transfer to another department or quit the organization.

5. *Distorting the Inputs or Outcomes of the Comparison Other:* Describe the other person's job as routine and unchallenging.

6. *Changing the Comparison Other:* Find someone in the organization more like himself or herself—another high-performing worker.

Equity Theory does not predict which method will be selected by the individual. The behavior chosen by the individual depends on the situation with the goal of maximum utility (see Case Study 6–2: I Don't Know What to Do). According to Mowday (1983), the easiest method is trying to distort the other's inputs and outcomes. Leaving the organization will be considered only in extreme cases. Managers need to be aware of how employees perceive inequities in the work environment. If subordinates perceive that they are not being dealt with fairly, it would be difficult, if not impossible, to motivate them.

Case Study 6–2 I Don't Know What to Do

Katie was so disgusted with the situation she was seriously thinking about applying for the open RN position in the hospital's ambulatory surgery center just to get away from Beth. Katie has been employed at Good Point Hospital for the past 10 years. She originally started in the housekeeping department, but she knew she wanted more. So Katie took advantage of the hospital's tuition reimbursement program and returned to school to earn her nursing degree. Katie didn't care that she was 39 years old at the time she returned to school and that it took her three long years to earn her Associate of Science (AS) degree. It was worth the time and effort. Although, sometimes she had to admit it was stressful working full time during the day in the housekeeping department, with three small children still at home. But her husband Mike supported her, taking care of the children and household chores at night and on weekends so she could attend class or study in the library. She felt very blessed that she could set an example for her children by being the first person in her family to earn a college degree! It has been four years since she became an RN and Katie has enjoyed the hospital's intensive care unit (ICU). That was until Beth joined the ICU nursing staff last year.

When Katie returned home that evening, Mike could see that Katie was very upset. When Mike asked her what was bothering her, she related, "Beth has been working at Good Point Hospital for two years and in the ICU for the past year. I am now convinced that Beth has absolutely no work ethics. Maybe it's part of her being from Generation X; her twenty-first birthday is next month. She spends half of her shift either on the phone or e-mailing her friends from the new computer at the nurses' station. She calls in sick almost every other Monday or Friday when she is not scheduled for the weekend shift. She's always complaining how busy she is and how can the hospital's administration think she can get all her work done in a 12-hour shift! Beth's workload is similar to mine; in fact, I have more responsibility than she does, but I always seem to get my work done. Because Beth never finishes her jobs, it causes more work for me. For example, Beth is always the first one off the floor at the end of our shift and never completes her patients' medical charts, so the nurses from the incoming shift have to ask me to bring them up-to-date on Beth's patients before they start their shift. I don't mind helping them out, but it usually takes at least 30 minutes, and since the hospital froze overtime, I don't get paid to cover for Beth's laziness! Today Beth started whining because I have seniority, I get first pick for vacation time and holidays. I tried to lighten the mood by saying when I'm gone, she will have the seniority. I had to remind her that I've had my share of non-holiday time off, and everyone has to work his or her way up the ladder. I've spoken to Terry, our manager, about Beth on numerous occasions, but I feel I'm wasting my time. Terry says he'll talk to Beth, but he never does. I think he's overwhelmed trying to manage the ICU along with the other two departments that were recently assigned to him.

"I just don't know what to do since I'm not Beth's supervisor. Beth has this attitude of 'I don't want to work, but pay me anyway.' I'm so frustrated with the situation, I'm ready to leave the ICU!"

Discuss Katie's motivation to quit the ICU using Adams' Equity Theory.

SATISFACTION–PERFORMANCE THEORY

One of the major criticisms of the Expectancy Theory is that it does not take into account the relationship between employee performance and job satisfaction. As such, Lyman Porter and Edward Lawler (1968a) extended the Expectancy Theory and incorporated the Equity Theory into a model to reflect the relationship of an employee's performance to job satisfaction. Job satisfaction is related to both absenteeism and turnover. This is a great concern to organizations because turnover and absenteeism have a direct influence on an entity's effectiveness (Lawler, 1983). Lawler (1983) points out that,

> absenteeism is very costly because it interrupts scheduling, creates a need for overstaffing, increases costs; turnover is expensive because of the many costs incurred in recruiting and training replacement employees. Because satisfaction is manageable and influences absenteeism and turnover, organizations can control them. By keeping satisfaction high and, specifically by seeing that the best employees are the most satisfied, organizations can retain those employees they need the most. (p. 87)

Interestingly, prior to Porter and Lawler (1968a), no motivational model had directly dealt with the relationship between satisfaction and performance (Luthans, 2002). The Porter and Lawler model does not predict who is satisfied; it simply gives the conditions that lead to employees experiencing feelings of satisfaction or dissatisfaction (Lawler, 1983). The researchers believe that performance leads to satisfaction rather than satisfaction to improved performance.

The Porter and Lawler model reflects that satisfaction results from performance itself, the rewards for performance, and the perceived equitability of those rewards (see Figure 6–4).

Porter and Lawler (1968a) stated that job satisfaction is generated when an employee receives rewards for his or her performance. These rewards can be intrinsic (e.g., sense of accomplishment) or extrinsic (e.g., bonus). An employee's degree of satisfaction will be proportionate to the amount of rewards he or she believes he or she is receiving.

An important aspect of Porter and Lawler's theory is the fact that the amount of the reward an employee receives may be unrelated to how well he or she has performed (e.g., pay increases based on seniority or labor union agreements). As such, for employees whose rewards are tied to factors that are beyond their control versus receiving rewards based on how well they perform, there will be little or no correlation between satisfaction and job performance. However, if an employee holds a position (e.g., manager) where

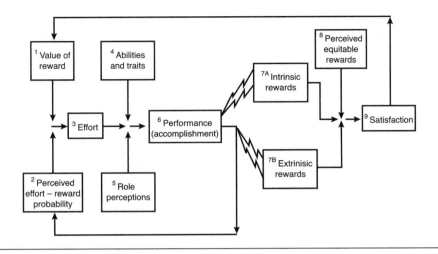

Figure 6–4 Porter–Lawler Satisfaction–Performance Motivation Model

rewards are received on the basis of the quality and quantity of his or her performance, there would be a correlation between satisfaction and performance. Porter and Lawler's (1968a, 1968b) research confirmed this hypothesis. The researchers found that managers who are ranked high by their supervisors report significantly greater satisfaction than do the low-ranked managers. More important is that, although the best performing managers did not report receiving any greater extrinsic rewards (e.g., pay and security) as compared to their counterparts, they did report receiving greater intrinsic rewards (e.g., expressed autonomy and the ability to obtain self-realization in the job). Therefore, the question asked is, "Does the organization actively and visibly give rewards directly in proportion to the quality of job performance for all of its employees?" If the answer is yes, then high satisfaction should be more closely related to higher performance, if the employees value the rewards distributed.

The Satisfaction–Performance Model tells us two things. First, if an individual is attracted by the value of the reward, if he or she perceives that a higher degree of effort on his or her part will lead to those rewards, and if the employee has the necessary abilities and accurate role perceptions, then higher performance will result. Second, if the intrinsic and extrinsic rewards an employee receives for higher performance are perceived as equitable, then satisfaction will result—satisfaction being the difference between perceived equity and actual rewards.

GOAL-SETTING THEORY

In the 1960s and 1970s, Gary Latham and Edwin Locke (1983) performed a number of laboratory and field research studies that determined that participants who were given specific, challenging goals outperformed those who were given vague goals such as "do your best." On the basis of their studies, Latham and Locke developed a goal-setting model. Although goal setting is a simple concept, it requires careful planning and forethought on the part of the manager (see Figure 6–5).

Latham and Locke suggest that there are three steps to be followed: (1) setting the goal, (2) obtaining goal commitment, and (3) providing support elements.

1. *Setting the Goal:* The goal set should have two main characteristics. First, it should be specific, rather than vague, and measurable. For example, a goal statement such as "increase elective outpatient surgeries by 5 percent within the next six months" is specific with a time limit for goal accomplishment. Second, the goal should be challenging yet reachable. Difficult goals lead to better performance. However, two points need to be made. For employees with low self-confidence or ability, goals should be set at a level that is easy and attainable by the employees. For employees with high self-confidence and ability, goals should be made difficult but attainable. In either case, if employees perceive the goals as unattainable, they will not accept them and performance will not improve. In fact, the employee will experience dissatisfaction and frustration. Managers need to be conscious that seeking unattainable goals may cause employees to view management with suspicion and distrust.

Latham and Locke stated that there are five possible methods, in addition to an employee's confidence and ability levels, for managers to use to determine goals for an employee. First, the manager could use time-and-motion studies to set the appropriate goal level. A second option, which would be more readily accepted, would be setting future goal levels on the basis of the average past performance of the employee. However, if the employee's past performance

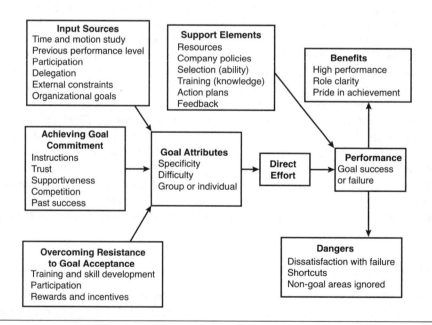

Figure 6–5 Latham and Locke's Goal-setting Model

was unacceptably low, upward adjustments need to be made. A third option would allow for the supervisor and subordinate to jointly set the goal. This participative approach has the advantages of being readily acceptable by both the manager and subordinate, and promotes role clarity. The fourth method may be determined by external sources. This is very common in the healthcare industry; because third parties determine reimbursements, the goal is to deliver service at the lowest possible cost without reducing quality. The fifth method is determining individual goals that correspond to the long-term goals of the health services organization as determined by the organization's board of trustees.

2. *Obtaining Goal Commitment:* If goal setting is to be successful, the manager needs to ensure that subordinates will accept and remain committed to the goals. Appropriate pay (i.e., rewards) with the manager's supportiveness is usually sufficient for goal acceptance and commitment by the employee. Employees receive a feeling of satisfaction for reaching challenging, fair goals, which tends to reinforce acceptance of future goals.

Generally, employees resist goals for two reasons. First, they may perceive themselves as being incapable of reaching the goals. To overcome this resistance, managers need to provide training to increase employees' skills and knowledge, therefore increasing their self-confidence that the goal can be achieved. Second, employees may not see any relationship between their personal benefits (i.e., feeling of accomplishment or external rewards) and obtaining the goals. Managers may use a participative approach so that employees have a feeling of control over the situation. Reward systems must be in place to directly compensate employees for obtaining the agreed-upon goals.

3. *Providing Support Elements:* Managers must ensure that employees have adequate resources (e.g., financial, equipment, time, assistance, etc.) to reach their goals. Furthermore, company policies and procedures must not create barriers to employees' goal attainment. Employees need to trust that management is supporting, not undermining, their efforts.

Managers need to provide employees with an action plan of agreed-upon goals and rewards so there is no ambiguity in the process. In addition, feedback is essential. Employees must have access to information as to the status in their goal attainment. Finally, Latham and Locke point out that goal setting is not a solution for poor management or the low/undercompensation of employees.

REINFORCEMENT THEORY

Reinforcement Theory is based primarily on the work of B.F. Skinner (1953), who experimented with the theories of operant conditioning. Skinner's research found that an individual's behavior could be redirected through the use of reinforcement. Reinforcement Theory suggests that an employee's behavior will be repeated if it is associated with positive rewards and will not be repeated if it is associated with negative consequences. Although Reinforcement Theory is not a motivation theory (at least not in the context we have been discussing in this chapter and in Chapter 5), it does help managers understand and influence, when necessary, behavioral change by the reinforcements used. Reinforcement is a behavioristic approach, which argues that reinforcement conditions behavior (Robbins, 2003). Since reinforcement is an important means of understanding what controls an individual's behavior, it is included in motivation discussions (see Figure 6–6) (Robbins, 2003; Tosi & Mero, 2003).

There are four types of reinforcement: positive, negative, punishment, and extinction.

Positive reinforcement occurs when a desirable outcome is associated with a behavior. Desirable outcomes can be simple and symbolic, such as words of praise, a certificate of accomplishment, or a month's use of the parking space directly outside the hospital's main entrance. To fully appreciate its effect, managers should use positive reinforcement only when an employee displays the desired behavior. For example, the Director of Nursing has attempted to reduce the turnover time [i.e., time required to set up an operating room (OR) after each surgical procedure] of the hospital's ORs to improve the efficiency of the department. The OR nurses formed a task group and after many months and careful planning with full cooperation of the physicians and support staff, the daily turnover time decreased by 15 percent within a six-month period. The decrease in OR turnover time allowed for one additional case to be scheduled per day. The Director of Nursing recognized the team's accomplishment by publishing it in the health system's newsletter and hosting a thank-you lunch for the department.

Negative reinforcement occurs when an unpleasant effect is eliminated or avoided, which, like positive reinforcement, encourages repeated positive behavior. We return to our OR example. The nurse responsible for ordering surgical supplies, by working with the hospital's technology department,

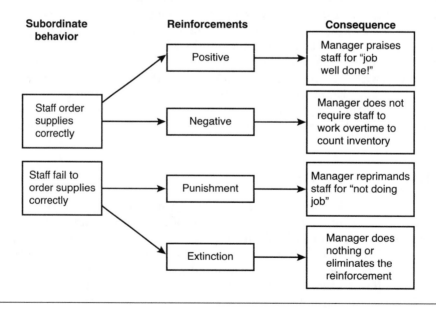

Figure 6–6 Reinforcement Theory and Types of Reinforcements

designs an inventory system using bar codes that alert her when supplies are at a reordering level. With the use of technology, the system automatically transmits a message that an order must be placed to the purchasing department. By designing and implementing the new inventory ordering system, the nurse has eliminated her need to work overtime counting inventory and has eliminated the negative consequences (e.g., unhappy patients and physicians, lost revenues) when a surgery case has to be canceled and rescheduled because the hospital did not have the necessary supplies on hand.

Punishment can come in two forms: negative consequences and positive consequences, both undesirable. A negative consequence is an undesirable response to an employee's behavior in the attempt to stop the behavior from being repeated. For example, the OR nurse who is responsible for ordering supplies was reprimanded by the department's manager when she failed to place an order for a required surgical instrument, causing an OR case to be canceled. (Because of this reprimand, the OR nurse was "motivated" to design an inventory system so the situation would not occur again.) A positive consequence occurs when something desirable is removed from the employee. For example, when the OR nurse failed to order the necessary surgical instrument, the department's manager required her to update the inventory supply list within 24 hours, which required her to work on her scheduled day off and cancel her trip to Disney World.

Extinction is defined as the removal of an established reinforcement (positive or negative) that was previously used to reinforce an employee's behavior. This removal may weaken an employee's future behavior. For example, in the hospital's OR department, if the room charge nurse's surgical cases started and ended on time (measured on a weekly basis), he or she would receive a $50 certificate to a local restaurant. Because of a change in the hospital's senior management, this positive reinforcement was eliminated with the following message: "It is your job to make sure the OR is run efficiently, which includes having the cases start and end on time. Therefore, we are eliminating the previously awarded gift certificate. If you have any questions regarding this new policy, please contact your manager."

Managers need to be very careful regarding the administrating of punishment reinforcements. Unless done carefully and appropriately, the effects can cause long-term consequences for the organization. It can cause employee resentment, hostility, and turnover. As a guide when administering punishments, the manager should only punish undesirable behavior and be very clear as to what constituted the undesirable behavior when discussing it with the employee; give reprimands or discipline actions as soon as possible after the behavior has occurred; administer punishment in private; and, when possible, combine negative and positive reinforcements.

Reinforcement schedules refer to the timing and frequency with which the consequences are associated with behavior. The scheduling of the reinforcement is important because the frequency will determine the time it takes to learn a new behavior (Tosi & Mero, 2003). Reinforcement schedules can be continuous, fixed interval, variable interval, fixed ratio, or variable ratio.

- When a continuous-reinforcement schedule is used, it requires the specific employee's behavior to be reinforced each time it occurs [e.g., the chief executive officer (CEO) rewards all employees every time the hospital passes its Joint Commission accreditation].

- When a fixed-interval reinforcement schedule is used, the reinforcement is administered at predetermined periods (e.g., annual performance appraisals). Fixed-interval schedules may cause irregular behavioral responses because an employee will usually work harder the closer it gets to his or her performance appraisal date.
- The variable-interval schedule allows reinforcements to be administered at irregular intervals (e.g., the hospital's CEO attends monthly departmental staff meetings on an impromptu basis).
- The fixed-ratio schedule requires the reinforcement to be administered after a predetermined number of behaviors have occurred (e.g., the pharmaceutical department's manager is awarded a bonus if the department's monthly revenues are greater than those of the previous month). Fixed-ratio schedules can produce high rates of responses that continue as long as the reinforcement has value to the employee.
- The variable-ratio schedule is evident when the number of behaviors necessary for reinforcement varies (e.g., managers who reward employee behavior on a haphazard basis) (Tosi & Mero, 2003).

Consider the following scenario:

A hospital CEO is discussing his facility's experiences at trying to effectively manage the ordering and tracking of supplies in the hospital's OR department.

"We started looking at some product line assessments. As an example, a couple of years ago we met with two different groups of ophthalmologists to look at their costs on a case-by-case basis. We then compared what they used and might use, and determined the areas in which we might be able to standardize products and equipment. . . . We had the ophthalmologists work with vendors and use a case supply cap, and we saved some money that way. Recently though, we've noticed that some of the ophthalmologists are drifting back to their old routines again, so I think this is something that you can't just do once and expect it to manage itself. . . ."

What reinforcement schedule would you advise the CEO to use in the future? Why?

Source: *Healthcare Financial Management Association's Executive Roundtable Series, July 2004., Improving OR throughput: Real world successes and challenges.* Reprinted with permission.

SUMMARY

In this chapter, we have discussed the various process theories of motivation. These motivation theories help healthcare managers predict employee behavior. Managers can then effectively influence that behavior, achieving organizational success through increased job satisfaction.

END-OF-CHAPTER DISCUSSION QUESTIONS

1. Discuss the various components of Expectancy Theory.
2. Explain Newsom's "Nine Cs."
3. Discuss the two components of Equity Theory.
4. Explain the methods of inequity resolution.
5. Discuss the significance of the Satisfaction–Performance Theory.
6. Explain how the Satisfaction–Performance Theory relates to Expectancy Theory and Equity Theory.
7. Discuss the three components of the Goal-setting Theory.
8. Explain how goals can be determined under the Goal-setting Theory.
9. Explain management's responsibilities under the Goal-setting Theory.
10. Explain why we include Reinforcement Theory in motivation discussions.
11. Discuss the types of reinforcements available to managers for changing an employee's behavior.
12. Discuss the various reinforcement schedules and why their timing and frequency are important.

END-OF-CHAPTER CASE STUDY

Case Study 1 All in a Day's Work (Part Two)[a]

Sarah Goodman, Senior Manager of Network Development for the Holy Managed Care Company, continues her day.

After her lunch meeting with the advisor for the MHSA (Master's of Health Services Administration) program at State University, she is back on the job attending more meetings! At 1:30 PM she has a meeting to discuss pay issues. The Human Resources Department has evaluated the salary picture for the entire organization and is concerned that women are not being paid as well as men. They want input on a strategy to bring the pay issue into line so as to avoid a gender discrimination charge. Personally, Sarah wondered if she got paid as well as Dave, her counterpart in Tampa. Certainly she has been there as long and worked about twice as hard as he seems to! He does seem to benefit from the "good old boy network," however.

Then at 3 o'clock there is a performance appraisal she'd scheduled with her assistant Maria. Sarah wasn't sure what to do about Maria. Her work was terrific from the standpoint of accuracy and amount. As long as she got a pat on the back pretty frequently, Maria was an ideal employee in a lot of ways. Sarah knew that Maria would be prepared for the interview, including her goals for the next six months. The problem was that Sarah really wanted to get Maria more involved with others in the department. If she wasn't able to get Maria ready to assume her position, how could Sarah ever hope to be promoted? Productive as she was, Maria just wasn't a "people person."

Then at 4:00 PM, there is another performance appraisal scheduled. This one was going to be difficult. Janine was a fairly new employee and Sarah loved the work she produced, but she didn't think she'd ever seen a more uptight person! She seemed to need to be told at each step what to do next and worried constantly about breaking the rules. Sarah had begun to think Janine had even invented some new rules that didn't even exist! There was that time last week, for example, when she'd ask Janine to stay a little late and finish up a project. She didn't discover until the next day that Janine had been late picking up her baby from the babysitter. Certainly overtime wasn't required and Sarah felt bad about causing the problem. She could have asked someone else to do the work, but thought it might be a way of encouraging Janine to "get out of the box" a little.

By the time that was over, Sarah figured she'd just have time to return her phone calls and scan the mail before it was time to go home. She'd promised Richard something special for dinner, mostly because she was planning to tell him about graduate school. The traffic would be awful and she needed to stop by the store on the way. "Oh well! It's all in a day's work," she thought.

Discuss the various motivation theories reflected in this case study.

AUTHOR : Pidge Diehl, EdD. Reprinted with permission.
[a]Part One was presented at the end of Chapter 5.

REFERENCES

Adams, J. S. (1963). Toward an understanding of inequity. *Journal of Abnormal and Social Psychology, 67,* 422–436.

Adams, J. S. (1965). Inequity in social exchange. In L. Berkowitz (Ed.), Advances in experimental social psychology (Vol. 2, pp. 267–300). New York: Academic Press.

Latham, G. P., & Locke, E. A. (1983). Goal setting—A motivational technique that works. In J. R. Hackman, E. E. Lawler & L. W. Porter (Eds.), *Perspectives on behavior in organizations* (pp. 296–304). New York: McGraw-Hill Book Company.

Lawler, E. E. (1983). Satisfaction and behavior. In J. R. Hackman, E. E. Lawler & L. W. Porter (Eds.), Perspectives on behavior in organizations (pp. 78–87). New York: McGraw-Hill Book Company.

Luthans, F. (2002). *Organizational behavior* (9th ed.). New York: McGraw-Hill Book Company.

Mowday, R. T. (1983). Equity theory predictions of behavior in organizations. In J. S. Ott (Ed.), *Classic readings in organizational behavior* (pp. 94–102). Albany, NY: Wadsworth Publishing Company.

Nadler, D. A., & Lawler, E. E. (1983). Motivation: A diagnostic approach. In J. R. Hackman, E. E. Lawler & L. W. Porter (Eds.), *Perspectives on behavior in organizations* (pp. 67–78). New York: McGraw-Hill Book Company.

Newsom, W. B. (1990, February). Motivate, now! *Personnel Journal,* 51–55.

Porter, L. W., & Lawler, E. E. (1968a). *Managerial attitudes and performance.* Homewood, IL: Irwin.

Porter, L. W., & Lawler, E. E. (1968b). What job attitudes tell about motivation. *Harvard Business Review, 46*(1), 118–126.

Robbins, S. P. (2003). *Organizational behavior* (10th ed.). Upper Saddle River, NJ: Prentice Hall.

Skinner, B. F. (1953). *Science and human behavior.* New York: Macmillan.

Tosi, H. R., & Mero, N. P. (2003). The fundamentals of organizational behavior: What managers need to know. London: Blackwell Publishing.

Vroom, V. H. (1964). *Work and motivation.* New York: John Wiley & Sons.

CHAPTER 7

Attribution Theory and Motivation

Paul Harvey, Ph.D. and Mark J. Martinko, Ph.D.

LEARNING OUTCOMES

After completing this chapter, the student should be able to understand:

- ☞ The basic premises of attribution theory.
- ☞ The differences between optimistic, pessimistic, and hostile attribution styles.
- ☞ The role of attributions, emotions, and expectations in motivating employees.
- ☞ Techniques managers can use to promote accurate and motivational attributions.

OVERVIEW

In this chapter we expand on the discussion of attribution theory introduced in Chapter 3, as well as the motivational topics described in Chapters 5 and 6. In this chapter's discussion, attribution theory is used to provide managers with a better understanding of the highly cognitive and psychological mechanisms that influence motivation levels. The chapter begins with an overview of attribution theory. We then discuss the different attribution styles that can bias the accuracy of causal perceptions, potentially undermining the effectiveness of motivational strategies. We then describe the impact of attribution-driven emotions and expectations on motivation. This is followed by an overview of techniques healthcare managers can use to promote motivational attributions among employees.

ATTRIBUTION THEORY

Before describing the basic tenets of attribution theory, it is useful to understand exactly what is meant by the term *attribution*. An attribution is a causal explanation for an event or behavior. To illustrate, if a nurse observes a colleague performing a procedure incorrectly on a patient, he is likely to try to form an attributional explanation for this behavior. The nurse might conclude that his colleague is poorly trained, meaning that the observer is attributing the behavior to insufficient skills. People also form attributions for their own behaviors and outcomes. For example, a physician might attribute her success in diagnosing a patient's rare disease to her intelligence and training, or to good luck.

As these examples might suggest, the attribution process is something that people are likely to engage in many times each day. For many of us, the process is so automatic and familiar that we do not notice it. However, a wide body of research indicates that the formation of causal attributions is vital for adapting to changing environments and overcoming the challenges we are confronted with in our daily lives. When we experience desirable outcomes, attributions help us understand what caused those events so we can experience them again. When we experience unpleasant outcomes, attributions help us identify and avoid the behaviors and other factors that caused them to occur.

As discussed in Chapter 3, Fritz Heider (1958) argued that all people are "naïve psychologists" who have an innate desire to understand the causes of behaviors and outcomes. Attribution theory holds that attributions for these behaviors and outcomes ultimately help to shape emotional and behavioral responses (Weiner, 1985). A simplified depiction of this attribution–emotion–behavior process is shown in Figure 7–1. In order to understand these relationships, however, it is important to be familiar with the various dimensions along which attributions can be classified.

First, attributions can be classified along the dimension of *locus of causality*, which describes the internality or externality of an attribution. If a physician misdiagnoses a patient and attributes this medical error to his own carelessness (i.e., ignored the patient's symptoms), he is making an internal attribution. If the same outcome is attributed to faulty laboratory results even though the patient's symptoms contradicted the lab results, the physician is making an external attribution. The locus of causality dimension is particularly relevant to emotional reactions. Internal attributions for undesirable events or behaviors are frequently associated with self-focused negative emotions, such as guilt and shame. External attributions for the same behaviors and outcomes are generally associated with externally focused negative emotions, such as anger and resentment (Gundlach, Douglas, & Martinko, 2002; Weiner, 1985).

Causal attributions can also be categorized along the *stability* dimension. Stable causes are those that tend to influence outcomes and behaviors consistently over time and across situations. Causes such as intelligence and physical or governmental laws are generally considered relatively stable in nature because they are difficult, if not impossible, to change. Unstable causal factors, such as the amount of effort exerted toward a task, are comparatively easy to change. Unlike the locus of causality dimension, which primarily influences emotional reactions to events and behaviors, the stability dimension affects individuals' future expectations (Kovenklioglu & Greenhaus, 1978). When an outcome such as poor performance is attributed to a stable cause, such as low intelligence, it is logical to expect that the employee's performance is not going to change in the future. If the same poor performance is attributed to a less stable factor, such as insufficient effort, we can expect that the employee could improve his or her performance by working harder in the future.

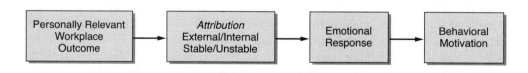

Figure 7–1 Attribution–Emotion–Behavior Process

Researchers have also classified attributions in terms of the intentionality and controllability of the cause (Weiner, 1995). However, for the purposes of understanding the basic impact of attributions on motivation, we will limit our discussion to the aforementioned dimensions of locus of causality and stability. Thus, we can consider attributions that are internal and stable (e.g., intelligence), external and stable (e.g., laws), internal and unstable (e.g., effort), or external and unstable (e.g., temporary organizational policies). Before examining the influence of these attributions on motivational states, however, it is useful to understand how attribution styles can bias the attributions individuals form.

ATTRIBUTION STYLE

It is important to recognize that, as with all perceptions, attributions are not always an accurate reflection of reality! We can probably all think of an instance where someone failed at a task because of his or her own actions, but erroneously blamed the failure on other people or circumstances. In fact, if we are totally honest with ourselves, we can each probably recall one or two instances where we made these false attributions ourselves.

Astute observers may also notice that some people make these attributional errors more frequently than others. These individuals are said to have a biased *attribution style*. An attribution style is defined as a tendency to consistently contribute positive and negative outcomes to a specific type of cause (e.g., internal or external, stable or unstable). The aforementioned tendency to attribute negative outcomes to external factors is often coupled with a tendency to attribute positive outcomes to internal factors. This self-serving attribution style is referred to as an *optimistic attribution style* (Abramson, Seligman, & Teasdale, 1978; Douglas & Martinko, 2001). This term reflects the fact that people with an optimistic attribution style often feel good about themselves and their capacity for success. An obvious downside, however, is the fact that this personal optimism may be unfounded and can set the individual up for disappointments in the future.

A second attribution style, known as a *pessimistic attribution style*, denotes the opposite tendency. Individuals who demonstrate this attributional tendency frequently attribute undesirable events to internal and frequently stable factors such as lack of intelligence, while attributing desirable outcomes to external and frequently unstable factors, such as bad luck. As the name suggests, people who exhibit this tendency often lack confidence in themselves and are pessimistic concerning their chances for success (Abramson et al., 1978). This tendency can also promote depression and a tendency toward learned helplessness (this is discussed in greater detail later in the chapter and Chapter 12).

A third attributional tendency, known as a *hostile attribution style*, also warrants discussion. This style is similar to the optimistic style just described in that it denotes a tendency toward external attributions for negative outcomes. The two styles differ in that the external attributions for undesirable events associated with a hostile style are also stable in nature. A study by Douglas and Martinko (2001) suggested that the stability of these attributions could promote anger toward the external "entity" (e.g., one's manager) and increase the likelihood of an aggressive response. It appears, for example, that a number of highly publicized incidents of workplace violence that have occurred in the United States were committed by individuals with a history of consistently external and stable causal explanations for the negative events in their lives. As such, we can conclude that hostile attribution styles in the workplace are not only unproductive but can also be dangerous as well.

Before discussing the implications of these attribution styles, and attributions in general, on employee motivation, one point should be clarified. In many situations the causes of an event are perfectly clear. For example, if a person is rear-ended at a traffic light well after coming to a complete stop, she is going to blame the other driver regardless of her attribution style. Thus, because attribution styles are only tendencies to make certain types of attributions, they are unlikely to have an effect in situations where the causes of an outcome are obvious. However, when the causes are ambiguous, attribution styles are more likely to have an effect. A manager's goal, therefore, should be to make (as well as to encourage) accurate and unbiased attributions so that employees' successes can be repeated and the causes of problems can be rectified.

ATTRIBUTIONS AND MOTIVATIONAL STATES

The discussion of attributions and motivational states is divided into four sections, each of which describes a desirable or undesirable motivational state and the capacity of specific attributions and attribution styles to bring about these states. Two undesirable states, learned helplessness and aggression, are discussed first. Two desirable motivations states, empowerment and resilience, are then discussed.

Table 7–1 Summary of Attribution Styles

Attributional Style	Impact on Attributions	Examples
Optimistic	Biased toward internal (often stable) attributions for positive outcomes, external (often unstable) for negative	Attribute successful diagnoses to personal ability, and misdiagnoses to inadequate information from patients.
Pessimistic	Biased toward internal (often stable) attributions for negative outcomes, external (often unstable) for positive	Attribute successful outcomes to good luck; poor outcomes are due to lack of personal ability.
Hostile	Biased toward external, stable attributions for negative outcomes	Attribute most workplace problems to a biased and vengeful manager

Learned Helplessness

After repeated punishments and failures, people often become passive and unmotivated and stay that way even after the environment changes so that personal or professional success is possible (Abramson et al., 1978; Martinko & Gardner, 1982). This phenomenon has been labeled "learned helplessness" because it describes a situation in which individuals come to believe that effort is futile because failure is inevitable. They have, in effect, learned to be helpless.

Learned helplessness is a consequence of the reinforcement process described in Chapter 6. When people see that behaviors lead to desired rewards and outcomes, they are motivated to repeat those behaviors. When specific behaviors do not achieve desired outcomes, the motivation to perform those behaviors is lost. Learned helplessness was first observed by Overmier and Seligman (1967) in dogs placed in a shuttle box with two sides. One side had an electric grid, the other side was safe. Initially, the dogs were tethered to the electrified half of the chamber. Before administering an unpleasant, but nonlethal, shock, a light flashed. The dogs quickly learned to associate the flash of light with the impending electrical shock, because of classic conditioning. After the conditioning was complete, the experimenters removed the tethers that had previously made escaping to the nonelectrified side of the chamber impossible. Instead of leaping to safety when the light flashed, however, most of the dogs froze, whimpered, and braced themselves for the shock. It was concluded that the dogs had "learned" helplessness, believing that the shock was inevitable regardless of their efforts.

More recent research suggests that this tendency toward learned helplessness is also common in people and that organizational rules and norms can cause learned helplessness among employees in the same way the experiments induced it in dogs (Martinko & Gardner, 1987). Specifically, organizational policies/norms and leaders' behaviors that cause employees to feel that success and/or recognition is unobtainable are likely to inhibit motivation. For instance, a manager who routinely takes credit for her subordinates' successes while blaming them for their failures may find herself with employees who see little reason to work any harder than is necessary to keep their jobs. Similarly, an organization that forces employees to follow outdated and ineffective procedures may find itself with employees who show little urgency or interest in their work, given that they expect the effort to fail. If you expect to fail, why bother trying?

The significance of organizationally induced learned helplessness is that, like the aforementioned dogs, it often remains even when the barriers to success are removed. To continue the previous examples, if the unfair manager is replaced or restrictive policies are removed, we might expect that employee motivation and performance would immediately improve. The reality, however, is that employees who work under such conditions for an extended period of time often retain their learned helplessness and remain unmotivated even after the situation and conditions change.

This tendency can be explained by the attribution process. External barriers to success in the workplace can, ironically, promote internal and frequently stable attributions for failures while promoting external attributions for successes. Over time, these attributions can manifest themselves in the form of a pessimistic attribution style, causing employees to accept blame for failures they did not contribute to, while attributing successes to their manager or to other external factors. To illustrate, a manager that consistently takes credit for departmental successes while blaming employees for failures can, over time, cause employees to believe and feel that they are incompetent at their jobs. This perception can remain even after the manager is removed if proper steps to restore employees' confidence are not taken. This example also illustrates one of the downsides of the aforementioned optimistic-attribution style. When organizational leaders demonstrate this tendency, they may feel good about themselves (at least in the short term), but their tendency to take credit for successes and attribute blame for failures to others may cause their employees to lose confidence and experience learned helplessness.

Aggression

Another undesirable motivational state discussed here differs from learned helplessness in several ways. Perhaps the most significant is that, unlike the diminished motivation associated with learned helplessness, aggression refers to a state of heightened motivation. The problem is that this motivation is focused on an undesirable behavior or goal.

Instrumental aggression describes behaviors targeted at obtaining a goal that the employing organization is not providing. For instance, an employee who feels he is underpaid and steals from his employer is performing instrumental aggression. Hostile aggression refers to behaviors aimed primarily at harming another person or entity. An employee who physically attacks a manager, for example, probably does so not to get anything from the manager, except the satisfaction of inflicting physical pain. Beyond the obvious surface-level differences in these forms of aggression, there are different underlying motivations (Martinko, Douglas, Harvey, & Joseph, 2005). Whereas instrumental aggression is primarily motivated by a desire to obtain something, hostile aggression is motivated by a desire to retaliate and harm others.

Both types of motivation may be sparked by the causal perceptions associated with hostile attribution styles. Case Study 7–1, at the end of the chapter, describes a study that indicated that individuals can more easily justify instrumental acts of deviance, such as forging paperwork or lying about their performance, in response to negative workplace events that were attributable to stable organizational factors (e.g., inadequate resources). Research has also shown that the attribution of undesirable workplace outcomes to external and stable causes can increase the likelihood of a hostile aggressive response. Similarly, research suggests that individuals with a hostile attribution style are more likely to engage in acts of hostile aggression than others (Douglas & Martinko, 2001). In addition to empirical research evidence, anecdotal reports suggest that a number of workplace shootings in the United States, such as those at several U.S. Post Office facilities, were perpetrated by individuals with external attributional tendencies.

From this evidence we can conclude that employees who attribute negative events at work to external and stable causes are more likely than others to become motivated to engage in aggressive behaviors. A key element in determining which form of aggression will occur, or if any aggression will occur at all, appears to be the perceived intent of the responsible party. In cases where an undesirable workplace event is deemed to be caused by factors beyond the control of any specific party (e.g., an economic downturn), aggression becomes less likely (Harvey, Martinko, & Borkowski, 2007). There is some evidence, however, that some individuals will remain motivated to engage in acts of instrumental aggression in these situations (see Martinko et al., 2005). When it is perceived that an external and stable factor caused a negative outcome and could have been prevented, hostile aggression toward the "guilty" party becomes more likely. This is probably due to the feelings of anger associated with such perceptions (Weiner, 1995). That is, when causality and intent can be attributed to a specific person or entity, people often feel anger, which, in turn, frequently motivates acts of hostility.

Empowerment

Turning our attention to desirable motivational states, we first discuss the notion of empowerment. Empowerment refers to a heightened state of motivation caused by optimistic effort-reward expectations (Conger & Kanungo, 1994). Put differently, empowered individuals expect their efforts toward their goals to succeed and are therefore motivated to exert high levels of effort. Empowerment is also associated with high levels of innovation and managerial effectiveness (Spreitzer, 1995).

Because empowerment among employees is generally good for overall organizational effectiveness, it is helpful to understand the cognitive processes that help foster this state of heightened motivation. Research has shown that the causal attribution process can tell us a lot about how employees become empowered. Unlike learned helplessness, empowerment appears to result from the attribution of negative workplace events to factors that are either internally controllable or that are external, unstable, and uncontrollable. Thus, a physician who misdiagnoses a patient's disease, but believes the error was under her control (e.g., "I didn't think to check for this disease, but I will know to do so in the future"), is less likely to experience strongly negative emotions and learned helplessness than a physician who attributes the error to his incompetence. Similarly, a physician who attributes a similar error to an external, unstable, and uncontrollable factor (e.g., the patient gave incomplete information and there was not enough time to run a full battery of diagnostic tests) is likely to feel optimistic about her future chances for successful diagnoses.

Naturally, we can also expect individuals who attribute positive events to internal factors, such as their intelligence, skill, and effort, to experience empowerment (Martinko & Gardner, 1987). It follows that individuals with an optimistic attribution style are more likely to demonstrate empowerment than those with pessimistic or hostile attribution styles. Recall, however, that attribution styles can cause individuals to form inaccurate perceptions of causality. A caveat, therefore, is that those with an optimistic attribution style may become disillusioned with themselves and feel empowered even when their skills and abilities are lacking. Thus, as we discuss later in the chapter, it is more important to promote attributions that are accurate than to encourage attributions that are optimistic.

Resilience

Resilience is defined as a "staunch acceptance of reality . . . strongly held values, and an uncanny ability to improvise and adapt to significant change" (Coutu, 2002, p. 47). Research suggests that resilient people are relatively good at developing accurate attributions (Huey & Weisz, 1997). More specifically, it appears that people with low levels of resilience have a tendency to be overly external or internal in their attributions for negative outcomes. Thus, people who are nonresilient are likely to err in the attributions and are prone to blame others or themselves for their failures. As we have discussed, either of these attributional errors can promote negative motivational outcomes. High levels of resilience have the opposite effect, helping people keep their attributions in line with reality (recall that resilience denotes a "staunch acceptance of reality").

Resilience, then, can be thought of as a factor that helps individuals avoid the attributional errors that can hurt motivation levels. By promoting accurate causal perceptions, resilience helps to keep people grounded in reality and helps to prevent pessimistic and hostile attributional tendencies. It is also likely that resilience can help prevent overly optimistic attributions, and the disillusionment and unfounded optimism noted in the previous section.

If we assume that resilience is good for promoting motivation through accurate attributions, the next logical question is, where does resilience come from? We begin the next section by addressing this question, after which we discuss some additional techniques for promoting empowerment while discouraging learned helplessness and aggression.

Table 7–2 Summary of Attributions Associated with and Motivational States

Motivational State	Associated Attributional Tendency
Learned Helplessness	Tend to favor internal and stable attributions for failures; external attributions for successes
Aggression	Tend to favor external and stable attributions for failures
Empowerment	Tend to favor internal and stable attributions for successes; external and unstable attributions for failures
Resilience	Tend to favor accurate attributions, not biased toward overly internal or external attributions for successes or failures

PROMOTING MOTIVATIONAL ATTRIBUTION PROCESSES

In this section, we summarize five techniques that can be used by managers to promote and maintain employee motivation. These techniques are grounded in the formation of accurate and empowering attributions.

Screening for Resilience

In the previous section, we discussed the benefits of resilience for forming attributions that are accurate and motivational. Unlike most of the suggestions in this section, however, our advice concerning resilience does not focus on increasing it among existing employees. This is because individuals' levels of resilience appear to form very early in life (Masten, 2001). With proper emotional support, children have shown remarkably high levels of resilience in dealing with undesirable circumstances, such as poverty and violence. Conversely, we are probably all familiar with both children and grown adults who break down in response to relatively minor problems. This suggests that resilience levels are formed early in life and are unlikely to change dramatically in the course of normal life events (note that drastic events such as war and serious disease appear to increase resilience levels in adults, but these do not fall under the umbrella of "normal life events").

Employers may determine that their organizations require a high level of resilience in their employees. Hospitals, for example, can provide a very stressful and emotionally draining working environment. If employees form overly hostile or pessimistic attributions in response to the negative events that are bound to happen in such settings, motivational problems are likely to arise. This type of organization, then, will probably benefit from a resilient workforce. A less stressful organization, on the other hand, might not require such resilience among employees.

Organizations such as hospitals that require high levels of resilience should, then, try to attract and hire individuals that demonstrate high levels of resilience. Although it is unlikely that managers can increase the resilience levels of employees, they can try to form a workforce that has high preexisting levels. This can be accomplished through the use of standardized measures of resilience (see Huey & Weisz, 1997, for an example) during the employee screening process, or through simple interview questions. Asking potential candidates to describe past hardships, and their responses to these hardships, is likely to shed light both on candidates' resilience levels and their attributional tendencies (Campbell & Martinko, 1998).

Attributional Training

Although resilience is a fairly stable and unchanging personal characteristic, accurate and optimistic attributional tendencies can be fostered in other ways. One technique for accomplishing this is attributional training (Martinko & Gardner, 1987). This can take several forms, one of which is measuring employees' attribution styles with an existing assessment device (see

Kent & Martinko, 1995; Lefcourt, 1991; Lefcourt, von Baeyer, Ware, & Cox, 1979; Peterson, Bettes, & Seligman, 1985; Peterson, Semmel, von Baeyer, Abramson, Metalsky & Seligman, 1982; and Russell, 1982 for examples of these instruments) and discussing their attributional biases with them. Often, by simply realizing that they favor overly optimistic, pessimistic, or hostile attributions, individuals can begin to deliberately adjust their "perceptual lenses" to correct for their biases. Over time, this correction can become subconscious, allowing employees to form accurate attributions without additional cognitive effort.

A second form of attributional training is less formal and involves discussing the causes of employees' successes and failures on a case-by-case basis. This can help employees understand both the internal and external factors involved with workplace outcomes, by helping them to understand the "big picture" in terms of the multiple personal and situational factors likely to contribute to positive and negative events. This promotes a more thorough causal search process and can help employees avoid the cognitive shortcuts that enable overly optimistic, pessimistic, or hostile attributions.

Immunization

Another technique recommended by Martinko and Gardner (1987) is to immunize against demotivational attributions by enabling successes early in an employee's career or tenure with an organization. If an employee fails miserably at the first few tasks she is assigned in a new position, she may quickly decide that she lacks the ability to succeed at the job (an internal and somewhat stable attribution). If she is allowed to tackle a number of more surmountable assignments before engaging in more difficult tasks, however, she is likely to see that she has the basic ability to succeed at the job. This will probably promote more optimistic attributions throughout the employee's tenure by providing a basic level of confidence at the beginning.

Increasing Psychological Closeness

In addition to individual attributional biases, employees can also become the unwitting victims of their managers' inaccurate attributional tendencies (Martinko, 1995). Managers provide an important, and often highly valued, source of feedback for employees. If this feedback consistently attributes blame for negative outcomes to employees' internal characteristics, employees might accept the feedback as accurate even if it is not, and experience organizationally induced learned helplessness (Martinko & Gardner, 1987).

Research suggests that people in observational capacities (which is often the case for managers) frequently tend to be overly dispositional in their attributions for others' performance (Jones & Nisbett, 1971). That is, they tend to focus on the influence of actors' effort and ability levels while overlooking situational factors that contribute to performance. As a result, managers can be overly hard on employees when their performance is low. Managers might also demonstrate an optimistic attribution style and take credit for the successes of their departments without giving credit to their subordinates, while also blaming employees when their department's performance suffers. Again, these tendencies can be demotivational, particularly if employees believe their managers' attributional explanations for their performance.

One technique for avoiding this tendency is to promote psychological closeness. Psychological closeness describes the extent to which two or more people form the same perceptions regarding their situation. Research has shown that managers who have direct experience with the work their employees perform are relatively less likely to form inaccurate attributions regarding employee performance. Managers who have little or no experience with their employees' tasks (or who have not performed them in a long time) appear to be less familiar with the situational challenges associated with the work and are more likely to blame employees' effort and ability levels when their performance in low (Fedor & Rowland, 1989).

To increase psychological closeness between managers and employees, then, organizations should work to ensure that managers have experience with the work their subordinates perform. This can be accomplished through internal promotions (i.e., selecting future managers from the pool of employees currently performing the job to be supervised) and by requiring existing managers to perform the jobs they are managing from time to time. These techniques will ensure that managers are familiar with both the internal and external factors associated with performance, allowing more accurate and motivational attributional feedback to be formed and communicated to employees.

Multiple Raters of Performance

A final recommendation for improving the accuracy and motivational capacity of employees' attributions is the use of multiple raters of performance, when possible (Martinko, 2002). As mentioned previously, managers can demonstrate attribution styles that bias them toward demotivational explanations for employee performance. This tendency can be offset by the use of multiple performance raters.

An illustrative example of this style of judging performance is the use of multiple judges to evaluate figure skaters in the Olympics. This system is used to help ensure that potential biases among one or more raters can be offset by the accuracy, or counteracting biases, of other judges. Similarly, organizations can use more than one individual to rate the performance of employees. An increasingly common example of this is the use of 360-degree evaluations, in which peers, managers, subordinates, customers, and the employees themselves rate performance. Although each of these parties may demonstrate some attributional inaccuracy, the hope is that through the use of multiple sources, an accurate picture of the causes of each employee's successes and failures will emerge. With this information, the proper steps can be taken to correct poor performance and encourage future successes, ultimately promoting empowerment among employees.

SUMMARY

Our overarching goal in this chapter was to illustrate the importance of attributional perceptions in predicting employee motivation. One of the key findings from research on this topic is that internal and stable attributions for successes in the workplace, as well as external and unstable attributions for negative workplace events, are associated with higher levels of empowerment. We have seen repeatedly, however, that such attributions are only desirable when they are accurate. If an employee fails at a task because the employee is simply not "cut out" for the type of work being performed, it is generally better for the employee to realize that to believe that the repeated failures are due to external factors. Similarly, if failures are caused by unstable internal factors such as insufficient effort, it is important for employees to make that attribution, even if it is not the most desirable short-term conclusion. These accurate attributions help steer employees down the path toward empowerment, and managers can assist in the process by providing honest and accurate assessments of the causes of employees' performance.

END-OF-CHAPTER DISCUSSION QUESTIONS

1. What is an attribution?
2. Differentiate between optimistic, pessimistic, and hostile attribution styles.
3. Why might an optimistic attribution style be undesirable?
4. How can different types of attributions and attribution styles encourage high or low levels of learned helplessness, aggression, and empowerment?
5. How does resilience promote motivational attributions?
6. How can organizational leaders promote accurate and motivating attributions among their employees?

END OF CHAPTER CASE STUDY

Case Study 7–1 "Unhealthy" Motivation: How Physicians Justify Deviant Behavior

We probably all know the feeling, something bad happens at work and there are a few choices for dealing with it. You can go "by the book," and potentially suffer some unpleasant consequences, or bend the rules just a bit to make the whole thing go away. For example, imagine a situation where you miss a deadline by a few hours and you can choose to tell your manager or, because your manager happens to be in a long meeting, finish the job late and slip it under some paperwork on her desk, claiming that it has been there all day. You know what you *should* do, but you also know that the sneakier alternative is probably the path of least resistance. What would you do?

Your answer to this question would probably depend, at least in part, on *why* you missed the deadline in the first place. If you missed the deadline because you procrastinated all week and then took an extended lunch break on the day the work was due, you might feel a degree of guilt over lying to your manager. Attribution theory suggests that this is because you are attributing the missed deadline to an internal and unstable/controllable factor, namely insufficient effort. This guilt might, depending on other factors, such as your values and the consequences of your manager learning of the missed deadline, reduce your willingness to lie about finishing the work on time.

Your response might change, however, if you feel that you missed the deadline because the amount of time your manager gave you to complete the work was unreasonably short. If you worked late and skipped lunch all week, but still needed a couple extra hours to get the work done, you are much less likely to blame yourself. Instead, you will probably attribute the missed deadline to an external and relatively stable factor—your manager. Such attributions are associated with anger, and anger is a strong motivator of deviant behavior. This attribution-driven anger might help you feel justified in sneaking the work onto your manager's desk—why should you get in trouble if the request was unreasonable?

To test the strength of attributions such as these to motivate deviant behaviors, Harvey et al. (2005) examined the relationship between attributions, emotions, and the justification of workplace deviance using a sample of physicians. The researchers gave the physicians a hypothetical scenario similar to the one just described and asked them whether they would feel comfortable altering dates on paperwork to disguise the fact that a nonlethal, but procedural, mistake had been made in diagnosing a patient. Each physician was given the same hypothetical scenario with one difference—the cause for the mistake (i.e., the attribution) was varied so that in some cases the mistake was due to internal and stable or unstable factors (i.e., the physician has poor attention to detail or was distracted), or to external and stable or unstable factors (i.e., the physician's department is chronically understaffed or an emergency meeting was called and the required test could not be ordered on time).

As you might expect, on the basis of the preceding discussion, physicians were more likely to say they would alter the paperwork when the cause of the mistake was beyond their control and was stable (i.e., likely to occur again) in nature. Before taking an overly dim view of these physicians, however, remember that the hypothetical mistake described in the scenarios was deliberately designed to be very minor and inconsequential. Still, this study provides some insight into the power of attributions to motivate behaviors we might not normally consider.

This justification process is an almost unavoidable part of life. There are always going to be times where it is tempting to break the rules because we feel that it is a justifiable response to a wrongdoing we have suffered. Indeed, many timeless stories are based on the notion of justifiable wrongdoing—Robin Hood returning the king's wealth to the peasants, for example.

There is a decidedly darker side to the justification process, however. Perpetrators of many serious crimes throughout history have, at least at the time of the crime, convinced themselves that they were justified in their behavior. In many cases, the justification can be traced to a desire for revenge resulting from the attribution of negative events to externally controllable, stable factors. Thus, we can see that there is more at stake than productivity when it comes to forming accurate attributions.

REFERENCES

Abramson, L. Y., Seligman, M. E. P., & Teasdale, J. D. (1978). Learned helplessness in humans: Critique and reformulation. *Journal of Abnormal Psychology, 87,* 49–74.

Campbell, C. R., & Martinko, M. J. (1998). An integrative attributional perspective of empowerment and learned helplessness: A multi-method field study. *Journal of Management, 24,* 173–200.

Conger, J. A., & Kanungo, R. N. (1994). Charismatic leadership in organizations: Perceived behavioral attributes and their measurement. *Journal of Organizational Behavior, 15,* 439–452.

Coutu, D. L. (2002). How resilience works. *Harvard Business Review, 80,* 46–55.

Douglas, S. C., & Martinko, M. J. (2001). Exploring the role of individual differences in the prediction of workplace aggression. *Journal of Applied Psychology, 86,* 547–559.

Fedor, D. B., & Rowland, K. M. (1989). Manager attributions for subordinate performance. *Journal of Management, 15,* 37–48.

Gundlach, M. J., Douglas, S. C., & Martinko, M. J. (2003). The decision to blow the whistle: A social information processing framework. *Academy of Management Review, 28,* 107–123.

Harvey, P., Martinko, M. J., & Borkowski, N. (2007). Unethical behavior among physicians and students: Testing an attributional and emotional framework. Presented at the 2007 Academy of Management Conference, Philadelphia, PA.

Heider, F. (1958). *The psychology of interpersonal relations.* New York: John Wiley & Sons.

Huey, S. J., & Weisz, J. R. (1997). Ego control, ego resiliency, and the five-factor model as predictors of behavioral and emotional problems in clinic-referred children and adolescents. *Journal of Abnormal Psychology, 106,* 404–415.

Jones, E. E., & Nisbett, R. E. (1971). The actor and the observer: Divergent perceptions of the causes of behavior. In E. E. Jones, D. E. Kanouse, H. H. Kelley, R. E. Nisbett, S. Valins, & B. Weiner. (Eds.), *Attribution: Perceiving the causes of behavior* (pp. 79–94). Morristown, NJ: General Learning Press.

Kent, R., & Martinko, M. J. (1995). The development and evaluation of a scale to measure organizational attribution style. In M. Martinko (Ed.), *Attribution theory: An organizational perspective* (pp. 53–75). Delray Beach, FL: St. Lucie Press.

Kovenklioglu, G., & Greenhaus, J. H. (1978). Causal attributions, expectations, and task performance. *Journal of Applied Psychology, 63,* 698–705.

Lefcourt, H. M. (1991). The multidimensional-multiattributional causality scale. In J. P. Robinson, P. R. Shaver, & L. S. Wrightsman (Eds.) *Measures of personality and social psychological attitudes* (Vol. 1, pp. 454–457). San Diego, CA: Academic Press.

Lefcourt, H. M., Von Baeyer, C. L., Ware, E. E., & Cox, D. J. (1979). The multidimensional-multiattributional causality scale: The development of a goal specific locus of control scale. *Canadian Journal of Behavioural Science, 11,* 286–304.

Martinko, M. J. (1995). The nature and function of attribution theory within the organizational sciences. In M. J. Martinko (Ed.), *Attribution theory: An organizational perspective* (pp. 7–16). Delray Beach, FL.: St. Lucie Press.

Martinko, M. J. (2002). *Thinking like a winner: A guide to high performance leadership.* Tallahassee, FL: Gulf Coast Publishing.

Martinko, M. J., Douglas, S. C., Harvey, P., & Joseph, C. (2005). Managing organizational aggression. In R. Kidwell & C. Martin (Eds.). *Managing organizational deviance: Readings and cases* (pp. 237–260). Thousand Oaks, CA: Sage.

Martinko, M. J., & Gardner, W. L. (1987). The leader-member attribution process. *Academy of Management Review, 12,* 23–249.

Masten, A. S. (2001). Ordinary magic: Resilience processes in development. *American Psychologist, 56,* 227–238.

Overmier, J. B., & Seligman, M. E. P. (1967). Effects of inescapable shock upon subsequent escape and avoidance learning. *Journal of Comparative and Physiological Psychology, 63,* 23–33.

Peterson, C., Bettes, B. A., & Seligman, M .E. P. (1985). Depressive symptoms and unprompted casual attributions: Content analysis. *Behavior Research and Therapy, 23,* 379–382.

Peterson, C., Semmel, A., Von Baeyer, C., Abramson, L., Metalsky, G., & Seligman E. (1982). The attributional style questionnaire. *Cognitive Therapy and Research, 6,* 287–300.

Russell, D. (1982). The causal dimension scale: A measure of how individuals perceive causes. *Journal of Personality and Social Psychology, 42,* 1137–1145.

Spreitzer, G. M. (1995). Psychological empowerment in the workplace: Dimensions, measurement, and validation. *Academy of Management Review, 38,* 1442–1465.

Weiner, B. (1985). An attributional theory of achievement motivation and emotion. *Psychological Review, 97,* 548–573.

Weiner, B., (1995). *Judgments of responsibility: A foundation for a theory of social conduct.* New York: Guilford Press.

OTHER SUGGESTED READING

Schermerhorn, J. R. (1987). Improving health care productivity through high-performance. *Health Care Management Review, 12*(4), 49–55.

Leadership

"Power is America's last dirty word. It is easier to talk about money—and much easier to talk about sex—than it is to talk about power. People who have it deny it; people who want it do not want to appear hungry for it; and people who engage in its machinations do so secretly." (Kantner, 1979)

Power is the ability to influence others' actions, thoughts, or emotions. When discussing power, the topic of leadership always enters into the conversation because the two terms are almost inseparable. In Part III, we attempt to answer the often-asked question, "What does it take to be an effective leader?" First, we begin our discussions with Chapter 8, in which we provide an overview of the definition of power and the types, sources, and uses of power. Chapter 9 discusses the early theories of leaderships, such as the great person and trait theory. In Chapter 10, we turn our attention to the next generation of leadership theories—the contingency theories. Contingency theories state that leaders apply different styles in different situations, depending on the factors involved. Chapter 11 provides us insight into some of the contemporary theories in leadership, such as transformational, visionary, and servant leadership. These contemporary theories of leadership look to the person and the organization's culture in the attempt to answer the question, "What does it take to be an effective leader?"

CHAPTER 8

Power and Influence

Nancy Borkowski, DBA, CPA, FACHE

LEARNING OUTCOMES

After completing this chapter, the student should understand the:

- ☛ Definition of power.
- ☛ Difference between potential and kinetic power.
- ☛ Different sources of power.
- ☛ Ways managers develop a power base.
- ☛ Definition of organizational politics and the various political behaviors.
- ☛ Definition of upstream influence and the various influence tactics categories.

OVERVIEW

Since 2002, *Modern Healthcare* has been publishing a list of the 100 most powerful people in health care annually. *Modern Healthcare*'s readers develop the list. The readers are first asked to nominate and then vote for individuals they believe have the greatest power to influence the US healthcare delivery system. When David Burda (2003), editor of *Modern Healthcare*, reviewed the 2003 list, the one theme that caught his attention was control. He stated that, "controlling something of value makes you powerful, and that's what the people on the list have in common" (p. 36). So then it would be no surprise to learn that almost 25 percent of the top 100 powerful people (and 40 percent of the top 25 people on the list) are elected or appointed federal employees (see Table 8-1). These individuals wield the most influence as to how the federal government's $650 billion health services budget will be spent, in addition to the power to impose, delay, or eliminate costly regulatory requirements on healthcare providers.

Power has been defined in a variety of ways. Thibaut and Kelley (1959) defined power as having behavioral or fate control over the behavior of another. Mechanic (1962) defined it as any force that results in behavior that would not have occurred if the force had not been present. Siu (1979) defined power as the influence over the beliefs, emotions, and behaviors of people, which is the definition adopted for our discussions.

Power exists only when there is an unequal relationship between two people and where one of the two is dependent upon the other (Emerson, 1962). Using the example of the 100 most powerful people in health care reflects these two components of power: unequal relationship and dependency. Healthcare providers are dependent on the federal government, specifically the Medicare and Medicaid programs, for reimbursements. Any change in the levels of reimbursement can have a dramatic effect on the industry. For example, the Balanced Budget Act of 1997 had a tremendous negative affect on the industry.

Table 8–1 2003's Top 25 of the 100 Most Powerful People in the Healthcare Industry

Name	Position
George W. Bush	President of the United States
Bill Friest	US Senator; Senate Majority Leader
Tommy Thompson	Secretary, Department of Health and Human Services (HHS), Washington
Edward Kennedy	US Senator; ranking minority member of the Health, Education, Labor and Pension Committee, Washington
John Ashcroft	US Attorney General, Justice Department, Washington
Tom Scully	Administrator, Consumer and Marketing Service (CMS), Washington (former)
Richard Gephardt	US Representative; presidential candidate (former)
Gail Wilensky	Senior Fellow, Project HOPE; former Health Care Financing Administration (HCFA) administrator
Dennis O'Leary	President, Joint Commission
Uwe Reinhardt	James Madison Professor of Political Economy; professor of economics and public affairs at Princeton University
Thomas Frist, Jr.	Retired chairman, Health Care Authority (HCA)
Neal Patterson	Chairman and CEO, Cerner Corp.
Donald Berwick	President and CEO, Institute for Healthcare Improvement; professor of health policy management at Harvard
Gary Mecklenberg	President and CEO, Northwestern Memorial Healthcare, Chicago
Tom Ridge	Secretary, US Department of Homeland Security
Pete Stark	US Representative; ranking minority member, Ways and Means Committee's health subcommittee
Jeff Goldsmith	President, Health Futures; associate professor of medical education, School of Medicine, University of Virginia
Newt Gingrich	Former Speaker of the House; founder, Center for Health Transformation, Washington
John Hammergren	Chairman and CEO, McKesson Corp., San Francisco
Pamela Thompson	CEO, American Organization of Nurse Executives, Washington
Barbara Blakeney	President, American Nurses Association, Washington
Donald Young	President, Health Insurance Association of America, Washington
Elias Zerhouni	Director, National Institutes of Health

SOURCE: "100 most powerful," by M. Romano, 2003. *Modern Healthcare, 33*(34), pp. 6–7 and 42–54. Reprinted with permission.

The situation was so severe (e.g., hospitals reporting financial deficits, managed care companies withdrawing from geographic areas) that the federal government restored funding under the Balanced Budget Reform Act of 1999. There is an unequal relationship because of the federal government's ability to enact new regulations that require major changes in how healthcare providers and suppliers conduct business (e.g., Stark I and Stark II regulations, Health Insurance Portability and Accountability Act of 1996).

Potential power exists when an individual has the ability to influence (e.g., a supervisor sitting at her desk completing paperwork, but without staff interaction). When the individual actually uses the power to influence, it is referred to as kinetic power (e.g., a supervisor awards a bonus to a subordinate for completing a challenging task on time and correctly) (Siu, 1979).

The concept of power is an integral part of the organizational behavior subjects we have discussed so far—attitudes, perception, and motivation. Power is also central to the topics we will discuss in upcoming chapters—leadership, group dynamics, and change management.

SOURCES OF POWER

John French and Betram Raven (1959) identified five bases or sources of social power: reward power, coercive power, legitimate power, referent power, and expert power. An individual is not limited to only one source of power; individuals may hold and exercise multiple sources of power simultaneously.

Reward power is defined as the ability to give rewards, something that holds value to another individual. Reward power has two components. First, the individual (P) must perceive that the other person (O) has the ability to reward. Second, the reward must have some value to P. If O offers a reward to P and then fails to deliver, future attempts by O to change P's behavior by using reward power have been diminished.

Coercive power is defined as the ability to punish either by administering a punishment or by withholding something that an individual needs or wants. Coercive power stems from P's expectation that O will administer a punishment if P fails to conform to the influence attempt. As with reward power, for coercive power to be effective, P must perceive that O has the ability to punish or sanction, and this negative valence must have some value (e.g., avoidance of punishment) to P.

Legitimate power is authority given to an individual on the basis of a given role or position. There are three bases of legitimate power: culture, social structure, and delegation of power. In some cultures, certain groups are granted the right to prescribe behavior for others. For example, in some cultures the aged or one sex is granted the power to demand conformity of behavior by others. Social structure is the second basis for legitimate power. In formal organizations, this power is granted by the title someone holds within the company's hierarchy. The third base of legitimate power is delegation of the power by the legitimizing agent. For example, a department manager may accept the authority of a vice president in certain areas because the organization's president has specifically delegated the authority to the vice president. It is important to remember that O only holds legitimate power if P accepts O as holding a legitimate power position.

Referent power stems from P's affective regard (i.e., attraction) for, or identification with, O. Interestingly, O has the ability to influence P even though O may be unaware of this referent power. Also, because P desires to be associated with or identified with O, P will assume attitudes, beliefs, or behavior displayed by O. Therefore, the greater the attraction, the greater the identification and the greater the referent power.

Expert power exists when P awards power to O on the basis of P's perception of O's knowledge within a given area. P evaluates O's expertness in relation to his or her own knowledge as well as against an absolute standard. The expert is seen as having superior knowledge or ability in very specific areas. Therefore, the attempt to exert expert power outside of the specific area will reduce that expert power and an undermining of confidence may take place.

OTHER SOURCES OF POWER WITHIN AN ORGANIZATION

David Mechanic (1962) found that employees without formally defined power positions exercise significant personal power within an organization by creating a sense of dependency. Employees create this dependency by controlling access to:

1. Instrumentalities, which includes any aspect of the physical plant of the organization or its resources (e.g., equipment, materials, budgets).
2. People, including anyone within the organization or anyone outside the organization upon whom the organization is in some way dependent.
3. Information, which includes knowledge of the norms, procedures, and techniques of doing business within the organization.

The most effective way for lower-level employees to achieve power is to have higher-ranking employees dependent upon them. Thomas Scheff's research (1961) provides us with an illustration of this dependency relationship and the power associated with it. Scheff's study involved a state mental hospital that failed to implement reforms because of the opposition of the hospital attendants. The failure was largely due to the ward physicians' dependency on the attendants. The dependency resulted from the physicians' short tenure, lack of interest in administration, and the large amount of administrative responsibilities the physicians had to assume. An implicit trading agreement developed between physicians and attendants, whereby attendants would take on some of the responsibilities and obligations of the ward physician in return for increased power in decision-making processes concerning patients. Failure of the ward physician to honor his or her part of the agreement resulted in information being withheld, disobedience, lack of cooperation, and unwillingness of the attendants to serve as a barrier between the physician and a ward full of patients demanding attention and recognition. When the attendants withheld cooperation, the physicians had difficulty in making graceful entrances and departures from the ward, in handling necessary paperwork (officially their responsibility), and in obtaining information needed to deal adequately with daily treatment and behavior problems. When the attendants opposed change, they could wield influence by refusing to assume responsibilities officially assigned to the physician.

Another example is new physician residents' dependency on the floor nurses in a large teaching hospital. These new physicians are dependent on the nurses for providing all the information regarding how to maneuver through the hospital maze to obtain the necessary care for their patients. How are tests ordered? What paperwork must be completed? Does the patient need an authorization from his or her insurance company? The new residents are dependent on the nurses' goodwill toward them. If the nurses withhold their cooperation, the physicians would have little or no alternative but to attempt to decipher the hospital's policies and procedures, which would be a very time-consuming process.

Increasing complexity within organizations has made the expert or staff person more powerful as a result of the organization's dependency on his or her specialization, knowledge, and skills. Experts have tremendous potentialities for power by withholding information or providing incorrect information. For example, Mechanic (1962) discusses the situation of a lay hospital administrator (as opposed to a hospital administrator who is also a physician) who makes an administrative decision that physicians oppose on the basis of medical necessity. A lay administrator is not in a position to contest these claims independently. To evaluate these claims, the administrator would need to engage medical consultants to serve as a buffer between the medical staff and the lay administration.

Employees also form coalitions that demonstrate power to get things done in a highly functionally structured organization, such as a hospital (see Chapter 21). Hospitals are complex entities organized into functional units such as medical, nursing, administration, and physical plant, which are controlled at high levels of authority. It is not unusual for coalitions to form at the intermediate and lower levels that overlap the functional units. For example, the hospital's orthopedic unit secretary knows the person in patient support services who schedules patient transport or the person in the centralized supply unit who coordinates deliveries to the various departments. The secretary can handle informally what would be very time-consuming if handled formally. As such, managers become dependent on employees who know how to get around the system, which gives those employees power.

Employees also gain power because others have delegated responsibilities to them, which they themselves do not want to do, but which are accompanied with a certain amount of power. For example, a physician usually delegates the responsibility of scheduling his or her appointments to a secretary. The secretary schedules both patient and nonpatient appointments and, as such, wields enormous power as to who will or will not see the physician this week. Ask any pharmaceutical representative trying to schedule an appointment to discuss a new drug with a physician! Or the administrative assistant in the primary care physician's (PCP's) office who issues patient referrals has the power of selecting what specialists the physician's patients will be referred to within the managed care network. A specialist could experience a decrease in his or her patient referrals by not cooperating with the PCP's administrative staff's requests (e.g., forwarding copies of medical records or seeing referred patients in a timely fashion).

DEVELOPING A POWER BASE

Managers are dependent on others because of two organizational factors: division of labor and limited resources (Kotter, 1977). Managers are dependent on subordinates, peers, supervisors, other units within the organization, outside suppliers, and many others. Managers are sensitive to this issue and they cope with their dependency by eliminating it, limiting it, or establishing power over others (Kotter, 1977). Kotter describes four ways managers have been successful in developing a power base.

- *Creating a Sense of Obligation:* Managers will go out of their way to do favors for people whom they expect will feel an obligation to return those favors.

- *Building a Reputation as an Expert in a Certain Area:* Managers will establish themselves as experts so that others will defer to them on those matters. This can be accomplished through visible achievement (i.e., professional reputation and track record).

- *Identification:* Managers will try to foster others' unconscious identification with them or ideas they stand for. Managers try to look and behave in ways that others respect. They go out of their way to be visible to their employees and give speeches about their organization's goals, values, and so on.

- *Perceived Dependence:* Managers will attempt to have others believe that they are dependent on the manager, either for help or not being hurt. The manager can accomplish this by securing resources that another person requires to perform his or her job. At the same time, the manager makes it known that he or she can also have the same resources removed. Managers may also resort to influencing others' perception of the manager's available resources, which may be more than, in reality, he or she possesses. In trying to influence people's judgments, managers pay attention to the trappings of power and to their own reputations and images. They associate with people and organizations that are known to be powerful.

Kotter notes that managers who build their power based on perceived expertise or on identification can often use it to influence attitudes as well as someone's immediate behavior, which would result in a lasting impact.

ORGANIZATIONAL POLITICS

Allen, Madison, Porter, Renwick, and Mayes (1979, p. 77) describe organizational politics as the intentional acts of influence to enhance or protect the self-interest of individuals or groups. On the basis of their research, eight types of political behaviors were identified. They are as follows:

- *Attacking or Blaming Others:* Attacking or blaming others is often associated with scapegoating—blaming others for a problem or failure. It may also include trying to make a rival look bad by minimizing his or her accomplishments.

- *Using Information as a Political Tool:* Using information as a political tool may include withholding important information when doing so might further an employee's political interests. This type of behavior can also include information overload, for example, to bury or obscure important (but potentially damaging) details that the employee hopes go unnoticed.

- *Creating and Maintaining a Favorable Image:* Creating and maintaining a favorable image includes drawing attention to one's successes and the successes of others, creating the appearance of being a player in the organization, and developing a reputation of possessing qualities considered to be important to the organization (i.e., impression management; see Chapter 3). The behavior also includes taking credit for the ideas and accomplishments of others.

- *Developing a Base of Support:* Examples of developing a base of support include getting prior support for a decision before a meeting is called and getting others to contribute to an idea to secure their commitment.

- *Ingratiation/Praising Others:* Ingratiation/praising includes praising others and establishing good rapport for self-serving purposes. Organizational jargon for this behavior includes buttering up the boss, apple polishing, and brown nosing.

- *Developing Allies and Forming Power Coalitions:* Developing allies and forming power coalitions includes developing networks of coworkers, colleagues, and/or friends within and outside the organization for purposes of supporting or advocating a specific course of action.

- *Associating with Influential People:* Associating with influential people includes developing professional connections with organizations and people that are known to be powerful individuals.

- *Creating Obligations and Reciprocity:* Creating obligations and reciprocity includes performing favors to create obligations from others, commonly known as "you scratch my back and I'll scratch yours."

From an organizational perspective, withholding and distorting information are the most dysfunctional and should be safeguarded against by the company. Note the similarities between Kotter's power bases and Allen et al.'s types of political behavior: creating a favorable image, developing allies and forming power coalitions, creating obligations, and associating with influential people. Although Kotter and Allen et al. developed their arguments 20 years ago, they are still valid today.

UPWARD INFLUENCE

There has been a growing recognition among organizational behavior researchers that a political influence perspective is a useful way to examine the effectiveness of managers (Falbe & Yukl, 1992; Farmer & Maslyn, 1999; Pfeffer, 1992). This perspective has focused on employees' influence tactics directed upward at those higher levels in the formal organizational structure. Kipnis, Schmidt, and Wilkinson (1980), on the basis of their research, grouped influence tactics into various categories, of which six relate to upward influence. These categories are as follows:

- *Assertiveness* includes such influence tactics as demanding compliance, ordering, and setting deadlines, as well as nagging and expressing anger.

- *Ingratiation* includes behaviors such as praising, politely asking, acting humble, making the other person feel important, and acting friendly.

- The *rationality tactic* consists of using reason, logic, and compromise in attempting to influence others. This also includes attempts to convince others that certain actions are in their own best interests.
- The *exchange category* refers to such behavior as offering to help others in exchange for reciprocal favors.
- *Upward appeal* is indicated by behavioral attempts to gain support from superiors in an organization.
- *Coalition formation* refers to attempts to build alliances with others.

Kipnis and Schmidt (1988) assessed the use of upward influence with hospital supervisors, clerical workers, and chief executive officers. Using the tactics of the six categories of upward influence, Kipnis and Schmidt identified four clusters:

- *Shotguns:* Individuals who use all tactics, but especially assertiveness and higher authority.
- *Tacticians:* Individuals with a high use of reason or rationality, but average use of other tactics.
- *Bystanders:* Individuals with lower than average scores on all tactics.
- *Ingratiators:* Individuals with the highest use of friendliness or ingratiation tactics, but average use of other tactics.

In the early stages, this research stream has been productive. There is a growing knowledge of how various employee tactics used to influence behaviors of those in higher positions within the organization work or do not work under certain circumstances (Farmer & Maslyn, 1999).

SUMMARY

In this chapter, we discussed what is meant by power and how individuals can use it to influence others. As noted, the concept of power is an integral part of organizational behavior. As you will see in Chapters 9, 10, and 11, power is central to the subject of leadership.

END-OF-CHAPTER DISCUSSION QUESTIONS

1. Discuss what is meant by the term power.
2. Explain the difference between potential and kinetic power.
3. Describe the different sources of power.
4. Explain what is meant by a manager's power base and the ways managers develop it.
5. Describe organizational politics and the resulting political behaviors.
6. Discuss what is meant by upstream influence and the various influence tactics categories associated with it.

END-OF-CHAPTER CASE STUDY

Case Study 1 Scott's Dilemma

Let's revisit the case study of Scott's Dilemma that was presented in Chapter 3.

Scott is a licensed physical therapist who works for a national rehabilitation company. The rehabilitation facility in which Scott works is located in an urban Southwest city. He has worked at this facility for four years and, up until recently, was satisfied with his working environment and the interactions he shared with his coworkers. In addition, Scott received personal fulfillment from helping his patients recover from their disabilities and seeing them return to productive lives.

Last year the health system went through reorganization, with some new people being brought in and others reassigned. Scott's new boss, George, was transferred from one of the system's Midwest facilities. Almost immediately upon taking his new position, George began finding fault with Scott's care plans, patient interactions, and so on. Scott began feeling as if he couldn't do anything right. He was experiencing feelings of anxiety, stress, and self-blame. Although his previous performance evaluations had been above average, Scott was shocked by his first performance review under George's authority—it was an extremely low rating.

Scott began trying to work harder, thinking that by working harder he could exceed George's expectations. Despite Scott's long hours and addressing George's critiques, George continued to find fault with Scott's work. Staff meetings began to be a great source of discomfort and stress because George would belittle Scott and single him out in front of his colleagues.

Scott began to feel alienated from his family, friends, and colleagues at work. His eating and sleeping habits were adversely affected as well. Scott's activities held no joy for him anymore and the career that he had once loved and been respected in became a source of pain and stress. He began to call in sick more often and started visualizing himself confronting and even hurting George, which created even more guilt and anxiety for Scott.

As time went on, George encouraged Scott's coworkers to leave Scott alone to do his work. The perception of the coworkers became more sympathetic to George's point of view. Scott's coworkers mused that perhaps Scott really was a poor worker and that George knew better because of his position as the supervisor of the rehabilitation department. Eventually, Scott's coworkers began to distance themselves from him, in order to protect their own interests. They began to see Scott as an outsider, with whom it was unsafe to associate.

In an effort to resolve the situation, Scott spoke to George directly, stating his feelings and expressing an interest in how they might improve the situation. Rather than making the situation better, what George perceived as Scott's insubordination served to enrage George, and the personal attacks against Scott intensified. Feeling frustrated and helpless, Scott then decided to take his problem to the Human Resources Department (HRD). A human resources manager listened to Scott's complaints and suggested that Scott return with documented evidence of what Scott perceived to be George's mistreatment. In an effort to help ease the situation, the HRD manager discussed the issue with George, which only stirred the flames of George's anger and his negative behavior toward Scott.

As a last resort, Scott decided to go to George's boss, Rebecca. Rebecca met with George to get his side of the story. George portrayed Scott as an unproductive employee with no respect for authority. The result was a strong letter of reprimand in Scott's file for insubordination.

Describe French and Raven's five sources of power. What power(s) did the individuals in Scott's Dilemma hold?

SOURCE: "Case discussion: Workplace bully," by J. Pinto, M. Vecchione, & L. Howard, October 2004. Presented at the 12th Annual International Conference of the Association on Employment Practices and Principles, Ft. Lauderdale, FL. Reprinted with permission.

REFERENCES

Allen, R. W., Madison, D. L., Porter, L. W., Renwick, P. A., & Mayes, B. T. (1979). Organizational politics: Tactics and characteristics of its actors. *California Management Review, 22,* 77–83.

Burda, D. (2003, August 25). Command and control: To make powerful list, you need to hold the purse strings or hire the workers. *Modern Healthcare,* p. 36.

Emerson, R. M. (1962). Power-dependence relations. *American Sociological Review, 27,* 31–40.

Falbe, C. M., & Yukl, G. (1992). Consequences for managers of using single influence tactics and combinations of tactics. *Academy of Management Journal, 35,* 638–652.

Farmer, S. M., & Maslyn, J. M. (1999). Why are styles of upward influence neglected? Making the case for a configurational approach to influence. *Journal of Management, 25*(5), 653–682.

French, J., & Raven, B. (1959). The bases of social power. In D. Cartwright (Ed.), *Studies in Social Power,* (pp. 150–167). Ann Arbor, MI: University of Michigan Press.

Kantner, R. M. (1979, July/August). Power failure in management circuits. *Harvard Business Review 57*(4), 65–75.

Kipnis, D., & Schmidt, S. M. (1988). Upward influence styles: Relationship with performance evaluations, salary, and stress. *Administrative Science Quarterly, 33,* 528–542.

Kipnis, D., Schmidt, S. M., & Wilkinson, I. (1980). Intraorganizational influence tactics: Explorations in getting one's way. *Journal of Applied Psychology, 65,* 440–452.

Kotter, J. P. (1977, July/August). Power, dependence, and effective management. *Harvard Business Review 55*(4), 125–136.

Mechanic, D. (1962, December). Sources of power of lower participants in complex organizations. *Administrative Science Quarterly, 7*(3), 349–365.

Pfeffer, J. (1992). *Managing with power: Politics and influence in organizations.* Boston, MA: Harvard Business School Press.

Scheff, T. J. (1961). Control over policy by attendants in a mental hospital. *Journal of Health and Human Behavior, 2,* 93–105.

Siu, R. G. H. (1979). *The craft of power.* New York: John Wiley & Sons.

Thibaut, J., & Kelley, H. H. (1959). *The social psychology of groups.* New York: John Wiley & Sons.

CHAPTER 9

Trait and Behavioral Theories of Leadership

Gloria J. Deckard, Ph.D.*

LEARNING OUTCOMES

After completing this chapter, the student should understand the:

- ☛ Difference between leaders and managers.
- ☛ Importance of early behavioral and trait studies.
- ☛ Role of behavioral and trait theories in the evolution of leadership research.
- ☛ Contributions of the early leadership studies at Ohio State and the University of Michigan.
- ☛ Design and application of Blake and Mouton's Managerial Grid.

OVERVIEW

What is leadership? *Leadership* can be described as a complex process by which a person sets direction and influences others to accomplish a mission, task, or objective and directs the organization in a way that makes it more cohesive and coherent (Winder, 2003). What makes an individual a leader, and what makes a leader effective? The answers to these questions have been the focus of organizational researchers for nearly a century. Numerous leadership theories have developed and evolved, and in the next three chapters we explore the findings and interpretations of various theories presented to us over time. In this chapter, we discuss some of the earlier studies in leadership, referred to as the trait and behavioral theories, that laid the foundation for the leadership theories described in Chapter 10 (contingency theories) and Chapter 11 (contemporary or transformational theories).

Often times when exploring leadership in organizations, the first question asked is, "Are managers leaders?" or "Is there a difference between managers and leaders?" Kotter (1988) believes that managers and leaders perform two distinctive but complementary activities. Winder (2003) and Hellriegel, Slocum, and Woodman (1995) point out that a manager is a person who directs the work of employees and is responsible for results. By contrast, a leader inspires employees with a vision and helps them cope with change. Leaders make people want to achieve an organization's goals and objectives, while managers direct people to accomplish a particular task or objective. In the words of Peter Druker

*We wish to acknowledge and thank Dr. Robert DeYoung, who was the contributing author of an earlier version of this chapter, which appeared in *Organizational Behavior in Health Care* (2005), Jones and Bartlett Publishers.

Table 9–1 Leaders vs. Managers

Leaders	Managers
Inspire employees with a vision	Direct the work of employees and devise systems to monitor employees' progress toward achieving preset goals
Help employees cope with change	Determine how to achieve preset goals and be responsible for achieving them
Make people want to achieve high goals and objectives	Tell employees to accomplish a particular task or objective
Articulate a direction or vision of what the future might look like	Handle activities through planning and budgeting
Develop strategies for producing changes needed to move in a new direction	Achieve their goals by organizing and staffing
Recruit and keep employees who understand and share their visions	Create an organizational structure and sets of jobs for accomplishing the organization's strategies

and Warren Bennis, "Management is doing things right; leadership is doing the right things." As noted, management and leadership are two separate behaviors that occur within an organization, but both are very necessary for an organization to achieve its goals (see Table 9–1). Note that the distinctions in the table are based on behaviors, that is, what an individual does, and are not based on particular characteristics, personality, or traits. Therein, we begin to discover the distinct contributions and applications of the theories presented in this chapter—trait and behavioral.

TRAIT THEORY

The belief that innate traits could be found and be the basis for identifying leaders is illustrated by the following quote from Henry Ford, "The question 'who ought to be boss' is like asking 'who ought to be the tenor in the quartet?' Obviously, the man who can sing tenor." One might conclude that not all of us are born to sing tenor, and not all of us are born to lead. Similar thoughts were expressed by sociologist Jerome Dowd, and at the time, many accepted his belief that individuals possess different degrees of intelligence, energy, and moral force and that the masses of society, in whatever direction they may be influenced, are always led by the superior few (Bass, 1990). Leaders, it was believed, were born with the personality, social, and physical characteristics that set them apart—traits that made them distinct from nonleaders.

The earliest trait studies of leadership reflect the social and psychological context of their times. These studies generally assumed that leaders were born—the Great Man Theory—and these born leaders possessed specific characteristics or traits that set them apart. More than 100 studies summarized by Stogdill (1948) and Mann (1959) sought to distinguish leaders from non-leaders on the basis of personality characteristics and individual traits, including intelligence, initiative, understanding of the task, and preference for a position of control and dominance. They suggest that traits such as intelligence, maturity and breadth, inner motivation, achievement drive, and employee centeredness are more likely to be found in midlevel and top managers than in team leaders or first-line supervisors. Leaders tend to be emotionally mature, have a broad range of interest, and are high achievers. They are able to work effectively with employees in a variety of situations, and they respect others and realize that to accomplish tasks they must be considerate of others' needs and values (Stogdill, 1974).

Study into leadership traits continued and a review by Grier (1967) of 20 different studies demonstrated the wide variance in the leadership traits chosen for investigation. Nearly 80 different traits were identified across 20 studies, and only five were common to four or more of the investigations. Thus, no clear set of traits upon which we can distinguish great leaders emerged. Despite the difficulties in linking traits to successful leaders, evidence does reveal that many successful leaders share some basic traits based on observed characteristics of both successful and unsuccessful leaders (see Exhibit 9–1). Other studies established differences in drive (achievement, ambition, energy, tenacity, and initiative), cognitive ability, honesty and integrity, self-confidence, knowledge of business, and desire to lead (Kirkpatrick & Locke, 1991). However, as noted by Robbins (2005), the power of these traits to predict leadership was modest. No consistent patterns between specific traits and effective leadership emerged.

Exhibit 9–1 Trait Theory

One researcher studied a large number of North American organizations and leaders and came to the conclusion that there were some traits that did appear commonly. If a leader possessed these traits, he or she could lead in different situations.

- Physical vitality and stamina
- Intelligence and action-oriented judgment
- Eagerness to accept responsibility
- Task competence
- Understanding of followers and their needs
- Skill in dealing with people
- Need for achievement
- Capacity to motivate people
- Courage and resolution
- Trustworthiness
- Decisiveness
- Self-confidence
- Assertiveness
- Adaptability/flexibility

SOURCE: *On leadership*, by J. Gardner, 1989. New York: Free Press.

Winder (2003) points out another criticism of trait theory related to its reference to leaders' physical characteristics such as appearance, physique, energy, and health. This is not surprising when one considers that the early leadership studies were conducted in the 1930s. How did the typical leader appear during that period? Leaders in the 1930s would have been male, Caucasian, authoritarian, and educated. Absent these traits, it would have been difficult to find minor differences from one organizational leader to the next. However, as we recognize today, physical characteristics are not requirements for leadership.

The failure of early studies to determine a clear set of leadership traits led a number of researchers to question the value of trait leadership theory and to explore another area of distinction—leader behavior. Rather than asking what traits distinguish leaders, behavioral theories of leadership ask the question "How do leaders act or behave differently than nonleaders?" The underlying assumption or hypothesis shifts from being born with innate leadership abilities to being able to acquire leadership behaviors. Can we identify and teach particular behaviors that promote effective leadership? Many would support the position that leadership can be learned, cultivated through work experience, training, education, opportunity, motivation, and even a little luck (Kotter, 1988).

LEWIN'S BEHAVIORAL STUDY

One of the earliest studies to examine the effect of leadership behavior was performed in the 1930s under the direction of Kurt Lewin, who is recognized as the father of group dynamics (see Chapter 14). Lewin (1951) and his colleagues observed the behavior of children under different leadership styles used by the adult participants. The 10-year-old boys, who were participating in an arts and craft club, were placed into groups matched on personal characteristics, for example, IQ and popularity, and all groups worked on the same project (produced the same item). Each group was exposed to three types of leadership styles:

- *Authoritarian:* The authoritarian leader remained aloof and used orders (without consultation) in directing the group's activities.
- *Democratic:* The democratic leader offered guidance and encouraged the children while actively participating in the groups' activities.
- *Laissez-faire:* The laissez-faire leader gave the children knowledge, but did not direct the activities, nor did this leader become involved or participate in the groups' activities.

The researchers measured and recorded both the amount of work produced and the levels of aggression displayed by the children. The results established that leadership style had a clear impact on group productivity as well as the behaviors and interpersonal relationships among group members. With the democratic leadership style, group morale was high and relationships between the group members and leader were friendly. When the group leader was absent, the children continued with their work. The group's work reflected levels of originality and quality; however, members of the group did not produce as many items as did the group under the autocratic leader. Under autocratic leadership, the group displayed two types of behavior: aggressive and apathetic. The aggressive children were defiant and continually wanted the leader's attention. They blamed one another when anything went wrong within the group. Although the apathetic children placed fewer demands on the leader, they displayed outbursts of aggression when the leader was absent. When groups experienced the laissez-faire leadership style, the children displayed low levels of satisfaction and a low tendency or ability to work independently. In addition, group members displayed little cooperation. Under the laissez-faire style, the group produced the least number of items and the items were of low quality.

Overall, the democratic leadership style appeared the most successful. However, some of the children reported that they preferred the authoritarian style. Thus, this study provided us with not only our initial examination of leadership behavior but also alerted us to the possibility that followers may exhibit a preference for specific leadership styles. In concert with the latter, Gladding (1995) suggested that different types of groups prefer specific styles of leadership. He contended that members' preference would be based on the leadership style they perceived as right or natural judging from their personal socialization process.

During the 1940s, comprehensive research projects were conducted at Ohio State University and the University of Michigan that focused attention on the identification of leader behaviors that are important for attaining organizational goals and measures of performance. These foundational studies greatly impacted future leadership theorists.

OHIO STATE LEADERSHIP STUDIES

The focus of the researchers at Ohio State University in the late 1940s was on the identification of independent dimensions of leadership behavior. The researchers developed an assessment tool, the Leader Behavior Description Questionnaire, which was used to discover how leaders carry out their activities. Leaders from the military, educational, manufacturing, and other sectors were included in the research project. The researchers found that two dimensions of leadership were consistent among the studied groups: consideration for people and initiating structure.

Consideration for people focused on the human side of the business and was also called relationship behavior. This dimension recognized that individuals have needs and require relationships. The initiating structure dimension put an importance on tasks and goals. These findings were important to the study of organizational behavior because it was the first time researchers recognized these concepts and that the two dimensions were independent. In other words, consideration for workers and initiating structure existed simultaneously and to different degrees. A matrix was created that showed the various combinations and quantities of the elements (see Figure 9–1).

Leaders who ranked high on both dimensions were more likely to influence the workforce to higher levels of satisfaction and performance. A weakness

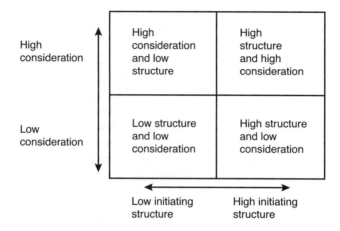

Figure 9–1 Ohio State Studies

noted in the Ohio State studies was that situational factors were absent from the research. Not all workplace situations require an emphasis on consideration for people or initiating structure. For example, healthcare professionals who are highly skilled and intrinsically motivated may not require initiating structure from their manager.

UNIVERSITY OF MICHIGAN STUDIES

During the same period of time as the Ohio State studies were being performed, researchers at the University of Michigan were also conducting research in an attempt to determine the most effective style of leadership based on two dimensions of leadership behavior: an employee-centered focus or a production-centered focus. Employee-centered leaders emphasized interpersonal relations, took a personal interest in the needs of their subordinates, and accepted individual differences among members. Production-centered leaders emphasized the technical aspects of the job, focused on accomplishing the tasks, and saw the members as a means to an end, that is, achievement of the tasks. The researchers found that general supervision (i.e., providing support and direction without being autocratic) created higher levels of productivity than did production-centered supervision and that low-producing supervisors placed an emphasis on production, displaying little concern for their employees. Years of research have confirmed the University of Michigan studies (Luthans, 2002). One particular note of interest from these studies was that productivity was not directly related to employee satisfaction.

Likert (1961) expanded on the Michigan studies with extensive research into what differentiates effective managers from ineffective managers. Likert related that job-centered managers were found to be the least productive, while employee-centered managers were found to be the most effective. In addition, effective managers set specific goals, but gave employees freedom in the way they achieved those goals (i.e., empowerment).

Blake and Mouton's Managerial Grid

The Ohio State studies discovered that two dimensions of leadership were consistently identifiable among managers: consideration for people and initiating structure. Blake and Mouton (1964) reexamined these dimensions by using "a two-factor framework, in which concern for production and concern for people are interdependent but uncorrelated" (Razik & Swanson, 1995, p. 53). The Managerial Grid is based upon the assertion that one best leadership style exists. The Managerial Grid provides the manager with a conceptual assessment as to what his or her current leadership style is and, theoretically, provides an avenue of development in becoming an ideal manager.

Although there is a possibility of being categorized in one of 81 possible positions on the grid, we will examine five positions on the grid to assist our understanding of the Managerial Grid. The Managerial Grid (see Figure 9–2) identifies a vertical axis, on a scale from one to nine, describing a concern for people. A horizontal axis, also on a scale from one to nine, identifies a concern for production. The five notable positions are the: impoverished manager (1,1); task manager (9,1); middle-of-the-road manager (5,5); country club manager (1,9); and ideal manager (9,9).

Let us examine leadership characteristics in each one of the five quadrants to better understand how the grid functions. At the lower left position on the grid (1,1), the impoverished manager exercises minimal effort on getting the

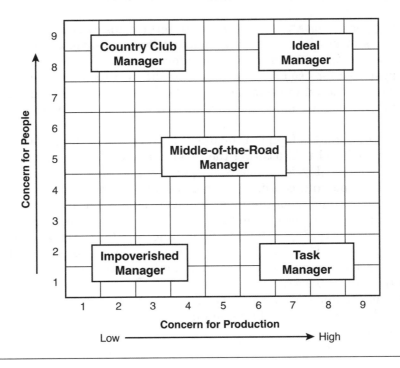

Figure 9–2 Blake and Mouton's Managerial Grid

task accomplished, doing only that amount of work that is required to sustain his or her position within the organization. Additionally, the impoverished manager is much more focused on his or her own well-being than on the subordinates he or she supervises. This manager possesses a low concern for people and a low concern for production.

The task manager is positioned at the lower right on the grid (9,1). This manager exhibits a true autocratic presence, often referred to as a dictator. The managerial focus in this quadrant is efficiency, with an ongoing effort to improve work processes to increase production. There is, at best, negligible concern for people. The task manager is unconcerned by the potential negative impact his or her leadership style might have on staff, such as conflict or stress.

Located directly in the middle of the grid, at the (5,5) position, is the middle-of-the-road manager. This manager appears to balance the concern for task and the concern for people in an effort to boost morale and satisfaction. On the surface this may seem to be a very effective approach to management, but this balancing act is often difficult to accomplish over time. One might consider the middle-of-the-road manager the perfect politician. These managers play both sides of the field, depending upon situational factors. They will tell you exactly what they think you want to hear and then, in contradictory fashion, tell someone else exactly what they want to hear despite their earlier stance. This is not to suggest that the middle-of-the-road manager operates exclusively on political alliances, but it should be clear that under the best of circumstances it is difficult to balance an equal concern for people and an equal concern for production.

At the upper left on the grid (1,9), we find the country club manager. This individual is most concerned with ensuring that employees' needs are met and that the work environment is comfortable and friendly. The lack of focus on concern for production diminishes the overall capacity for employees to meet or exceed organizational goals. This style of management will probably not lead to many successful ventures based upon production expectations.

The final quadrant is found in the upper right corner of the grid (9,9). Blake and Mouton labeled this position the ideal manager. As this label suggests, the ideal manager develops a sense of purpose and accomplishment in both concern for people and concern for task. This is not a balancing act as was described in the middle-of-the-road manager, but is a theoretically perfect infusion of concern for people and concern for task. One might ask, "what is the likelihood of scoring a 9,9 on Blake and Mouton's Managerial Grid?" Although possible, it is very unlikely. One should presume that there is always room for improvement, thereby diminishing the possibility of attainment of the elusive 9,9 score.

Blake and Mouton's Managerial Grid is a useful tool in identifying leadership style, both perceived and real. Managers are often surprised at where he or she scores on the grid.

SUMMARY

Trait and behavioral theories focused attention on the individual. Were differences found? Yes. Were the researchers able to produce a clear set of traits or behaviors upon which to definitely distinguish leaders? No. Examining the findings across numerous studies, we uncover a lack of consistency and modest relationships. One, however, would not want to diminish the importance of the early leadership research or of the contribution these efforts made. And, as we will see in Chapter 11, traits and behaviors have reemerged in contemporary leadership theories and behavioral competencies.

First, however, the theoretical evolution of leadership leads us to the next generation of research: contingency theories. Some suggest the questionable reliability and disputed validity of early leadership research efforts may be attributed to the absence of a single important dimension known as the contingency factor, which we will examine in Chapter 10. Contingency refers to the leader's contextual situation. "Effective leaders analyze the factors pertaining to the situation, task, followers, and the organization, and then choose the appropriate style" (Osland et al., 2001, p. 290).

What worked in the 1930s would not necessarily work in the 1940s. Why? The situation changed dramatically from one decade to the next. What impact does this statement have on today's work environment? Recognizing the phenomenal rate of change faced by today's healthcare organizations, one would conclude that what worked last year would not necessarily work today. Consider if you will, the economic, social, technological, and political environments in context with a newly emerging diverse workforce, and you have compelling reasons to incorporate the application of contingency leadership theory in attaining organizational goals.

END-OF-CHAPTER DISCUSSION QUESTIONS

1. Is leadership synonymous with management, or is leading just one of the many things that a manager does? In what ways are they the same or different?
2. Explain the findings of Lewin's behavioral studies regarding leadership styles and behaviors.
3. Discuss the contributions and the weaknesses of trait theory.
4. Discuss the results of the Ohio State studies in regard to their significant impact on leadership research.
5. Explain the difference between the University of Michigan studies and the Ohio State studies.
6. Explain Blake and Mouton's Managerial Grid in relationship to previous leadership research.

END OF CHAPTER CASE STUDY

Case Study 9–1 Leadership Style

A small group of nurses, employed at a large community hospital, were unhappy about their work environment and would meet daily during lunch to discuss the situation. There had been a recent change in the hospital's senior management, which caused a high level of uncertainty and anxiety among the nursing staff. The nurses felt overworked as a result of the industry's current nursing shortage. Their wages and benefits had been stagnant with no salary market adjustments for the past two years. The nurses saw the situation as management requiring them to do more work with fewer resources, with no appreciation or recognition of their efforts. Whenever the nurses approached management with their concerns, they perceived them as falling on deaf ears since no changes were made.

Feeling like they had no other choice, the nurses contacted a labor union. The labor union began an organizing effort in the hospital shortly thereafter, holding an aggressive campaign over a six-week period. There was tremendous peer pressure, as some of the well-respected nursing staff became active leaders for unionization, although they were not part of the initial group of nurses who had first contacted the union. The election was held and the union was voted in by two-thirds of the nursing staff. In the weeks that followed, the original group of nurses remarked that they were surprised by the union's victory; they had only wanted to scare management into making changes to their work environment.

Using Blake and Mouton's Managerial Grid, explain the leadership style displayed by management to the nursing staff.

EXERCISE 9–1

Think of some individuals whom you feel are really exceptional leaders. What, if anything, do they have in common?

Think of some individuals whom you believe are truly poor leaders? What, if anything, do they have in common?

Do your answers identify traits or behaviors? Which, traits or behaviors, do you personally view as dominant in effective leadership?

EXERCISE 9–2

Have you ever known people who were successful leaders in one situation and failures in another? Why is this so?

Exercise 9–3 Leadership Questionnaire

INSTRUCTIONS

Objective: To determine the degree that a person likes working with tasks and other people.
Time: 45 Minutes

Instructions

1. Complete the 18 items in the questionnaire section.
2. Transfer your answers to the two respective columns provided in the scoring section. Total the score in each column and multiply each total by 0.2. For example, in the first column (people), if you answer 5, 3, 4, 4, 3, 2, 5, 4, 3, then your final score is 5 33 3 0.2 5 6.6.
3. The total score for the first column (people) is plotted on the vertical axis in the matrix section, while the total score for the second column (task) is plotted on the horizontal axis. Intersect the lines to see which leadership dimension you normally operate out of:

   - Task Manager (Authoritarian)
   - Impoverished
   - Ideal Manager (Team Leader)
   - Country Club

Questionnaire

Below is a list of statements about leadership behavior. Read each one carefully. Then, using the following scale, decide the extent to which it actually applies to you. For best results, answer as truthfully as possible.

	Never		Sometimes		Always
	0	1	2	3	4	5

1. _____ I encourage my team to participate when it comes to decision-making time and I try to implement their ideas and suggestions.
2. _____ Nothing is more important than accomplishing a goal or task.
3. _____ I closely monitor the schedule to ensure a task or project will be completed in time.
4. _____ I enjoy coaching people on new tasks and procedures.
5. _____ The more challenging a task is, the more I enjoy it.
6. _____ I encourage my employees to be creative about their jobs.
7. _____ When seeing a complex task through to completion, I ensure that every detail is accounted for.
8. _____ I find it easy to carry out several complicated tasks at the same time.
9. _____ I enjoy reading articles, books, and journals about training, leadership, and psychology, and then putting what I have read into action.
10. _____ When correcting mistakes, I do not worry about jeopardizing relationships.
11. _____ I manage my time very efficiently.
12. _____ I enjoy explaining the intricacies and details of a complex task or project to my employees.
13. _____ Breaking large projects into small manageable tasks is second nature to me.
14. _____ Nothing is more important than building a great team.
15. _____ I enjoy analyzing problems.
16. _____ I honor other people's boundaries.
17. _____ Counseling my employees to improve their performance or behavior is second nature to me.
18. _____ I enjoy reading articles, books, and trade journals about my profession, and then implementing the new procedures I have learned.

(Continued)

Scoring Section

After completing the questionnaire, transfer your answers to the spaces below:

People Question	Task Question
1. _____	2. _____
4. _____	3. _____
6. _____	5. _____
9. _____	7. _____
10. _____	8. _____
12. _____	11. _____
14. _____	13. _____
16. _____	15. _____
17. _____	18. _____
TOTAL _____	TOTAL _____
× 0.2 = _____	× 0.2 = _____

(Multiply the Total by 0.2 to get your final score)   (Multiply the Total by 0.2 to get your final score)

Matrix Section

Plot your final scores on the graph below by drawing a horizontal line from the approximate people score (vertical axis) to the right of the matrix, and drawing a vertical line from the approximate task score on the horizontal axis to the top of the matrix. Then, draw two lines from each dot until they intersect. The area of intersection is the leadership dimension that you operate out of.

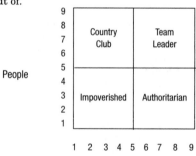

The Results

This chart will give you an idea of your leadership style. But, like any other instrument that attempts to profile a person, you have to take in other factors, such as how do your manager and employees rate you as a leader, do you get your job done, do you take care of your employees, are you GROWING your organization, etc.

You should review the statements in the survey and reflect on the low scores by asking yourself, "If I scored higher in that area, would I be a more effective leader?" And if the answer is yes, then it should become a personal action item.

SOURCE: Available at http://www.nwlink.com/~donclark/leader/leader.html. Created January 27, 1998; last update February 24, 2002. Copyright 1998 by Donald Clark. Reprinted with permission.

REFERENCES

Bass, B. M. (1990). *Bass & Stodgill's handbook of leadership* (3rd ed.), New York: The Free Press.

Blake, R. R., & Mouton, J. S. (1964). *The managerial grid*. Houston, TX: Gulf Publishing Co.

Gladding, S. T. (1995). *Groupwork: A counseling specialty*. Englewood Cliffs, NJ: Prentice-Hall Inc.

Geier, J. G. (1967). A trait approach to the study of leadership in small groups. *Journal of Communications*, Dec(4), 316–323.

Hellriegel, D., Slocum, J. W., & Woodman, R. W. (1995). *Organizational behavior*. New York: West Publishing Company.

Kotter, J. (1988). *The leadership factor*. New York: Free Press.

Kirkpatrick, A., & Locke, E. (1991). Leadership: Do traits matter? *Academy of Management Executive, 5*(2), 48–60.

Lewin, K. (1951). *Field theory in the social sciences*. New York: Harper and Row.

Likert, R. (1961). *New patterns of management*. New York: Garland Science Publishing.

Luthans, F. (2002). *Organizational behavior* (9th ed.). Boston, MA: McGraw-Hill.

Mann, R. D. (1959). A review of the relationship between personality and performance in small groups. *Psychological Bulletin, 66*(4), 241–270.

Osland, J., Kolb, D., & Rubin, I. (2001). *Organizational behavior: An experiential approach* (7th ed.) (p. 290). Upper Saddle River, NJ: Prentice Hall.

Razik, T. A., & Swanson, A. D. (1995). *Fundamental concepts of educational leadership and management* (1st ed.) (pp. 51–52). Upper Saddle River, NJ: Prentice Hall.

Robbins, S. P. (2005). *Organizational behavior* (8th ed.) Upper Saddle River, NJ: Prentice Hall.

Stogdill, R. M. (1948). Personal factors associated with leadership. A survey of the literature. *Journal of Psychology, 25,* 35–71.

Stogdill, R. M. (1974). *Handbook on leadership*. New York: Free Press.

Winder, R. (2003). Organizational dynamics and development. *Futurics, 27,* 1 & 2, 5.

CHAPTER 10

Contingency Theories of Leadership

*Gloria J. Deckard, Ph.D.**

LEARNING OUTCOMES

After completing this chapter, the student should be able to:

- ☛ Appreciate the contributions of contingency theories in understanding leadership.
- ☛ Distinguish between the various contingency theories.
- ☛ Apply the various contingency theories of leadership to today's work environments.

OVERVIEW

Leadership is truly a complex concept and related to a multitude of factors that extend beyond the individual to include situation factors. The simplicity of examining leadership on the basis of individual traits and behaviors becomes more complex as we add the interrelationships of leadership style, personal and professional values, one's ability to control by means of influence, subordinate relationships, subordinate development, and the variability of other situational factors. In contingency theories, the critical component becomes the characteristics of the situation rather than the individual. Analyzing contingent factors and properly matching leadership style can allow an individual, in the right context, to effectively move an organization toward its strategic goals by influencing other organizational members to participate in the collaborative effort to achieve corporate success and economic sustainability.

Understanding the development and application of leadership theory prepares the healthcare manager to fulfill three explicit administrative responsibilities: predict, explain, and control. Successful leaders must have the capability to predict how, when, where, and why things happen. Prediction permits the leader to enhance opportunities and diminish threats that are constantly arising in the workplace. The ability to explain these occurrences instills a sense of confidence on the part of peers and subordinates, further augmenting the legitimacy of one's ability to lead in a variety of situations. Finally, a leader recognizes and accepts the role of control, whereby individuals are influenced to participate in the achievement of strategic goals and organizational sustainability.

Contingency, by definition, means an event that may occur but that is not likely or intended; a possibility that must be prepared for; the condition of being dependent on chance or uncertainty. As such, contingency is about

---

*We acknowledge and thank Dr. Robert DeYoung, who was the contributing author of an earlier version of this chapter, which appeared in *Organizational Behavior in Health Care* (2005), Jones and Bartlett Publishers.

possessing the knowledge, skills, and abilities to respond to a changing situation. Analyzing and responding to the contingencies that influence leader effectiveness may provide one with the ability to succeed in an ever-changing healthcare environment. Healthcare leadership is about stepping up in times of uncertainty and moving forward to minimize potential threats and exploit opportunities.

In this chapter, we will discuss the various contingency leadership theories and their implications for the leader, the employee, and the healthcare organization. To maximize your understanding of these theories, consider how they apply to you and your work environment. Developing knowledge and a working application of contingency theories will enhance your ability to successfully accomplish your managerial responsibilities to predict, explain, and control.

FIEDLER'S CONTINGENCY THEORY

In studies of the relationship between leadership style and situation variables, Fiedler and his associates (1965; 1967; 1974) posit that individuals possess dominant leadership characteristics that are well established and generally inflexible. Leaders are characterized into one of two styles, either task-oriented (active, controlling, and structuring) or human relations–oriented (passive, permissive, and considerate). Fiedler believed that an individual's leadership style was grounded and somewhat inflexible; thus, leaders would improve their overall effectiveness by being placed in situations that best suited their orientation. Situations which display more variability and provide "contingencies" are analyzed across three dimensions:

- *Leader–Member Relations:* The degree of certainty, trust, and deference between the subordinate and the leader (Rating: good or poor).
- *Task Structure:* The extent to which job assignments are clear through the implementation of formalization and policy (Rating: high or low).
- *Leader Position Power:* The degree of control and influence the leader legitimately possesses in dealing with organizational activities (see Chapter 8); highly dependent upon the support the leader receives from senior management (Rating: strong or weak).

A leader's contribution to the successful performance by his or her group is determined by the leader's style (i.e., task or relations) in conjunction with situational variables (i.e., relationships, task structure, and power position). Effective leaders seek or are placed in situations that best match their leadership style.

Fiedler's research and the identification of leadership style were based upon a questionnaire known as the Least Preferred Coworker (LPC) Scale. Fiedler (1970) developed the LPC by asking the participants to describe their most and least preferred coworkers. Each participant was asked to think of all others with whom he or she had ever worked and then to describe the person with whom he or she worked best (i.e., most preferred coworker) and then the person with whom he or she worked least well (i.e., least preferred coworker or LPC). From the items identified, Fiedler created a scale that contains contrasting adjectives (such as pleasant/unpleasant, supportive/hostile, considerate/inconsiderate, and agreeable/disagreeable) to measure whether a person was task- or relations-oriented. Fiedler believed that the ratings individuals ascribed to their least preferred coworker, a person they least enjoyed working with, reflected more about themselves than the person they chose to describe. Thus, individuals who scored the LPC in relatively positive terms were labeled relations-oriented, while individuals who scored the LPC in relatively unfavorable terms were labeled task-oriented.

In assessing the three situational dimensions (leader–member relations, task structure, and position power), four levels of situational favorableness can be determined. Figure 10–1 identifies these four levels in a continuum of situational favorableness from Very Unfavorable to Unfavorable and Favorable to Very Favorable. Fiedler's research suggests that aligning the leadership style with the favorableness of the situation determines the effectiveness of the leader regarding a group's performance. If the leader is generally accepted and trusted by subordinates (good leader–member relations), if the tasks for which individuals are responsible are clear and fully understood through formalization and direction (high task structure), and the leader's power is recognized by senior management (strong position of power), then the situation is very favorable. On the opposite side of the coin, if the leader lacks acceptance or trust by subordinates (poor leader–member relations), if the tasks for which individuals are responsible are unclear and not fully understood because of a lack of formalization and an absence of direction (low task structure), and the leader's power is not recognized by senior management (weak position power), then the situation is very unfavorable. In either scenario, the leader with a task-oriented leadership style would be the most effective. When the situation variables are determined to be mixed (i.e., moderately unfavorable or moderately favorable), the human relations–oriented leadership approach would be most effective.

In a very unfavorable situation (i.e., leader–member relations are poor, there is low task structure, and leader has little position power), one can understand the importance of a task-oriented leadership approach. But why would a task-oriented leadership approach be best suited for a very favorable situation? In a very favorable situation the leader–member relationship is good, the task structure is high, and the position power is strong. This combination provides an environment in which individuals are prepared to be guided and expect to be told what to do. For example, Fiedler suggests one consider the captain of an airliner in its final landing; we would hardly want him to turn to his crew for a discussion on how to land the plane!

Fiedler's Contingency Theory made a tremendous contribution toward contingency theories for three reasons. It was the first theory to systematically account for situational factors (i.e., relationships, task structure, and position power). Second, the theory considers the leader's dominant orientation (i.e., a function of a leader's needs and personality), not the leader's behavior (Tosi & Mero, 2003). As Tosi and Mero (2003) point out, although this orientation may affect the leader's behavior, it is the leader's orientation toward his or her group that determines how effective the group will be. Third, because the leader's orientation is relatively stable, it is not likely that a leader will

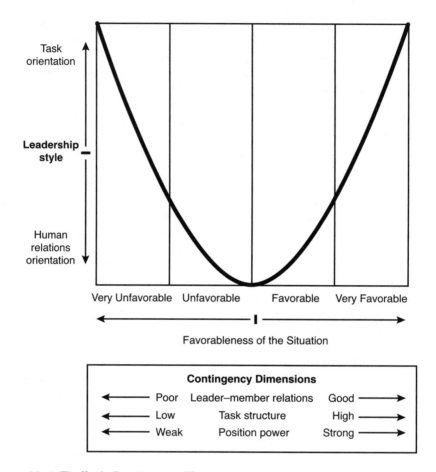

Figure 10–1 Fiedler's Contingency Theory

change orientations when confronted with different situations, though the leader can change his or her behavior when necessary and when the leader wants to (Tosi & Mero, 2003). Fiedler believed that it would be easier to change the situation (i.e., work environment) to fit the leader's style. As such, an organization should not choose a leader who fits a situation, but should change the situation to agree with the style of its leader, since the leader's personality is not likely to change (Fiedler, 1970). (See Case Study 10–1: "The New Chief Safety and Compliance Officer Position.")

Over the past 20 years, Fiedler (1995; Fiedler, Potter, Zais, & Knowlton, 1979; Fielder & Garcia, 1987) has introduced other variables into the original Contingency Theory. Fiedler (1996) suggests that when leaders are under stress, their intelligence and experience tend to interfere with each other, diminishing the leader's ability to think rationally, logically, and analytically. Fiedler and Garcia (1987) refer to this reconceptualization as cognitive resource theory. Cognitive resource theory states that: (1) a leader's intellectual abilities correlate positively with performance under low stress but negatively under high stress and (2) a leader's experience correlates negatively with performance under low stress but positively under high stress. For example, leaders under stress will fall back on their previously learned knowledge and behavior (e.g., relying on intuition and hunches); therefore, the greater the range of their experience, the better their performance. Under low-stress conditions, more experienced leaders are not challenged and tend to be bored and cut corners (Fiedler, 1996). Although this theory is relatively new, it is developing a solid body of research support (Robbins, 2001).

Case Study 10–1 The New Chief Safety and Compliance Officer Position

Ben Allrod, chief executive officer of a 300-bed community hospital located in Midwest suburbia, received a call from the hospital's Director of Nursing, Paul Muir, to ask whether they could meet immediately to discuss a problem. It was unlike Paul to make such a request, so Ben agreed to meet immediately.

When Paul arrived, Ben could see that he was distressed. His face was pale and he appeared nervous. Ben asked, "What's up?" Paul related, "A few hours ago a patient received the wrong blood type during a transfusion. The nurse realized something was wrong when the woman began reacting adversely to the transfusion. Although this type of a mistake is not automatically fatal, the patient died a few minutes ago. However, we cannot be certain that the wrong blood type was the cause of her death because 60 percent of people who receive the wrong blood type would not exhibit any symptoms of the problem. The patient may have expired because of other reasons; she was very sick with multiple diagnoses." Paul reminded Ben that, in addition to the family, the state's Medical Error Oversight Board would need to be notified of this medical error.

Ben was very shocked to hear this news, considering that two months ago the hospital had to report to the state's Medical Error Oversight Board that a metal clamp was left inside a patient after surgery because the surgeon forgot to order a postsurgical X-ray. Thank goodness the patient was not injured. At that time, the hospital's chief operating officer, Harry Benson, stated that new procedures were implemented so the problem should not happen again.

Ben thanked Paul for the information and instructed him to notify the state's Medical Error Oversight Board and that he would personally meet with the family to express his sympathy for the loss of their loved one and inform the family that "we" will be looking into the matter.

After Paul left, Ben knew he had to do something immediately. Although Harry Benson had been responsible for developing and implementing all the necessary policies and procedures to prevent medical errors, Harry was not doing enough and things were going to have to change—now! He would deal with Harry later, but his first priority was creating a new position—Chief Safety and Compliance Officer. This new position would report directly to him and would have full authority to do whatever was needed to ensure that these problems did not occur again. He immediately drafted the job description.

> The selected candidate will play a key role in the development of the organization's compliance culture with a focus on prevention. This position will be responsible for developing, implementing, and communicating the organization's compliance and safety standards, policies, and procedures. The position will oversee the design, organization, and implementation of systemwide compliance education and training programs. The position is responsible for monitoring and evaluating compliance activities to ensure program goals are being met across all functional areas. The position is responsible for establishing and participating in internal disciplinary actions for compliance violations.
>
> The candidate must have an MHA or related degree, 10 years of experience in the safety and compliance area, including seven years in the healthcare industry and five years in a managerial role. The position offers a competitive compensation package with excellent benefits.

Using Fiedler's Contingency Theory, analyze the situational factors and determine what type of individual would be the most effective for Ben Allrod to hire. Could Ben change situational factors instead of hiring a new leader? If so, what changes would you recommend?

HOUSE'S PATH–GOAL LEADERSHIP THEORY

Path–Goal Leadership Theory (House, 1971) suggests that effective leaders provide the path, the support, and resources to assist subordinates in attaining organizational goals. This theory combines elements of the Ohio State studies (i.e., consideration and initiating structure) with expectancy theories of motivation. (See Chapters 6 and 9.)

Four separate, but fully integrated, components make up House's Path–Goal Leadership Theory: Leadership Behaviors, Environmental Contingency Factors, Subordinate Contingency Factors, and Outcomes (see Figure 10–2). The first component, Leadership Behavior, identifies four specific leadership styles:

1. The *directive* leader provides employees a detailed understanding of expectations, a plan to accomplish those expectations, and the resources to achieve the tasks. The directive leadership style can increase employee motivation and satisfaction where role ambiguity exists.

2. The *supportive* leader shows concern for people, ensuring the work environment does not impede specific tasks that lead toward organizational goals, and creates a supportive atmosphere. The supportive leadership style may increase employee motivation and satisfaction where tasks are routine or stressful.

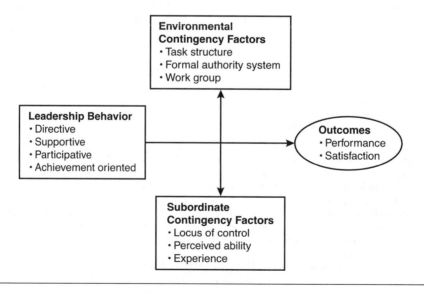

Figure 10–2 House's Path–Goal Theory

3. The *participative* leader seeks input from a multiplicity of internal sources, including the technical core of employees, to assist in the decision-making process. The participative leader maintains responsibility for the final decision, but includes the workforce in the process, ultimately enhancing buy-in from affected parties. The participative leadership style can improve motivation and satisfaction in environments that are uncertain or in the process of change.

4. The *achievement-oriented* leader establishes stimulating goals and expects high levels of performance in achievement of the stated goals. The achievement-oriented style of leadership creates an environment of trust, where the leader acknowledges the workforce's abilities to accomplish organizational goals.

Whereas Fiedler proposed that leadership styles were grounded and inflexible, House proposed that leadership styles are adaptable and that managers may be called upon to utilize any one of the four identified styles of leadership, depending on the situation (Razik & Swanson, 1995; Robbins, 2001).

Leadership style is dependent on two contingency factors: environmental and subordinate. House considered external dynamics, which are referred to as environmental contingency factors. These factors include: (1) clarity of the task to be performed, (2) hierarchical authority systems, and (3) group dynamics (i.e., work-group members' relationships). These factors are generally considered to be outside the control and influence of the worker and the manager. The second set of contingency factors, considered internal dynamics, are referred to as subordinate contingency factors. These factors include the employee's locus of control; knowledge, skills, and abilities (real or perceived); and experience. Subordinate contingency factors are characteristics exhibited by the employees (Robbins, 2001).

The integration of leadership style, environmental contingency factors, and subordinate contingency factors leads to outcomes (performance and satisfaction). According to House and Mitchell (1974), a leader's role is to influence subordinates' perceptions and motivate them toward achieving the desired outcomes (i.e., performance and satisfaction). To be effective, managers should:

1. Increase personal payoffs to subordinates for work goal attainment;
2. Provide coaching and direction, when needed;
3. Clarify expectations of workers;
4. Reduce frustrating barriers;
5. Increase opportunities for personal satisfaction contingent on effective performance.

The appropriate leadership style that a manager should use is the one that compensates for any item absent from the employee (i.e., experience, ability) or the work setting (i.e., task structure). The leadership style should not duplicate what the employee already has available to him or her. For example, the nurse manager should not provide direction (i.e., directive leadership style) as to how to complete a patient's history and physical to a nurse with 20 years of experience. However, the nurse manager should provide direction and/or training to a nurse with 20 years of clinical experience but no experience with technology or electronic medical records as to how to complete a patient's history and physical if they are being done for the first time electronically.

TANNENBAUM AND SCHMIDT'S CONTINUUM OF LEADERSHIP BEHAVIOR

Tannenbaum and Schmidt (1958, 1973) conducted one of the first studies that indicated a need for leaders to evaluate the situational factors prior to the implementation of a particular leadership style (Ott, 1996). The Continuum of Leadership Behavior model is based on the variety of behaviors noted in earlier leadership studies, particularly the distinction of task versus employee or human relations orientations. This model identifies two styles of leadership that occur across a continuum, from boss-centered (task) through subordinate-centered (relationship).

As illustrated in Figure 10–3, the Tannenbaum and Schmidt (1958) model covers a range of leadership behaviors. The model identifies the amount of authority (boss-centered) used by the manager and the amount of freedom afforded to employees (subordinate-centered). At one end of the continuum (boss-centered), the manager takes complete control of the situation, makes a decision, and announces it to the employees. There is no effort to solicit feedback, ideas, or input. At the other end of the continuum (subordinate-centered),

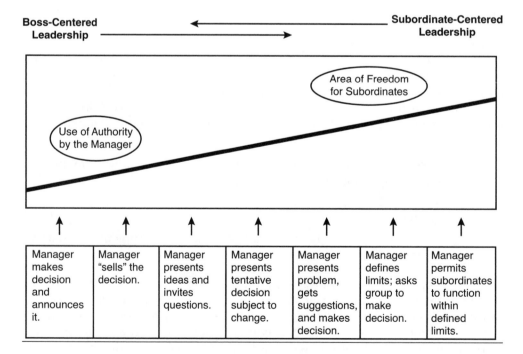

Figure 10–3 Tannenbaum and Schmidt Continuum of Leadership Behavior

the managers and the employees collaboratively make decisions within clearly defined organizational constraints. Within the two extremes of the continuum lie a multitude of managerial options to either include or exclude employee involvement in decision-making processes. The appropriateness of the behavior is dependent upon situational (contingent) factors.

How do managers determine where on the continuum they should position themselves? Determinants may include (1) the manager's style of leadership, (2) the culture of the organization, (3) the complexity of the task at hand, or (4) the relationship between the manager and the employee, specifically the level of confidence the manager has in the employee and the level of comfort in delegating a task or seeking participation in the decision process. Another situational factor important to the process is the level of acceptance by the employee to participate and acknowledge responsibility for delegated tasks. When an employee conveys a desire to participate, the subordinate-centered leadership is appropriate. Conversely, when a manager is faced with an employee who avoids involvement beyond what is minimally expected, the boss-centered leadership style would be the suitable approach.

One approach is not preferred over the other. The situational factors will determine appropriateness. Today's healthcare managers are faced with an onslaught of ongoing critical decisions for which they are accountable and responsible. With this in mind, it is imperative that managers function effectively at each placement on the leadership continuum. Attempts to maintain a subordinate-centered position on the continuum will not meet the needs of the organization when a manager is faced with making a decision that requires information that employees may not possess or when the situation is so critical that it prevents time to collaborate with employees.

Given appropriate time to seek involvement in a decision, the subordinate-centered approach is preferred for obvious reasons. Employees who are permitted to participate in the decision-making process most often are less threatened by the impending change by feeling more a part of the solution rather than as an observer who has no control over what may or may not happen. Unnecessary exclusion from a participatory effort can create an environment of distrust, fear, hopelessness, and anger. A manager's decision as to where on Tannenbaum and Schmidt's continuum he or she should be positioned is unquestionably critical to both the task and how he or she is perceived by those affected by the positioning.

HERSEY AND BLANCHARD'S SITUATIONAL LEADERSHIP ROLE

The work of Hersey and Blanchard (1988) suggests leaders should adapt their leadership style based on three dimensions: (1) task behavior, (2) relationship behavior, and (3) the level of maturity of the subordinate. *Task behavior* refers to a leader who clearly defines work roles and responsibilities while ensuring task clarity. The *relationship behavior* refers to the development of personal relationships, as well as emotional and psychological contracts between the leader and the subordinates. These two dimensions, task behavior and relationship behavior, are shaped by the final dimension, the level of maturity of the subordinate. The *level of maturity* or development of the subordinate is characterized by three specific criteria:

1. The level of motivation exhibited by the subordinate.
2. The willingness of the subordinate to assume responsibility.
3. The experience and educational level of the subordinate.

According to Hersey and Blanchard's Situational Leadership Model (see Figure 10–4), as the employee cultivates knowledge, skills, and abilities to perform at increasing levels of expectations, the manager modifies his or her leadership style. As the subordinate passes through different stages of com-

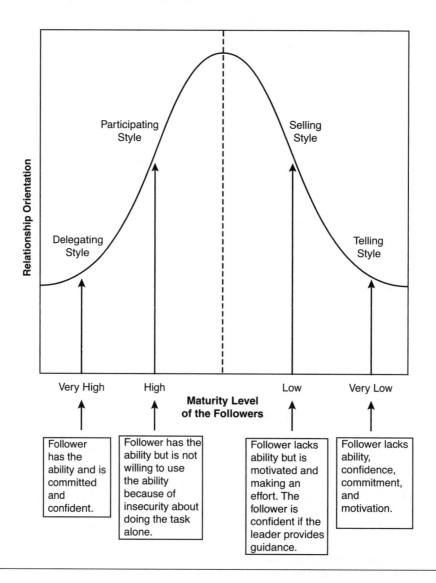

Figure 10–4 Hersey and Blanchard's Situational Leadership Model

mitment and competence, the leader varies the amount of direction and support given. The leader plays various roles of directing, coaching, supporting, and delegating as the subordinate "matures" and becomes able to perform more activities. The varying amounts of direction and support given are conceptualized into four leadership styles: Telling, Selling, Participating, and Delegating.

The Situational Leadership Model identified that when the level of maturity of the follower (i.e., subordinate) is very low, a high-task, low-relationship style of leadership is most effective. As an example, this situation occurs when an employee is new to an organization, attempting to learn task expectations while assimilating into a new culture. The employee, new to the environment, seeks direction by being told what to do; hence, the effective leader uses a telling style of leadership.

As the new employee better develops knowledge, skills, and abilities, thereby increasing his or her level of performance, the leader can incorporate a selling style of leadership. This method of leadership (high-task, high-relationship) is effective when the employee becomes increasingly confident and is willing to accept additional responsibilities. The leader no longer merely directs the employee as to what must be done, but makes the effort to tell the employee what to do and how his or her role is important to achieving departmental objectives and organizational goals. It is important that the leader recognize the importance of both the task behavior and the relationship behavior at this stage of maturity development.

As the maturity of the employee continues to increase to higher levels, the leader is required to place less of an emphasis on the task, but continues to advance the relationship (low-task, high-relationship). At this level of maturity the employee has demonstrated the ability to perform to organizational expectations with minimal managerial influence, allowing the leader to function most effectively using a participative style of leadership. In this stage of the model, the leader seeks input from the subordinate in areas concerning processes, tasks, and productivity concerns. The leader still makes the decision and ensures compliance, but the employee participates in the decision-making process through an exchange of information between the leader and employee.

Upon full maturity, the employee has fully developed by exhibiting an unquestionable ability to perform expected tasks. This subordinate's maturity level is very high (low-task, low-relationship), creating an environment conducive to a delegating style of leadership. At this point in the model, the leader modifies his or her own behavior to a level where the leader is comfortable to not only delegate, but to allow the employee to identify innovative ways to accomplish the task.

Empirical research, as in other leadership studies, is critical of the Situational Leadership Model. Critics question the coherence of the results of the model, where a questionnaire identifies 12 situations that are supposed to represent levels of subordinate maturity and that managers have only one of four styles of leadership. Hersey and Blanchard admit the model may be oversimplified, yet, one can clearly apply the model in a practical workplace environment (Luthans, 2002).

LEADER–MEMBER EXCHANGE THEORY

Whereas the contingency theories discussed thus far relate leadership style with general situational and subordinate factors across a group of employees, Leader–Member Exchange (LMX) directs us to the differentiated relationships that arise between individual subordinates and their supervisors.

The foundation for LMX comes from the work of Graen and Cashman (1975), who coined the phrase Vertical Linkage Dyad (VDL) to describe how leaders develop dyadic (two-person) relationships with subordinates that affects the behavior of the leader and the subordinate. Over time, the leader identifies with subordinates as belonging to an in-group or an out-group. The leader cognitively assigns an individual membership to either the in-group or the out-group. Individuals assigned to the in-group are perceived by the leader as being more committed to organizational goals and more likely to fulfill responsibilities with higher levels of performance. The in-group is "rewarded with more of the leaders' positional resources (i.e., information, confidence, and concern) than individuals assigned to the out-group" (Luthans, 2002, p. 583).

Not surprisingly, in-group members report fewer problematic issues with leader–member interactions and higher levels of responsiveness with the leader than do members of the out-group. Additionally, it is noted that the in-group is more often led with less emphasis on formal authority to control and influence, while the out-group is more often supervised with a much stronger emphasis on formal authority to control and influence. The mere nature of the high quality of the leader–member relationship that occurs with the in-group generates individuals who accept greater responsibility and exhibit higher levels of contribution to organizational goals (Graen & Ginsburgh, 1977; Liden & Graen, 1980).

A more recent application of VDL is known as the Leader–Member Exchange (LMX) Theory. Taking VDL one step further, LMX examines the characteristics of individuals belonging to the in-group, noting similarities that exist between in-group members and the leader in the dyadic relationship. Individuals with high self-efficacy will tend to form in-group relationships with the leader. In this dyadic relationship, the leader perceives the followers to be more friendly, approachable, and similar in personality to the leader him or herself. The perception of similarity becomes a very important factor for the inclusion in the in-group and the resultant development of relationships and contributions to task accomplishment.

According to Robbins (2005, p. 163), "studies confirm many of the LMX predictions that leaders do differentiate among followers and those with in-group status have higher performance ratings, lower turnover intentions, and higher satisfaction with superiors than those in the out-group."

SUMMARY

Contingency theories provide us with the understanding that one leadership style is not effective across all the variable situations that exist in organizations. The leader who is able to respond to ever-increasing levels of environmental uncertainty through the utilization of more than one style of leadership will be most likely to increase employees' levels of motivation, satisfaction, and productivity. One should not underestimate the importance of the interrelationship of applying the appropriate leadership style of leadership based upon the accurate analysis of situational factors.

END-OF-CHAPTER DISCUSSION QUESTIONS

1. Describe Fielder's Contingency Model. What is the impact of his assumption that leadership style is "fixed"?
2. Summarize the path–goal model of leadership. What theories of motivation (Chapters 5 and 6) can you tie to the assumptions of the model?
3. Identify healthcare situations in which the Tannenbaum and Schmidt's Continuum of Leadership would suggest the autocratic leadership style as the most appropriate.
4. Discuss the role of leadership style in response to follower maturity (development) as presented in the work of Hersey and Blanchard.
5. What impact does the assignment of followers to the "in" or "out" group (LMX) have on worker performance and satisfaction?
6. Apply the contingency theories discussed in this chapter as they relate to your work environment to assess the appropriate style of leadership and the implications for motivation, satisfaction, and productivity.

EXERCISE 10–1

Write a brief description of a personal experience as either the leader or follower when:

- A "telling" style of leadership was used.
- A "selling" style of leadership was used.
- A "participating" style of leadership was used.
- A "delegating" style of leadership was used.

Examine the effectiveness of the style by answering some questions about it, such as: Did it work? Could a different style have worked better? Which style do you prefer your supervisor to use with you? Which style are you most comfortable using yourself? Why?

Form a group of 3 to 4 individuals, and share and discuss your questions with your group.

Case Study 10–2 A New Employee Scheduling System

You are the Director of Human Resources of Baptist Health System, an integrated network of nonprofit hospitals, physician clinics, and home medical services with over 4,000 employees. You wish to implement a new software application to upgrade and automate employee-related scheduling. You estimate that replacing the organization's antiquated system and automating this labor-intensive, time-consuming task can save the health system thousands of dollars each year. Frank is a person in the organization's Office of Technology (OT) who has the skill set you need. However, Frank does not report to you and you know that OT is understaffed and overworked. You have permission from Frank's boss, Jane, to use some of his time only if it doesn't interfere with his regular duties.

Scenario One:

Upon obtaining Jane's permission, you send Frank an e-mail stating "I need you to assist staff in my department with the implementation of a new software application to upgrade and automate the organization's employee-related scheduling. This needs to be completed within two weeks. My assistant will contact you tomorrow to discuss the specific details of this project so you can start immediately."

Scenario Two:

You schedule a meeting with Frank for the next day to discuss your situation. "Frank, I want to talk to you about this project I am working on because I understand that you have experience with database conversions and Jane told me that you were the best person to talk to about this subject. This project is very important to the organization because, like most healthcare organizations, we are facing ongoing challenges of labor cost control and maintaining the appropriate staff levels necessary to maintain high levels of patient care. Baptist has been using an antiquated application to manage staffing and scheduling for several years; the software is outdated and no longer fulfills the needs of the organization. We need a new employee scheduling system that is flexible and scalable enough to accommodate continued organizational growth.

"Frank, let me tell you what I'm trying to accomplish in the next 30 days. The system has to integrate with our existing time and attendance system so information can be shared between our facilities. We also want to get a handle on our data in real time, not 14 days after the pay period. Additionally, the Joint Commission on Accreditation of Healthcare Organizations requires high levels of tracking and reporting, so the organization has to find a way to deal with these reporting expectations. Frank, how can you help us reach our goal?"

Using Hersey and Blanchard's Situational Leadership Model, discuss how Frank will react under each of the preceding scenarios. Why?

REFERENCES

Fiedler, F. E. (1965). Engineer the job to fit the manager. *Harvard Business Review, 43,* 115–122.

Fiedler, F. E. (1967). *A theory of leadership effectiveness.* New York: McGraw-Hill Book Company.

Fiedler, F. E. (1970). The contingency model: A theory of leadership effectiveness. In C. W. Backman, & P. F. Secord (Eds.), *Problems in social psychology* (pp. 279–289). New York: McGraw-Hill Book Company.

Fiedler, F. E. (1995). Cognitive resources and leadership performance. *Applied Psychology—An International Review, 44,* 5–28.

Fiedler, F. E. (1996). Research on leadership selection and training: One view of the future. *Administrative Science Quarterly, 41*(2), 241–250.

Fiedler, F. E., & Chemers, M. M. (1974). *Leadership and effective management.* Flenview, IL: Scott, Foresman.

Fiedler, F. E., & Garcia, J. E. (1987). *New approaches to effective leadership: Cognitive resources and organizational performance.* New York: John Wiley & Sons.

Fiedler, F. E., Potter, E. H., Zais, M. M., & Knowlton, W. (1979). Organizational stress and the use and misuse of managerial intelligence and experience. *Journal of Applied Psychology, 64,* 635–674.

Graen, G., & Ginsburgh, S. (1977). Job resignation as a function of role orientation and leader acceptance: A longitudinal investigation of organizational assimilation. *Organizational Behavior and Human Performance, 19,* 1–17.

Hersey, P., & Blanchard, K. H. (1988). *Management of organizational behavior.* Upper Saddle River, NJ: Prentice Hall.

House, R. J. (1971). A path-goal theory of leader effectiveness. *Administrative Sciences Quarterly, 16*(3), 321–338.

House, R. J., & Mitchell, T. R. (1974). Path–goal theory of leadership. *Journal of Contemporary Business, 3*(4), 81–97.

Liden, R. C., & Graen, G. (1980). Generalizability of the vertical dyad linkage model of leadership. *Academy of Management Journal, 23,* 451–466.

Luthans, F. (2002). *Organizational behavior* (9th ed.). Boston, MA: McGraw-Hill Book Company.

Ott, J. S. (1996). *Classic readings in organizational behavior* (2nd ed., p. 168). Albany, NY: Wadsworth Publishing Company.

Razik, T. A., & Swanson, A. D. (1995). *Fundamental concepts of educational leadership and management* (1st ed., pp. 51–52). Upper Saddle River, NJ: Prentice Hall.

Robbins, S. P. (2001). *Organizational behavior* (6th ed.). Upper Saddle River, NJ: Prentice Hall.

Robbins, S. P. (2005). *Organizational behavior* (8th ed.). Upper Saddle River, NJ: Prentice Hall.

Tannenbaum, R., & Schmidt, W. (1958). How to choose a leadership pattern. *Harvard Business Review, 36*(2), 95–101.

Tannenbaum, R., & Schmidt, W. (1973). How to choose a leadership pattern. *Harvard Business Review, 51*(3), 1–10.

Tosi, H. L., & Mero, N. P. (2003). *The fundamentals of organizational behavior: What managers need to know* (p. 254). Malden, MA: Blackwell Publishing.

Exhibit 10–1 Leadership Style Survey

Directions

This questionnaire contains statements about leadership style beliefs. Next to each statement, circle the number that represents how strongly you feel about the statement by using the following scoring system:

- Almost Always True - 5
- Frequently True - 4
- Occasionally True - 3
- Seldom True - 2
- Almost Never True - 1

Be honest about your choices as there are no right or wrong answers—it is only for self-assessment.

Leadership Style Survey

1. I always retain the final decision-making authority within my department or team. 　　5　4　3　2　1
2. I always try to include one or more employees in determining what to do and how to do it. However, I maintain the final decision-making authority. 　　5　4　3　2　1
3. I and my employees always vote whenever a major decision has to be made. 　　5　4　3　2　1
4. I do not consider suggestions made by my employees, as I do not have the time for them. 　　5　4　3　2　1
5. I ask for employee ideas and input on upcoming plans and projects. 　　5　4　3　2　1
6. For a major decision to pass in my department, it must have the approval of each individual or the majority. 　　5　4　3　2　1
7. I tell my employees what has to be done and how to do it. 　　5　4　3　2　1
8. When things go wrong and I need to create a strategy to keep a project or process running on schedule, I call a meeting to get my employees' advice. 　　5　4　3　2　1
9. To get information out, I send it by e-mail, memos, or voice mail; very rarely is a meeting called. My employees are then expected to act upon the information. 　　5　4　3　2　1
10. When someone makes a mistake, I make a note of it and tell them not to ever do it again. 　　5　4　3　2　1
11. I want to create an environment where the employees take ownership of the project. I allow them to participate in the decision-making process. 　　5　4　3　2　1
12. I allow my employees to determine what needs to be done and how to do it. 　　5　4　3　2　1
13. New hires are not allowed to make any decisions unless it is approved by me first. 　　5　4　3　2　1
14. I ask employees for their vision of where they see their jobs going and then use their vision where appropriate. 　　5　4　3　2　1
15. My workers know more about their jobs than me, so I allow them to carry out the decisions to do their job. 　　5　4　3　2　1
16. When something goes wrong, I tell my employees that a procedure is not working correctly and I establish a new one. 　　5　4　3　2　1

Exhibit 10–1 Leadership Style Survey 201

Exhibit 10–1 *(Continued)*

17. I allow my employees to set priorities with my guidance.	5	4	3	2	1
18. I delegate tasks in order to implement a new procedure or process.	5	4	3	2	1
19. I closely monitor my employees to ensure they are performing correctly.	5	4	3	2	1
20. When there are differences in role expectations, I work with them to resolve the differences.	5	4	3	2	1
21. Each individual is responsible for defining his or her job.	5	4	3	2	1
22. I like the power that my leadership position holds over subordinates.	5	4	3	2	1
23. I like to use my leadership power to help subordinates grow.	5	4	3	2	1
24. I like to share my leadership power with my subordinates.	5	4	3	2	1
25. Employees must be directed or threatened with punishment in order to get them to achieve the organizational objectives.	5	4	3	2	1
26. Employees will exercise self-direction if they are committed to the objectives.	5	4	3	2	1
27. Employees have the right to determine their own organizational objectives.	5	4	3	2	1
28. Employees seek mainly security.	5	4	3	2	1
29. Employees know how to use creativity and ingenuity to solve organizational problems.	5	4	3	2	1
30. My employees can lead themselves just as well as I can.	5	4	3	2	1

On the fill-in lines below, mark the score of each item on the questionnaire. For example, if you scored item one with a 3 (Occasionally), then enter a 3 next to Item One. When you have entered all the scores for each question, total each of the three columns.

Item	Score	Item	Score	Item	Score
1	_____	2	_____	3	_____
4	_____	5	_____	6	_____
7	_____	8	_____	9	_____
10	_____	11	_____	12	_____
13	_____	14	_____	15	_____
16	_____	17	_____	18	_____
19	_____	20	_____	21	_____
22	_____	23	_____	24	_____
25	_____	26	_____	27	_____
28	_____	29	_____	30	_____
TOTAL	_____	TOTAL	_____	TOTAL	_____
Authoritarian Style (autocratic)		Participative Style (democratic)		Delegative Style (free reign)	

This questionnaire is to help you assess what leadership style you normally use. The lowest score possible for a leadership style is 10 (Almost never) while the highest score possible for a stage is 50 (Almost always).

The highest of the three scores indicates what style of leadership you normally use. If your highest score is 40 or more, it is a strong indicator of your normal style. The lowest of the three scores is an indicator of the style you use least. If your lowest score is 20 or less, it is a strong indicator that you normally do not use this leadership style.

Exhibit 10–1 *(Continued)*

If two of the scores are close to the same, you might be going through a transition phase, either personally or at work, except:

If you score high in both the participative and the delegative, then you are probably a delegative leader.

If there is only a small difference between the three scores, then this indicates that you have no clear perception of the leadership style you use, or you are a new leader and are trying to feel out the correct style for you.

SOURCE: Available at: http://www.nwlink.com/~donclark/leader/survstyl.html. Created July 15, 1998; last update February 24, 2002. Copyright by Donald Clark. Reprinted with permission.

CHAPTER 11

Contemporary Leadership Theories

*Gloria J. Deckard, Ph.D.**

LEARNING OUTCOMES

After completing this chapter, the student should be able to:

☛ Define transformational leadership.

☛ Identify the similarities and differences between transformational and transactional leadership approaches.

☛ Discuss the appropriate application of transformational leadership style in the contemporary work environment.

☛ Examine transformational leadership in the health management setting.

☛ Define charismatic, visionary, and servant leadership.

☛ Identify characteristics common to charismatic, visionary, and servant leaders.

☛ Describe the effect of charismatic, visionary, and servant leadership on organizational outcomes and the attainment of strategic organizational goals.

☛ Discuss the development of behavioral competencies for healthcare leaders.

OVERVIEW

In this chapter, we will examine contemporary leadership theories, including transformational, charismatic, visionary, and servant. These theories build upon both the individual trait and behavior theories presented in Chapter 9 and the contingencies theories presented in Chapter 10. When one first attempts to examine leadership, the focus is typically on an individual who possesses sufficient sources of power to exert influence and control over members of the organization in the effort to achieve organizational goals. In general, the flaw in using this approach is that the narrow perspective is on the individual. More appropriate assessment of leadership includes the characteristics of the leader, as well as subordinates, peers, supervisors, and the organization itself. This broader perspective provides a more detailed examination of the leader, the external environment, and the situation—all factors that determine appropriateness of leadership style. Contemporary theories also emphasize emotion, vision, and values.

While contemporary theories recognize the complexities and expand the multiplicity of variables impacting leadership, they also return us to the examination of individual characteristics and behaviors. Novick, Morrow, and Mays (2008) suggest that transformational leadership seemingly appears as

*We acknowledge and thank Dr. Robert DeYoung, who was the contributing author of an earlier version of this chapter, which appeared in *Organizational Behavior in Health Care* (2005), Jones and Bartlett Publishers.

the reemergence of trait-based theories. Indeed, numerous studies in recent years have focused on personality traits of effective transformational, transactional, and charismatic leaders (De Hoogh, Den Hartog, & Koopman, 2005). Many credit this resurgence to the work of Judge, Bono, Ilies, and Gerhardt (2002), who group the numerous traits identified in leadership studies into to a Big Five personality framework (see Chapter 3). By organizing similar traits into five categories (Extroversion, Agreeableness, Conscientiousness, Emotional Stability, and Openness to Experience), stronger and more consistent relationships emerged. This five-factor view of personality provided a new framework for linking personality and leader behavior and effectiveness in studies on charistmatic, transformational, and transactional leadership (Bryman, 1992; Den Hartog & Koopman, 2001, Digman, 1990). A second individual trait that has received considerable attention is Emotional Intelligence (EI). Emotional Intelligence involves the ability to monitor one's own and other's feelings and emotions, to discriminate among them, and to use this information to guide one's thinking and actions (Salovey & Mayer, 1990).

While innate personality traits play a role in leadership, the variance explained by personality remains limited. A leader may have intrinsic traits that enhance or allow leadership to emerge, but he or she must also have knowledge, skills, vision, and values to effectively influence followers and facilitate individual and organizational performance. Therefore, we will conclude this chapter with a brief review of the development of behavioral competencies for healthcare leadership.

TRANSFORMATIONAL VERSUS TRANSACTIONAL LEADERSHIP

It is helpful to define the terms *transformational* and *transactional* to establish a foundation in regard to how each approach is appropriate and vital to organizational success.

In general terms, transactional leadership is directed toward task accomplishment and the maintenance of good relations between the leader and subordinates through consideration of performance and reward. Transformational leadership is directed toward the influence and management of institutional change and innovation through revitalization and vision (Dessler, 1998, p. 350).

Recalling from the Ohio State studies discussed in Chapter 9, leader behaviors included characteristics identified as consideration and initiating structure. *Consideration* is the recognition that individuals have needs and require relationships; *initiating structure* denotes an emphasis on tasks and goals. Burns (1978) reported that transactional leadership style is based on both consideration and initiating structure. Transactional behaviors are "largely oriented toward accomplishing the task at hand and maintaining good relations with those working with the leader by exchanging promises of rewards for performance" (Dessler, 1998, p. 350). Transactional leaders seek to maintain the status quo and reward subordinates for doing what is expected from them. Expectations of performance and the resultant rewards are clearly identified and delivered upon completion of the agreement. As De Hoogh, Den Hartog, and Koopman (2005, p. 840) put it, "transactional leaders influence followers through task-focused behaviors; they clarify expectancies, rules and procedures, emphasizing a fair deal."

In contrast, the transformational style of leadership incorporates emotion, values, and vision to motivate individuals and seeks to change the status quo. Transformational leadership is all about change, innovation, improvement, and entrepreneurship through vision and inspiration. Osland, Kolb, and Rubin (2001, p. 297) state that, "transformational leaders are value-driven change agents who make followers more conscious of the importance of task outcomes. They provide followers with a vision and motivate them to go beyond self-interest for the good of the organization."

Transformational leadership establishes subordinate effort and performance that extends beyond that which occurs as a result of transactional leadership. These two approaches to leadership are not mutually exclusive; most leaders exhibit both transactional and transformational behaviors in different intensities and amounts (Bass, 1990b; Luthans, 2002). According to Bass (1990b) and Luthans (2002, p. 592), each leadership approach differentiates itself in the identification of four specific characteristics unique to each style:

Transactional Leadership

- *Contingent Reward:* Contracts exchange of rewards for effort; promises rewards for good performance; recognizes accomplishments.
- *Management by Exception (an active approach):* Watches and searches for deviations from rules and standards; takes corrective action.
- *Management by Exception (a passive approach):* Intervenes only if standards are not met.
- *Laissez-Faire:* Abdicates responsibilities; avoids making decisions.

Transformational Leadership

- *Charisma:* Provides vision and sense of mission; instills pride; gains respect and trust.
- *Inspiration:* Communicates high expectations; uses symbols to focus efforts; expresses important purposes in simple ways.
- *Intellectual:* Promotes intelligence, rationality, and careful problem solving.
- *Individualized Consideration:* Gives personal attention; treats each employee individually; coaches; advises.

Transformational leadership elevates the level of insight about the importance and value of outcomes through the growth of subordinates by encouraging followers to question their own way of doing things. Transactional leadership constitutes behavior that operates through consideration and covenants between the leader and the follower, focusing on the needs of current subordinates. These considerations include economic, political, and/or psychological issues.

TRANSFORMATIONAL LEADERSHIP: A CONTRADICTORY VIEW

Kotter (1995) provided a contradictory view as to the success of incorporating transformational efforts. Kotter noted that transformational change (through transformational leadership) is conducted under many banners: cultural change, reengineering, and total quality management, to name a few. The purpose of transformational leadership is to address the essential changes necessary to respond to an ever-changing, globally competitive environment.

Kotter (1995) added that transformational leadership resulting in successful change is best executed in phases and that failure to address each phase to the fullest significantly diminishes the capacity to succeed. As illustrated in Table 11–1, Kotter identified eight transformational phases to enhance the success of the leader. Tichy and Devanna (1986), cited in Luthans (2002, pp. 591–592), found that transformational leaders shared the following seven characteristics:

1. They identified themselves as change agents.
2. They exhibited courage.
3. They trusted people.
4. They were value driven.
5. They valued life-long learning.
6. They possessed the capability to face complexity, ambiguity, and uncertainty.
7. They were imaginative, creative, innovative, and visionary.

OTHER CONTEMPORARY LEADERSHIP APPROACHES

Over 50 years ago, the Office of Strategic Services published a book titled *The Assessment of Men*, in which two types of leadership were described: (1) the leader in articulation, who was forceful and inspirational in expression and who spelled out clearly what was needed and how it was to be accomplished; and (2) the leader in action who, by setting himself in motion, demonstrated how to accomplish a goal and whose successes encouraged others to join in the pursuit of the goal(s). In either case, "the leader—by words or action—inspired others to achieve something beyond the ordinary by appealing to a goal worthy of human effort" (Curtin, 1997, p. 7).

Although the primary focus of this chapter is transformational leadership, other leadership styles and their respective characteristics also focus on transformation or change. Here we examine some of these styles and their conceptual similarities.

Bolman and Deal (1997) offer for consideration the *symbolic leader*. Symbolic leaders interpret and reinterpret experiences, developing the capacity to impart purpose and meaning. Recall that transactional leadership is directed toward task accomplishment and good relations between the leader and subordinates through consideration of performance and reward, while transformational leadership is directed toward the influence and management of institutional change and innovation through revitalization and vision

Table 11–1 Eight Specific Errors That Diminish the Transformational Effort

Phase	Transformational Errors	Processes to Enhance Transformational Success
1	Failure to create a true sense of urgency	Establish a sense of urgency by examining market/competitive realities and conducting a SWOT analysis (strengths, weaknesses, opportunities, and threats)
2	Failure to create a powerful guiding coalition	Form powerful coalitions by assembling groups of teams with the power to effect change
3	Failure to create a clearly understood vision	Create a vision with direction and focus consistent with organizational strategies
4	Failure to adequately communicate the vision	Use all available channels of communication to convey the change and lead by example
5	Failure to remove obstacles in moving toward transformational change	Remove obstacles, change systems and structures, encourage creativity and innovation through empowerment
6	Failure to systematically plan for or create short-term successes	Plan for and recognize visible, short-term improvements through established reward systems
7	Proclaiming success prematurely	Utilize credibility to change systems, structures, processes, and policies to arrive at the vision
8	Failure to anchor the transformational change in the organizational culture	Institutionalize the change by infusing appropriate behaviors that will lead to development and succession

SOURCE: "Leading change: Why transformational efforts fail," by J. P. Kotter, 1995. *Harvard Business Review, 73*(2), p. 61. Reprinted with permission.

(Dessler, 1998). Symbolic leaders use symbols to seize attention. They frame experiences in an uncertain environment, providing reasonable interpretation and understanding of events. Symbolic leaders disseminate information through persuasive communication, especially through the use of stories, rites, and rituals, both current and past. Symbolic leaders are consistent in their use of rules and customs (Bolman & Deal, 1997).

Another contemporary view of leadership is the *superleadership* perspective. Because today's leaders are required to function effectively in an ever-changing, fast-paced, global environment, traditional leadership approaches lack the depth of knowledge, skill, and ability required of today's leaders. As contemporary work environments increasingly develop and implement new and innovative structural designs, there is an unprecedented level of employee participation, and the myriad of prevailing management practices make it difficult, at best, to identify an appropriate leadership approach. In response to these issues, the superleader willingly shares power and control with the employees, and instills a sense of empowerment that redirects the basis of vision and direction from the leader to the follower. Like transformational leadership, superleadership encourages followers to do or become more—to discover, use and maximize their abilities. The superleader continues to lead, but recognizes the value of vision and direction that can be assembled by individuals at all levels of the organization. The superleader approach is effective in that the leader creates a positive atmosphere, promotes self-leading teams, provides appropriate reward and constructive reprimand, and fosters a corporate culture that contributes to high levels of performance (Osland et al., 2001).

The Charismatic Leader

Charismatic leaders are individuals who exhibit high levels of self-confidence and trust in subordinates, high expectations for subordinates, and ideological vision and purpose through personal example. In return, followers of charismatic leaders demonstrate loyalty to, confidence in, and trust in the charismatic leader's values, behaviors, and vision. This relationship and connectedness are critical elements between the followers and the charismatic leader. The effect is profound, often producing performance results that exceed established expectations (Luthans, 2002).

In light of the high esteem in which the charismatic leader is held, one would expect that the charismatic leader exhibits high ethical standards. This presumption, in most cases, would be correct. The ethical charismatic leader will, in general, exhibit the characteristics outlined in Exhibit 11–1. Yet, not all charismatic leaders are, in fact, ethical. The standard is not always met.

Exhibit 11–1 Characteristics Exhibited by the Ethical Charismatic Leader

The ethical charismatic leader:

- Uses power to serve others;
- Aligns vision with followers' needs and aspirations;
- Considers and learns from criticism;
- Stimulates followers to think independently and to question the leader's view;
- Uses open, two-way communication;
- Coaches, develops, and supports followers; shares recognition with others;
- Relies on internal moral standards to satisfy organizational and societal interests.

SOURCE: Organizational Behavior (9th ed., p. 591), by F. Luthans, 2002. Boston, MA: McGraw-Hill. Reprinted with permission.

Howell and Avolio (1992) noted that charismatic leaders "deserve this label only if they create transformations in their organizations so that members are motivated to follow them and to seek organization objectives not simply because they are ordered to do so, and not merely because they calculate that such compliance is in their self-interest, but because they voluntarily identify with the organization, its standards of conduct and willingly seek to fulfill its purpose" (Luthans, 2002, p. 590).

Though the components of transformational leadership and charismatic leadership differ somewhat (Yukl, 1999), these theories are often seen as equivalent. As discussed earlier in the chapter, research supports the position that transformational leadership qualities can be learned as long as the individual is comfortable and confident in the controlling and influencing roles. Combining the desire to lead with learning and understanding the position and responsibility in becoming a transformational leader allows individuals the capacity to transform organizations. Which brings us to the question: Can an individual acquire charismatic characteristics sufficient to develop a following based on trust, expectations, and purpose?

Benton (2003) describes a six-step plan for developing executive charisma. He suggests that many people accept the fact that, given organizational constraints and the competition among organizational leaders, many potential change agents acquiesce to acknowledge that they will only achieve a certain level of success. It is further presented that the one missing component to assuming charismatic positioning—beyond one's exemplary character, instincts, judgment, integrity, and positive energy—is *executive charisma*. Benton defines executive charisma as "the ability to gain effective responses from others by using aware actions and considerate civility in order to get useful things done" (p. x). Benton's (2003, p. 10) six steps to developing executive charismatic qualities are as follows:

Step 1: Be the First to Initiate
Step 2: Expect and Give Acceptance to Maintain Esteem
Step 3: Ask Questions and Ask Favors
Step 4: Stand Tall, Straight, and Smile
Step 5: Be Human, Humorous, and Hands On
Step 6: Slow Down, Shut Up, and Listen

It is important to recognize that being the first to initiate action establishes your willingness to accept uncertainty head-on; to acknowledge a situation can be either a problem or an opportunity to initiate transformation. This first step requires a consistent willingness to act. Recognition, both as a giver and a receiver, fulfills the second step of the plan to provide a sense of esteem, to oneself and others. This provision of esteem provides a cyclical optimism that can pervade others involved in the transformative effort.

The third step proffers an exchange of information as required to meet organizational objectives. Choosing one's words and tone carefully while being specific and concise is important to ensuring that information is timely, relevant, and accurate. Do not be too timid to ask questions or solicit favors. Be mindful to recall favors provided and extend thanks in return. Perception is important when exhibiting charismatic qualities. Step four demands that the executive leader not only play the role, but that looking the role is equally important. Standing tall with a relaxed confidence enhances one's charismatic appearance.

Interestingly, step five mandates that charismatic leaders take on responsibilities that others won't—but don't overdo it! By this Benton suggests that being human is imperative to being charismatic, but don't be too human. Be humorous with a sense of appropriateness. Do not cross social, ethnic, or gender boundaries; stepping across acceptable boundaries into indefinable territory can quickly distinguish one's effort to create charismatic leadership qualities. The final step involves maintaining a pace that permits decision making, implementation, and focus. Not talking (or shutting up) allows one the opportunity to listen. Listening provides the time to hear what others have to say, develop a response to the information, and gain the trust necessary to initiate transformational efforts. "Executive charisma isn't as much about you as about your effect on others and that comes not just from what you say and do but from what you don't say and don't do" (Benton, 2003, p. 153).

Visionary Leadership

Visionary leaders are able to develop, communicate, and foster change or transformational ideas toward the accomplishment of organizational goals through the commitment of resources and infusion of available talent. The creation of a strong sense of community facilitates the visionary change. Employees buy in to the leader's vision because they are provided sufficient information and resources to see how their efforts will become instrumental to the cause. The visionary leader manages the transformational change. "The key steps in managing the dream are communicating vision, recruiting carefully, rewarding appropriate results, and training and reorganizing when necessary" (Mello, 2003, p. 348).

What characteristics are necessary to effect visionary change? Visionary leaders seek out contrasting perspectives and values and modify their own views to better align the viewpoints of those affected by impending change. They also possess the capacity to empathize, exhibit competence, and provide a supportive setting (Mello, 2003). Visionary leaders don't step outside the box; instead, they make the box bigger!

Servant Leadership

Some scholars in the leadership area, such as Peter Senge, Warren Bennis, Peter Block, and Margaret Wheatley, see servant leadership as the emerging leadership paradigm for the twenty-first century for all corporations and institutions. The concept of servant leadership is captured in the following quote from Disraeli "I must follow the people. Am I not their leader?"

The term servant leadership was first used by Robert K. Greenleaf in 1969 as a way to describe a type of leadership that seeks to serve. Today, it is also referred to as dependent directorship or principled leadership. Servant leadership is an approach to managing people that "begins with a clear and compelling vision that excites passion in the leader and commitment in those who follow" (Blanchard & Hodges, 2003). A servant leader values others' strengths and talents and encourages the use of these strengths and talents for the betterment of the organization.

Servant leadership recognizes the importance of performance coaching while acknowledging that individual development and performance are strongly related. According to Blanchard and Hodges (2003, p. A2), instrumental to the implementation of servant leadership are three components of performance coaching:

1. *Performance Planning:* The servant leader sets goals and objectives.
2. *Day-to-Day Coaching:* Providing the resources and an environment conducive to the accomplishment of established goals.
3. *Performance Evaluation:* The timely and relevant evaluation of individual performance and the identification of professional developmental needs.

Anderson (2003) believes that servant leadership can build effective hospital–physician relationships. He states that servant leaders accept as their responsibility the need to invest in the lives of their followers, believing that they are "not superior to the follower and also know that on any given day or in a given circumstance the follower may become the leader. It is the servant leader's hope that the follower will indeed one day become a servant leader and, therefore, will make an investment in the follower's career to better ensure that indeed this happens" (Anderson, 2003, p. 45).

Although empirical research in the area of servant leadership is limited, Ornelas (2003) found a positive correlation between organizational outcomes and perception of servant leadership characteristics among departmental leaders within a large health system. The results of Ornelas' study showed that employees working in departments that reported managers with servant leadership characteristics reported lower turnover rates, higher job satisfaction, and increased commitment to the organization than those employees working in departments whose managers did not embrace the servant leadership philosophy.

In their studies of healthcare leadership, Pelote and Route (2007) concluded that the most successful leaders, whom they refer to as masterpiece leaders, displayed a form of servant leadership. These leaders viewed themselves as the leader–coach first and the leader–expert second. "Masterpiece leaders create, energize, and motivate the healthcare climate; exhibit a high level of passion, excitement, and drive to perpetuate their success" (p. 282).

The Implications of Transformational Leadership on the Healthcare Industry

Research relates that healthcare organizations will transform in many ways in the years to come. The healthcare manager must acquire the skills, abilities, and knowledge necessary to understand effective leadership processes and anticipated environmental change. Changes facing the healthcare manager necessitate a stronger focus on results, creativity, and innovation (Gummer, 1995). This results-oriented viewpoint will be a major challenge, given the process orientation of healthcare settings. The vanguard healthcare manager will experience increased levels of stress in balancing increased patient caseloads and additional discharges (Gellis, 2001).

Another study provides an interesting insight into the symptoms of a transactional approach to healthcare leadership. Thyler (2003) reported that "healthcare leadership continues to run under a transactional style of leadership that may be causing nurses to leave the system. Nurses no longer wish to remain in the profession, perhaps because they struggle ideologically with the system in which they work" (p. 73). Yet, Thyler also notes that nurses themselves hold the key to transforming the healthcare system, in that the transformational approach to leadership is well suited to the healthcare profession, which functions best in a team-based setting using high levels of communication.

Another study reported that staff nurses in acute care hospitals perceived their head nurses as demonstrating both transformational and transactional leadership styles. The factors related to transformational and transactional leaderships are in conflict with those reported by Bass (1990a) when compared to professions. This conflict is probably due to the fact that the very nature of work performed in human service organizations differs significantly from work performed in other public- and private-sector organizations. The main difference observed between nursing and other types of organizations involves the issue of contingent rewards. Staff nurses related contingent rewards with the transformational leadership approach, not the transactional leadership approach. The healthcare industry, especially as it applies to nursing, provides little recognition or tangible reward for exceptional performance. This lack of recognition provides support to the numerous studies conducted, noting the relationship between style of leadership and job satisfaction (or dissatisfaction). A similar relationship is reported between leadership style and retention (Medley & Larochelle, 1995).

Not surprisingly, Medley and Larochelle's (1995) research reported no significant relationship could be established between transactional leadership style and job satisfaction. "Since management by exception was the only factor nurses associated with transactional leadership, it is clear that staff nurses view behaviors associated with transactional leadership (e.g., negative feedback) unfavorably in relation to their jobs. This study indicated that head nurses with high transformational scores were more likely to have staff nurses with higher job satisfaction scores and longer association with their staff nurses than transactional leaders" (p. 64JJ). These results provide strong support that a transformational leadership approach advances retention efforts and diminishes turnover rates—a conclusion that has significant fiscal implications for healthcare facilities.

Chaffee (2001) recently addressed the implications of transformational leadership in a military healthcare environment. The purpose of Chaffee's study was to identify the ideal characteristics of a Navy healthcare executive of the future. Sixty-seven respondents reported most frequently the following ideal, transformational leadership characteristics:

- Possesses an ability to organize teamwork.
- Possesses a clear vision.

- Teaches others to succeed and mentors others.
- Takes risks and encourages others to do so.
- Develops and maintains excellent interpersonal relationship skills.
- Possesses credibility, honesty, and integrity.
- Embraces and drives change.
- Strives for excellence and continuous improvement.
- Possesses excellent communication skills.
- Exhibits a passion for work.
- Maintains a focus on the organizational mission.

"The characteristics identified by respondents describe leadership traits rather than management skills. None of the respondents identified the traditional managerial skills of planning, organizing, coordinating, directing, and controlling. Additionally, the most frequently identified characteristics fit the definition of transformational leadership" (Chaffee, 2001). These leadership characteristics support four managerial competencies sustained by successful leaders:

1. *Management of Attention:* The ability to get the attention of a group through a compelling vision that brings others to a place they have not been before.
2. *Management of Meaning:* The ability to make a vision clear to others and the ability to communicate ideas and create meaning.
3. *Management of Trust:* The ability to inspire trust through reliability and constancy.
4. *Management of Self:* Knowing one's skills and deploying them effectively. (Bennis, 1984; Chaffee, 2001)

Globalization has affected the healthcare industry as it has all other organizational environments. The strategic focus of healthcare administration is, and will continue to be, improved quality associated with cost controls. Transformation leaders possess the flexibility and multitasking capabilities to respond to this competitive, emergent venue. The explicit constraints placed on healthcare workers must not become an obstacle to the transformational effort. Clearly, the sustainability of the healthcare industry will depend upon mandating a broad focus, to include not only the leader and those led, but that the view must remain comprehensive, "reaching out to staff and suppliers with the single purpose of joining intellects and efforts in a common sense of purpose, to satisfy clients/customers" (Trofino, 2000).

World-class healthcare organizations, created through transformational leadership and change, will support the implementation of nurse case-management programs; the infusion of new technology will be embraced as beneficial to the quality of services provided; client education and alternate therapies will be evaluated and incorporated for appropriate delivery and use; healthcare workers will not feel they are merely holding a job, but the corporate culture will seek to make workers a part of the solution; and finally, successful healthcare organizations will transform a new paradigm to "meet both the stringent demands of the marketplace and the inner needs of the workforce" (Trofino, 2000).

Transformational leadership is, without question, very well suited to the needs of today's economic, social, political, and technological conditions. Why? Transformational leadership thrives on change and innovation. Transformational leadership provides the knowledge, skills, and abilities to facilitate innovation and transformation, beyond that which is available through a traditional approach. Doing things because that is the way it was always done will be replaced with dynamic solutions to old and new problems (Sofarelli & Brown, 1998).

Bennis and Nanus (1985), while noting the importance of both management and leadership, recognized a philosophical dissimilarity between the two approaches: "Managers are people who do things right and leaders are people who do the right things" (p. 21). The implications of this statement provoke questions as to how the healthcare industry will respond to an environment where leadership focuses less on managing technical skills and more on managing knowledge processes. Technical skills are controlled through clearly stated goals and measurable performance objectives. It is the mental processes, now replacing the mechanistic tasks that must be carefully monitored and managed, in that critical decisions are arrived at through cognitive processes not controlled through clearly stated goals and measurable performance objectives. This is an area that has been rarely traveled by managers and leaders until now. The transformational leadership approach is well suited to serve this new environment, addressing health care within the context of globalization, technology, and empowerment (Trofino, 1995).

ANOTHER LOOK AT TRAITS AND BEHAVIOR

As mentioned in the Overview section, many see contemporary theories of leadership as a resurgence of interest in individual traits and behaviors. Two such theoretical constructs currently receiving considerable attention are the Big Five personality factors (Judge et al., 2002) and Emotional Intelligence (EI) (Salovey and Mayer, 1990). Following an examination of these constructs, we return to behaviors. Bass (1990a, b) emphasized that leadership can be learned and suggested that one of the most significant applications of transformational theory is in the training of individuals to become transformational leaders. The success of transformational leadership training appears to be based on actual increases in leader uses of transformational behaviors. Identifying behaviors that define competent healthcare leaders has captured the attention of both scholars and practitioners.

Big Five Personality Factors

The Big Five personality framework, as introduced in Chapter 3, posits that the multitude of personality characteristics identified in theory and research can be organized into five factors that underlie all others. These factors as identified (De Hoogh et al., 2005; Robbins, 2005) include:

Extroversion: Extraverts tend to be social, assertive, active, and gregarious.
Agreeableness: Agreeable individuals are warm, generous, cooperative, and trusting.

Conscientiousness: Conscientious individuals are dependable, responsible, achievement oriented, organized, and proficient.

Emotional Stability: The dimension captures an individual's ability to withstand stress. Positive emotional stability people are calm, self-confident, and secure. Some researchers measure this factor as *Neuroticism*, which reflects the tendency to be anxious, insecure, and defensive.

Openness to Experience: Individuals open to experience are characterized by imagination, unconventionality, a range of interests, and fascination with novelty.

Robbins (2005) suggests that the studies of the Big Five approach resulted in consistent and strong support for traits as predictors of leadership. A different conclusion is drawn by DeHoogh et al. (2005). These authors suggest considerable variability in both the strength and direction of the relationships between the personality factors and transformational and transactional leadership. Such variances, they conclude, result in weak support for the Big Five factors.

The inconsistency of findings leads DeHoogh et al. (2005) to suggest that it is not the personality itself that is important in leadership style, but the interaction of the personality characteristics and the context. Their research examined both the direct measure of the Big Five personality factors and interactive relationship with emphasis on perceived leader effectiveness (transformational and charismatic leader styles were considered equivalent and contrasted with transactional). The context variable, the work environment, was defined as either dynamic environment (i.e., characterized by a high degree of challenge and opportunities for change), or stable (i.e., more structured, and orderly). Results from this study established that the relationships between personality and leadership style did indeed differ depending on the context.

Emotional Intelligence

Emotional intelligence (EI) is relatively new to the field of organizational behavior. Emotional intelligence involves assessing one's own feelings, as well as the feelings of others, then using those assessments to guide personal thought and action. EI has five distinct characteristics:

1. Self-awareness
2. Self-management or regulation
3. Self-motivation
4. Empathy or social awareness
5. Social skills

Coleman (1998, p. 318) describes self-awareness as involving self-understanding and knowledge of one's true feelings at any given moment. Self-management ensures that a manager can control his or her emotions to assist the task at hand while focusing on the problem's solution. Self-motivation allows the manager to stay focused on the goal and desired outcome, overcoming negative emotional stimulus and accepting delayed gratification. Empathy is the possession of the sense of what others feel and want while being sensitive to their needs. Finally, social skills relate to one's ability to read and react to social situations while interacting with others and guiding and influencing the behavior of others.

Coleman (1998), as cited by Luthans (2002, p. 306), noted that EI is not the "end all" in determining leadership characteristics and competencies, but nonetheless, he concludes:

- At the individual level, elements of emotional intelligence can be identified, assessed, and upgraded.
- At the group level, it means fine-tuning the interpersonal dynamics that make groups smarter.
- At the organizational level, it means revising the value hierarchy to make emotional intelligence a priority—in the concrete terms of hiring, training and development, performance evaluation, and promotions.

Coleman (1998) believes that EI is more important than IQ, proposing that EI is a better predictor of success in both personal and professional endeavors. Gibbs (1995) provided the following evidence as to the importance of EI: "IQ gets you hired, but EI gets you promoted" (p. 64).

Healthcare organizations are just beginning to recognize the importance of developing a manager's EI (Grossman, 2000). Only select progressive healthcare facilities have recognized the value of EI training and have incorporated programs that emphasize its principles. However, as Freshman and Rubino (2002) point out, the applications of EI fit well within the industry, as reflected in Table 11–2.

Behavioral Competencies

In general, behavioral competencies define the skills, knowledge, abilities, and actions that distinguish superior performance. Spencer and Spencer (1993) describe a competency as "what outstanding performers do more often, in more situations, with better results, than average performers." There has been a growing interest in the development of competencies since McClellan (1961, 1985) published his work on achievement and motivation (see Chapter 5). In the past decade, leadership competency models have proliferated in healthcare education and professional development. Numerous consulting organizations, professional associations, healthcare organizations, and educational programs have created leadership competency lists (Dye & Garman, 2006). The acceptance and implementation of competency-based education and training across healthcare systems may be viewed as acknowledgment that at least a significant portion of leadership may be learned, and as the desire to assure exceptional leadership and performance in health care.

The vast numbers of competency models preclude an exhaustive review. However, students in healthcare management programs should examine the competencies incorporated into their programs of study. The National Center for Healthcare Leadership (NCHL) in conjunction with the Robert Wood Johnson

Table 11–2 Healthcare Administration Application to Emotional Intelligence

Component	Definition	Examples of Application
Self-awareness	Having a deep understanding of one's emotions, strengths, weaknesses, needs, and drives	1. Confidently making decisions when budgets must be trimmed in medical areas 2. Knowing that the values of the healthcare system are not congruent with yours 3. Recognizing that the late-night committee meetings are affecting your family relations
Self-regulation	A propensity for reflection, ability to adapt to changes, saying no to impulsive urges	1. Knowing when to step away if having an argument with a provider 2. Acting to correct medical billing compliance issues rather than ignoring them 3. Accepting responsibility over additional healthcare facilities
Self-motivation	Driven to achieve, being passionate about enjoying challenges in the profession	1. Setting up a senior manager retreat to allow the best environment for planning 2. Being optimistic even when consensus is low 3. Embracing diverse populations of patients and employees
Social awareness	Thoughtfully considering someone's feelings when acting	1. Thinking of the family's perspective when involved in bioethical decisions 2. Being compassionate when dealing with employees and their personal problems affecting their work 3. Being patient-centered
Social skills	Moving people in the direction you desire	1. Being able to negotiate a favorable managed care contract 2. Having employees satisfied with their performance evaluation 3. Using good listening skills when talking with governing board members

SOURCE: "Emotional intelligence: A core competency for healthcare administrators," by B. Freshman, and L. Rubino, 2002, *The Health Care Manager, 20*(4), p. 6. Reprinted with permission.

Foundation has developed a framework to implement competency-based learning and assessment curricula in healthcare management education. The NCHL project relies on academics and experts in the field to define the technical and behavioral characteristics that leaders must possess to be successful across the health professions. The full model, which may be found on NCHL's Web site at www.nchl.org, contains levels for each competency that distinguish leaders at each career stage (early careerist, midcareerist, and senior executive). Future and current healthcare executives may be guided by the competencies set forth by the American College of Healthcare Executives (ACHE), the international professional organization for the more than 30,000 healthcare executives who lead hospitals and healthcare organizations around the world (see www.ache.org). ACHE offers a Healthcare Executive Competencies Assessment Tool derived from the Healthcare Leadership Alliance (HLA) (see www.healthcareleadershipalliance.org). The competencies were developed by HLA through job analyses and research. Three hundred competencies are categorized under five major domains: (1) leadership, (2) communications and relationship management, (3) professionalism, (4) business knowledge and skills, and (5) knowledge of the healthcare environment. The ACHE self-assessment is designed to assist executives in identifying areas of strength as well as areas in which they may wish to improve performance.

Do competencies create effective leaders? Dye and Garner (2006) suggest that competency is most accurately described as the *capacity* to perform (p. xxxi). Translating competency into success requires both motivation and opportunity. Further, competencies are not just learned but "are more accurately described as improving slowly over time as a result of mindful practice, feedback, and more practice" (p. xx). Pelote and Route (2007) also present a broader view of leadership competencies in the Healthcare Causal Flow Leadership Model. As the model demonstrates, individual characteristics do not exist in a vacuum and, of themselves, are not a source of success. Leadership competencies are viewed as one of the variables within a context (e.g., healthcare climate) that ultimately impacts performance outcomes (i.e., patient outcomes, patient satisfaction, and financial results).

SUMMARY

Contemporary theories recognize the complexity of leadership, and yet also bring us back to examining the role of traits and behaviors as the more simplistic, traditional leadership theories of the past. Today, leadership theorists acknowledge the presence of a symbiotic relationship between the leader's traits and behaviors, the follower, the environment, the situation, and the strategic organizational objectives. In response to an ever-changing, external environment, contemporary leadership approaches allow interactions between the leader and the follower that are not possible with traditional leadership approaches. A common thread among contemporary leadership models is an integration of ideological, moral, and value applications.

It is important to recognize that organizations require both transactional and transformational styles of leadership if strategic goals are to be met. One approach is not necessarily preferred over the other. Imagine an organization that has only transactional leaders. Despite the fact that tasks and processes would be accomplished, it is unlikely that the organization would have the ability to transform itself to respond to an ever-changing environment or redirect its efforts into new markets. At the same time, an organization that had only transformational leaders would certainly have the vision to change and innovate, but would not have the capacity to do so because of an absence of transactional agreements between managers and employees. Fortunately, this scenario is unlikely, but it does portray the importance of balance of leadership styles within organizations.

It is essential to create the proper blend of leadership that is flexible and adaptable to differing situational factors. The formula for balance is difficult. In a time of crisis, which style of leadership is most important: transactional or transformational? You can see there is not a simple answer to this question because of the multitude of situational factors. One could argue that in a time of crisis, transactional leadership would be more effective if control and efficiency were the primary concerns. Likewise, transformational leadership would be most effective in a time of crisis if change and innovation were the dominant interest.

There is supportive research that suggests that transformational, charismatic, and other contemporary leadership attributes can be learned. This finding is valuable to individuals who find that they have reached a plateau in their professional development plan. Leaders at all levels of the organization can enhance, modify, and develop leadership skills to increase their ability to influence, control, and manage by identifying personal leadership strengths and weaknesses.

Today's healthcare managers can move beyond transactional leadership into areas that create opportunities for ever-increasing levels of performance and connection to the workforce through visionary and servant approaches to leadership. Contemporary managers should look closely within themselves to determine appropriateness of leadership styles on the basis of situational, environmental, and personal factors. Understanding the need for aligning one's leadership approach with these factors can generate higher levels of workplace commitment and performance.

END-OF-CHAPTER DISCUSSION QUESTIONS

1. Identify the similarities and differences between transactional and transformational leadership. Discuss the appropriateness of each style dependent upon situational factors.

2. Discuss the type of leadership style—transactional, transformational, visionary, and servant—that occurs in your specific professional environment. List the positive and negative outcomes that exist as a result of the leadership approach used.

3. Debate the position that transformational and charismatic leadership can (or cannot) be learned. Be specific in your support (or opposition).

4. Discuss Benton's six-step plan for executive charisma. Would the plan work for you in your current healthcare setting?

5. Deliberate the need for transformational or charismatic leadership in the next five to ten years as the healthcare environment transforms as a result of globalization, technology, and empowerment.

EXERCISE 11–1

It has been stated that to lead people through the complex changes facing the healthcare industry, "transformational leadership" is required (i.e., leaders creating an environment in which staff can best apply their knowledge, skills, and efforts, engaging commitment and developing potential). As such, you are engaged as the consultant for Beltway Healthcare System to develop a management development program that will be the vehicle that managers can use to develop the necessary skills and knowledge to drive organizational change and improve the system's performance. What would you propose as the goals of the management development program? What learning methods would be best suited to achieve these goals?

EXERCISE 11–2

Access a leadership competency assessment tool of your choice. Review your scores to identify strengths as well as areas to further develop. Given your current strengths, how would you conceptualize your leadership style?

REFERENCES

Anderson, R. J. (2003). Building hospital–physician relationships through servant leadership. *Frontiers of Health Services Management, 20*(2), 45–47.

Bass, B. M. (1990a). *Bass and Stogdill's handbook of leadership: Theory, research and managerial applications* (3rd ed.). New York: The Free Press.

Bass, B. M. (1990b). From transactional to transformational leadership: Learning to share the vision. *Organizational Dynamics, 18*(3), 19–31.

Bennis, W. (1984). The four competencies of leadership. *Training and Development Journal*. August, 144–149.

Bennis, W., & Nanus, B. (1985). *Leaders: The strategies for taking charge*. New York: Harper & Row.

Benton, D. A. (2003). *Executive charisma*. New York: McGraw-Hill Book Company.

Blanchard, K., & Hodges, P. (2003, May 12). The journey to servant leadership in work, life. *San Diego Business Journal*, A2.

Bolman, L. G., & Deal, T. E. (1997). *Reframing organizations: Artistry, choice, and leadership* (2nd ed.). San Francisco: Jossey-Bass.

Bryman, A. (1992). *Charisma and leadership in organizations*. London: Sage.

Burns, J. M. (1978). *Leadership*. New York: Harper & Row.

Chaffee, M. W. (2001). Navy medicine: A health care leadership blueprint for the future. *Military Medicine, 166* (3), 240–247.

Coleman, D. (1998). *Working with emotional intelligence*. New York: Bantam Books.

Curtin, L. L. (1997). How—and how not—to be a transformational leader. *Nursing Management, 28*(2), 7–8.

De Hoogh, A., Den Hartog, D., & Koopman, P. (2005). Linking the big five-factors of personality to charismatic and transactional leadership; perceived dynamic work environment as a moderator. *Journal of Organizational Behavior, 26,* 839–865.

Den Hartog, D., & Koopman, P. (2001). Leadership in organizations. In N. Anderson, D. Ones, H. Kepir-Sinangil, & C. Viswesvaran (Eds). *International handbook of industrial, work & organizational psychology* (Vol 2). London: Sage.

Dessler, G. (1998). *Management: Leading people and organizations in the 21st century* (1st ed.). Upper Saddle River, NJ: Prentice Hall.

Digman, J. (1990). Personality structure: The emergence of the five-factor model. *Annual Review of Psychology, 41,* 417–440.

Dye, C. F., & Garman, A. N. (2006). *Exceptional Leadership: 16 Critical Competencies for Healthcare Executives*. Chicago, IL: Health Administration Press.

Freshman, B., & Rubino, L. (2002). Emotional intelligence: A core competency for health care administrators. *The Health Care Manager, 20*(4), 1–9.

Gellis, Z. D. (2001). Social work perceptions of transformational and transactional leadership in health care. *Social Work Research, 25*(1), 17.

Gibbs, N. (1995, October 2). The EQ factor. Time. Available at: http://www.time.com/time/magazine/article/0,9171,983503,00.html

Grossman, R. J. (2000). Emotions at work. *Health Forum Journal, 43*(5), 18–22.

Gummer, B. (1995). Go team go: The growing importance of teamwork in organizational life. *Administration in Social Work, 19,* 85–100.

Howell, J. M., & Avolio, B. J. (1992, May). The ethics of charismatic leadership: Submission or liberation. *Academy of Management Executive,* 43–54.

Judge, T., Bono, J., Ilies, R., & Gerhardt, M. (2002). Personality and leadership: A qualitative and quantitative review. *Journal of Applied Psychology, 87,* 755–768.

Kotter, J. P. (1995, March/April). Leading change: Why transformational efforts fail. *Harvard Business Review, 73,* 59–67.

Luthans, F. (2002). *Organizational behavior* (9th ed.). Boston, MA: McGraw-Hill Book Company.

McClelland, D. C. (1961). *The achieving society*. New York: The Free Press.

McClelland, D. C. (1985). *Human motivation*. Glenwood, IL: Scott-Foresman.

Medley, F., & Larochelle, D. R. (1995). Transformational leadership and job satisfaction. *Nursing Management, 26*(9).

Mello, J. A. (2003). Profiles in leadership: Enhancing learning through model and theory building. *Journal of Management Education, 27*(3), 348–349.

Novick, L., Morrow, C., & Mays, C. (2008). *Public health administration: Principles for population-based management*. Sudbury, MA: Jones and Bartlett Publishers.

Ornelas, J. (2003). The effect of servant leadership on organizational outcomes. Poster Presentation at the American College of Healthcare Executives 2003 Congress, Chicago, IL.

Osland, J., Kolb, D., & Rubin, I. (2001). *Organizational behavior: An experiential approach* (7th ed). Upper Saddle River, NJ: Prentice Hall.

Pelote, V., & Route, L. (2007). *Masterpieces in health care leadership*. Boston, MA: Jones and Bartlett.

Robbins, S. P. (2005). *Organizational behavior* (8th ed.) Upper Saddle River, NJ: Prentice Hall.

Romm, C., & Pliskin, N. (1999). The role of charismatic leadership in diffusion and implementation of e-mail. *The Journal of Management Development, 18*(3), 273–291.

Salovey, P., & Mayer, J. (1990). Emotional intelligence. *Imagination, Cognition, and Personality, 9,* 185–211.

Sofarelli, D., & Brown, D. (1998). The need for nursing leadership in uncertain times. *Journal of Nursing Management, 6*(4), 201–207.

Spencer, L., & Spencer, S. (1993). *Competency at work models for superior performance*. New York: John Wiley & Sons.

Thyler, G. (2003). Dare to be different: Transformational leadership may hold the key to reducing the nursing shortage. *Journal of Nursing Management, 11*(2), 73–79.

Tichy, N. M., & Devanna, M. A. (1986). *The transformational leader*. New York: John Wiley & Sons.

Trofino, A. J. (1995). Transformational leadership in health care. *Nursing Management, 26*(8), 42–47.

Trofino, A. J. (2000). Transformational leadership: Moving total quality management to world-class organizations. *International Nursing Review, 47*(4), 232–242.

Yukl, G. (1999). An evaluation of conceptual weaknesses in transformational and charismatic leadership theories. *Leadership Quarterly, 10,* 285–305.

OTHER SUGGESTED READING

Conger, J. A., & Kanungo, R. N. (1988). Behavioural dimensions of charismatic leadership. In J. A. Conger and R. N. Kanungo (Eds.), *Charismatic leadership* (pp. 79 – 91). San Francisco: Jossey-Bass.

Dixon, D. L. (1998). The balanced CEO: A transformational leader and capable manager. *Healthcare Forum Journal, 41*(2), 26–29.

Yukl, G. (1989). Managerial leadership: A review of theory and research. *Journal of Management, 15*(2), 266.

Intrapersonal and Interpersonal Issues

In Part IV, we discuss stress and conflict and how the negative effects of both can be avoided. Having an optimal level of stress and conflict in our lives is good. It can lead us to work efficiently and effectively with creativity. However, when we experience too much of either stress or conflict, levels of productivity may decrease and problems may be created with our physical and mental health.

CHAPTER 12

Stress in the Workplace and Stress Management

Nancy Borkowski, DBA, CPA, FACHE

LEARNING OUTCOMES

After completing this chapter, the student should understand:

- The definition of stress.
- The process model of stress and coping.
- How stress can negatively affect individuals and organizations.
- The various forms of stress.
- The three stages of the General Adaptation Syndrome.
- How personalities, race, and gender affect an individual's level of stress.
- The definition and phases of burnout.
- The four categories of stress in the workplace.
- The various coping strategies available to organizations and individuals.
- The concepts of learned optimism and hardiness training.
- The definition of stress management and the various programs used by organizations.

OVERVIEW

Stress is a complex and highly personalized process. As such, stress levels in individuals can vary widely, even in identical situations, because of people's abilities to cope with different forms and levels of stress. The ways in which people are affected depends on a number of factors, such as their level of self-efficacy, adaptability, and resources available.

Cognitive-transactional theory defines stress as "a particular relationship between the person and the environment that is appraised by the person as taxing or exceeding his or her resources and endangering his or her well being" (Schwarzer, 2004, p. 343). Lazarus and his associates (Lazarus, 1991; Lazarus & Folkman, 1984; Lazarus, DeLongis, Folkman, & Gruen, 1985) argue that individuals may perceive the same stressful situation differently on the basis of their cognitive appraisal; some individuals see a specific situation as a threat, whereas other individuals see the same situation as a challenge or opportunity.

As illustrated in Figure 12–1, an individual's assessment of the situation includes demand appraisals or resource appraisals. Demand appraisals relate to the person's perception as to (1) physical demands, (2) task demands, (3) role demands, and (4) interpersonal demands (see Table 12–1). Resource appraisals

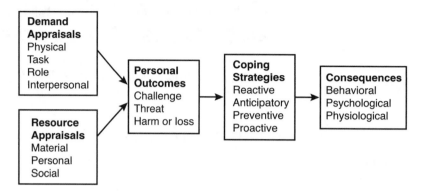

Figure 12–1 A Process Model of Stress and Coping

Table 12–1 Demand Appraisals

Physical Demands
- Indoor climate and air quality
- Temperature
- Illumination and other rays
- Noise and vibrations
- Office design

Task Demands
- Occupational category
- Routine jobs
- Job future ambiguity
- Interactive organizational demands (e.g., interface with various constituencies, such as with boundary spanning)
- Work overload

Role Demands
- Role conflict
    Interrole
    Intrarole
    Person/role (i.e., conflicting values or beliefs)
- Role ambiguity
- Work/home demands

Interpersonal Demands
- Status incongruity
- Social density (i.e., interpersonal need for space and distance)
- Abrasive personalities
- Leadership style
- Team pressures
- Diversity

SOURCE: *Preventive Stress Management in Organizations* (p. 22), by J. C. Quick, J. D. Quick, D. L. Nelson, and J. J. Hurrell, 1997. Washington, DC: American Psychological Association. Reprinted with permission.

may be material, personal, or social. Material appraisals ask the question: Do I have the necessary resources to complete this task? Personal resource appraisal refers to an individual's internal coping options. Individuals who are affluent, healthy, capable, and self-confident are less vulnerable to stressful events. Social resource appraisals relate to external coping options available to an individual, such as availability of obtaining assistance from others, receiving emotional support (reassurance), and/or advice or additional information necessary to complete the task (Lazarus, 1991; Schwarzer, 2004).

As a result of the person's appraisal of the situation, one of three perceptual outcomes occurs. These perceptual outcomes are: challenge, threat, or harm/loss. When a situation is viewed positively, the person sees the situation as a challenge and an opportunity to achieve personal growth. When the situation is viewed as a threat, the person perceives danger, either by physical injury or a blow to the self-esteem. For example, a task demand that is perceived to be difficult, ambiguous, unexpected, or time-consuming with an unrealistic deadline is more likely to induce a threat outcome than an easy task that can be thoroughly prepared for and solved at a convenient pace without time constraints. If the appraisal is viewed to be harm or loss, the person has determined that damage has already occurred, such as loss of self-worth, social standing, or physical injury (Lazarus, 1991; Schwarzer, 2004). Building on Lazarus' work, Schwarzer's (2004) process model illustrates that, on the basis of an individual's perception of the situation, he or she may engage in various coping strategies to manage the experience of stress. The combination of an individual's perception of the situation (appraisals) and the coping strategies employed (reactive, anticipatory, preventive, or proactive) will determine the resulting consequences, which may be behavioral, psychological, physiological, or combinations of the three (see Table 12–2).

In this chapter, we first examine the factors that contribute to a person experiencing stress in the workplace. Although many extraorganizational factors contribute to an individual's experience of stress, such as a pending divorce, housing conditions, and the general economy, this chapter focuses primarily on stress in the workplace. Second, we examine the various methods of coping with stress from both an organizational perspective and an individual perspective, which is referred to as stress management.

WORK-RELATED STRESS

Stress is a common phenomenon in today's workplace. Numerous surveys and studies confirm that occupational related pressures are the leading source of stress for adults. According to the American Institute of Stress (2004), job stress costs US industry approximately $300 billion annually in terms of accidents; absenteeism; employee turnover; loss of productivity; direct medical, legal, and insurance costs; workers' compensation awards; as well as tort and Federal Employers' Liability Act judgments.

The National Institute for Occupational Safety and Health (NIOSH), the federal agency within the US Department of Health and Human Services

Table 12–2 Individual Distress: Behavioral, Psychological, and Physiological Consequences

Behavioral Consequences
- Tobacco use
- Alcohol use
- Drug abuse
- Accident proneness
- Violence
- Eating disorders

Psychological Consequences
- Burnout
- Family problems
- Anxiety disorders
- Sleep disturbances
- Sexual dysfunction
- Depression
- Conversion reaction and somatization

Physiological Consequences
- Hypertension, heart disease, and stroke
- Cancer
- Back pain, arthritis, and other musculoskeletal conditions
- Peptic ulcer disease and other gastrointestinal conditions
- Headache
- Diabetes mellitus
- Liver cirrhosis and other alcohol-related diseases
- Lung disease
- Skin disease
- Other diseases (e.g., HIV, chronic fatigue syndrome)

SOURCE: *Preventive Stress Management in Organizations* (p. 66), by J. C. Quick, J. D. Quick, D. L. Nelson, and J. J. Hurrell, 1997. Washington, DC: American Psychological Association 66. Reprinted with permission.

responsible for conducting research and making recommendations for the prevention of work-related injury and illness, found that:

- 40 percent of workers reported that their jobs were very or extremely stressful;
- 25 percent viewed their jobs as the number one stressor in their lives;
- 75 percent of employees believed that workers have more on-the-job stress than a generation ago;
- 29 percent of workers felt quite a bit or extremely stressed at work;
- 26 percent of workers said they were "often or very often burned out or stressed by their work";
- Job stress was more strongly associated with health complaints than financial or family problems. (NIOSH, 1999)

Furthermore, stress may lead to physical violence in one out of ten work environments. According to a recent study of "desk rage" by Integra Realty Resources (2001), almost half of those surveyed said yelling and verbal abuse were common in their workplaces. Desk rage can include behaviors or acts of aggression, hostility, rudeness, and physical violence. Violence in the workplace is estimated to cost US industry between $6 billion and $36 billion in lost productivity, diminished image, insurance payments, and increased security costs. Integra's survey also reported that:

- 65 percent of workers said that workplace stress had caused difficulties, and more than 10 percent described these as having major effects;
- 10 percent said they work in an atmosphere where physical violence has occurred because of job stress, and of this group, 42 percent reported that yelling and other verbal abuse is common;
- 29 percent had yelled at coworkers because of workplace stress, 14 percent said they worked where machinery or equipment had been damaged because of workplace rage, and 2 percent admitted that they had actually personally struck someone;
- 19 percent, or almost one in five respondents, had quit a previous position because of job stress, and nearly one in four had been driven to tears because of workplace stress;
- 62 percent routinely found that they ended the day with work-related neck pain, 44 percent reported stressed-out eyes, 38 percent complained of hurting hands, and 34 percent reported difficulty in sleeping because they were too stressed-out;
- 12 percent had called in sick because of job stress;
- Over half said they often spent 12-hour days on work-related duties, and an equal number frequently skipped lunch because of the stress of job demands.

Desk rage is a common problem within the healthcare industry. For example, almost one-third of physician executives participating in a recent national study conducted by the American College of Physician Executives reported that serious problems erupted within their organization on either a monthly or weekly basis as a result of disruptive behavior by physicians (Weber, 2004). Furthermore, two-thirds of the nurses responding to a nurse/physician communication survey reported that they have suffered verbal, mental, or physical abuse by a physician. The most common complaints related to physicians yelling, cursing, and abruptly hanging up on the nurse during telephone conversations. Other comments cited were berating the nurse in front of patients, family members, or other staff. The highest number of desk rage responses came from nurses working in hospital operating rooms, and the incidents included throwing of surgical instruments (Homsted, 2003).

Stressors

Everyone encounters stress in their daily lives, but the effects on an individual depend on a number of factors. Causes or sources of stress, known as stressors, can take on a number of forms, such as positive or negative, external or internal, or short-term (acute) or long-term (chronic).

Positive and Negative Stressors

A certain degree of stress is necessary for good mental and physical health; it can be viewed as constructive stress, which compels us to act with optimum performance, whereby we achieve our goals. Hans Selye (1956, 1974), a Canadian physiologist referred to as the grandfather of stress research, coined the term eustress to describe good or positive stress. Eustress is from the Greek root eu for "good." Selye suggested thinking of eustress as euphoria + stress. It is only when stress is poorly managed or becomes overwhelming that the negative effects appear, which is referred to as distress (see Figure 12–2).

Distress refers to the unhealthy, negative, destructive outcomes of stressful events (Quick, Quick, Nelson, & Hurrell, 1997). Distress may have behavioral, physiological, and/or psychological effects on the individual. For example, as early as the 1930s, physiologists were studying the physiologic changes of individuals when confronted with a negative stimulus or environmental change. This is referred to as an individual's "fight-or-flight" response. The fight-or-flight response is when the brain and certain chemicals within the brain cause

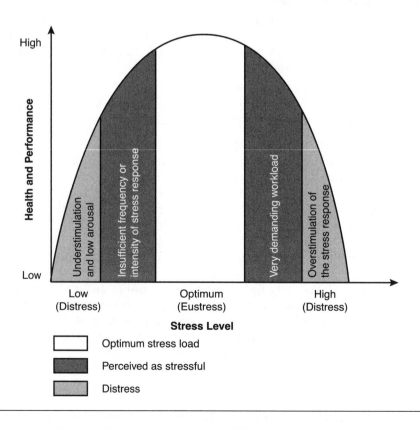

Figure 12–2 Distress–Eustress (An Expanded Yerkes–Dodson Curve)

a reaction to potentially harmful stressors or warnings (e.g., danger, harassment, noise). Selye (1956) studied the physiologic effects of the fight-or-flight response, which resulted in his description of the General Adaptation Syndrome (GAS). GAS describes the three phases an individual undergoes when a stressful situation is encountered: the alarm phase, the resistance phase, and the exhaustion phase.

The first stage of GAS, the alarm phase, is when an individual's fight-or-flight response is elicited for mobilization and geared for a fight or flight. The second stage, resistance, is when the individual fights the stressor and the acute fight-or-flight response ceases. The third stage, exhaustion, is when the individual can no longer adapt to the stressor (Jacobs, 2001).

In the first two stages, alarm and resistance, bodily responses are adaptive and beneficial (see Exhibit 12–1).

Exhibit 12–1 The Physiology Side of Stress

The initial physiological response to stress is the same for all: increased heart rate and blood pressure, followed shortly by sweating and faster breathing. These are a result of the hormonal surge that occurs to prepare us for action. What happens in our body when we perceive a situation as stressful? This requires knowledge of how the nervous system works.

Nervous System

There are two branches of the nervous system. The voluntary system controls conscious movement, whereas the autonomic nervous system (ANS) controls involuntary and automatic bodily activity. It is the latter that is involved in the stress response. The ANS comprises the parasympathetic system, which continuously maintains the resting state of all organs and processes, and the sympathetic system, which is excited mainly in difficult situations. It is the sympathetic system that prepares the body and mind for action through the secretion of hormones.

Stress Hormones

The hormones involved in the stress response include adrenaline, noradrenaline, and cortisol. These are secreted by the adrenal glands. The inner region of the adrenal glands is part of the sympathetic nervous system and the body's first line of defense and response to physical and emotional stress.

Noradrenaline and Adrenaline

Adrenal glands release adrenaline and noradrenaline, at the same time as noradrenaline is being released all over the body as a result of the action of the sympathetic nervous system. These chemical messengers activate two different types of receptors at various sites, preparing the body for action. For example, by activating beta receptors on the heart muscle, they help "it" beat faster and stronger, so it can pump blood containing oxygen and nutrients to the muscles. Their action on the receptors in the walls of the coronary arteries allows the arteries to dilate, allowing more blood and oxygen through to the heart.

Adrenaline prompts an increase in the hormone glucagon, which is responsible for mobilizing glucose normally stored in our muscle and liver as glycogen. This results in a sudden increase in energy for immediate action. Energy, which is not utilized in sedentary situations, contributes to unhealthy fluctuations of blood sugar levels, which has consequences for cardiovascular disease, diabetes, anxiety, and insomnia.

Exhibit 12–1 *(Continued)*

Cortisol

Cortisol is released from the adrenal glands following a sequence of events initiated by the production of corticotropin-releasing hormone in the brain. Cortisol stimulates the production of extra nutrients such as glucose and fatty acids to help cope with the stress. Raised cortisol levels are associated with a suppressed immune system, heart disease, cancer, osteoporosis, and aging.

What Else?

Besides the dominance of the sympathetic nervous system and the release of hormones, other physiological processes occur in response to stress. The digestive system slows and the pituitary gland and brain secrete endorphins to reduce pain. These reactions are part of the survival function, concentrating energy on essential short-term processes, such as heart beating, rather than comparatively unnecessary digestion, and to prepare the body to cope with possible ensuing pain. The latter is why people in accidents and soldiers in battle can suffer injuries but report feeling little discomfort.

Although the physical reactions to stress have evolved for survival purposes, their repeated occurrence in inappropriate situations, such as today's sedentary lifestyle, results in compromised health and ultimately disease.

Physical Reactions	Reasons
Dry mouth	Parasympathetic nervous system inhibited—stops producing saliva
Pounding heart/ fluttering or irregular beats	Sympathetic nervous system causes heart to beat faster and blood pressure rises to enable blood to reach parts of body that need it
Sweating	Cools the body, which in turn allows it to burn more energy
Tense muscles	Muscles contract when they are primed for action. In the absence of action, stiff neck and painful back can be experienced
Tiredness	Depleted energy levels when stress is constant because of the parasympathetic nervous system diverting from the digestive process and storing energy, and the sympathetic nervous system taking over and effectively drawing on stored nutrients
Loose stools/diarrhea/ irritable bowel syndrome (IBS)	Muscle contractions that move food along the gut either slow down, because of the parasympathetic system diverting its actions from digestion, or start working overtime to try and compensate

---

SOURCE: 50plusHealth, Ltd. Available at http://www.50plushealth.co.uk.

It is only in the final stage, exhaustion, that an individual may reflect behavioral, physiological, and/or psychological illnesses. Physiological illnesses may include chronic headaches or fatigue, hypertension, ulcers, and heart disease. Psychological illnesses or the emotional symptoms of stress in the exhaustion stage relate to frustration and/or depression. According to von Onciul (1996), these emotional symptoms are the behavioral consequences of the exhaustion stage, which may include emotional outbursts, violent or anti-social behavior, eating disorders, and general indifference and reduced attention to personal issues such as exercise and appearance. The individual may exhibit other mental dysfunctions in the exhaustion stage, such as the inability to concentrate and poor memory retention. This leads to impaired performance, poor judgment, and indecisiveness, as well as a negative attitude toward life and work, with the possibility of this leading to the misuse of alcohol and drugs (von Onciul, 1996).

Internal or External Stressors / Acute or Chronic

Individuals can experience two categories of stressors: external or internal. External stressors can be physical conditions, such as excessive temperatures, or psychological environments, such as abusive relationships. Internal stressors can be physical illnesses or psychological tendencies, such as an individual's personality type. These stressors can be described as either short-term (acute) or long-term (chronic). Short-term acute stress is the reaction to a real or perceived immediate threat (the fight-or-flight response). Long-term chronic stressors are those that are continuous, such as work pressures, relationship problems, and financial concerns (see Table 12–3).

INDIVIDUALS AND STRESS

Stress comes in all forms and affects all people. Although there are no external standards that can be applied to predict stress levels in individuals, research has provided us with some insight as to those who are more prone to experience higher levels of stress, such as certain personality types, belonging to a minority group, and gender.

Personalities

Drs. Rosenman and Friedman, along with their colleagues (Rosenman, Friedman, Wurm, Jenkins, Messinger, & Strauss, 1966), discovered the first relationship between stress and personality by linking coronary heart disease (CHD) and personality profiles. Starting in the 1950s, the Mount Zion's Harold Brunn Institute studied the role of personality in CHD and found that participants with Type A behavior patterns (TABP), such as aggressiveness, anger/hostility, competitiveness, time urgency, impatience, tenseness, and intense commitment to goals, were at higher risk for developing CHD than people with Type B personality traits (e.g., patient, low-key, noncompetitive) (Young, 1974). Although Type B individuals are equally intelligent and may be just as ambitious as those who are Type A, they approach life in a different way (Quick et al., 1997). Friedman and Rosenman (1974) define TABP as an "action-emotion complex that can be observed in any person who is aggressively involved in a chronic, incessant struggle to achieve more and more in less and less time, and if required to do so, against the opposing efforts of other things or other persons" (p. 84).

Table 12–3 External and Internal Stressors (Acute and/or Chronic)

External	*Internal*
Environment—Noise, poor lighting or bright lights, extreme temperatures of hot or cold, confined spaces, violence and other threats to personal safety, general economy, globalization, technology, war, and terrorism	Lifestyle—Unhealthy lifestyles, such as excessive caffeine, smoking, drinking, drugs, lack of sleep, trying to do too much (e.g., supermom)
Others—Rude, domineering, aggressive, peer pressures, and discrimination	Mental State—Pessimistic, self-critical, self-helplessness, unrealistic expectations, and lack of flexibility
Work—Excessive rules and policies, poor interpersonal relationships, lack of communication, mergers, downsizing, long and/or irregular hours, unrealistic deadlines, retraining, discrimination, and promotion or demotion	Personality—Perfectionist, workaholic, perceived expectation of others and ourselves, and other Type A personality characteristics
Major Life Events—Death of loved one, poor health and/or disability, loss of job, new job, marriage, divorce, bankruptcy or other financial worries, relocation, new baby, caring for aging parents, and pending retirement	
Everyday Hassles—Commuting, misplacing keys or other important items, poor customer service, standing in lines, dealing with teenagers at home	

Recent studies suggest that rather than the entire set of Type A characteristics, only particular dimensions, such as tenseness, may be related to CHD (Kim et al., 1998). For example, Barefort, Dahlstrom, and Williams (1983) found that anger and hostility were the lethal dimensions of TABP when they studied 255 physicians over a 25-year period. At this time, researchers are still unsure what component or components of TABP constitute(s) the greatest factor leading to CHD for Type A individuals.

Another dimension of a person's personality related to stress is the perception of control (Rotter, 1966). Employees with a high need for autonomy and control over their environments, such as the personality traits displayed by Type A individuals, will experience a higher degree of stress when they perceive a lack of control. For example, Kushnir and Kasan (1991) found that high-demand jobs combined with high workload and low perceived control were stressful for Type A but not Type B individuals.

Perceived control is defined as the amount of control that an individual believes he or she has over the environment, whether direct or indirect, to make it less threatening or more rewarding (Ganster & Fusilier, 1989). Within the work setting, this concept is reflected in the extent to which an individual is free to decide how to accomplish a task or the goals of the job. Very low levels of personal control have been found to be psychologically harmful, whereas greater control has been associated with better mental health (Evans & Carrere, 1991; Ganster & Fusilier, 1989). High levels of perceived control have been found to increase an employee's job satisfaction, commitment, and performance (Spector, 1986).

Much of the research on perceived control stems from Robert Karasek's (1979) job demands–decision latitude model. This model proposes that the effects of job demands (psychological stressors in the work environment) on employee well-being are influenced by job decision latitude (i.e., the degree to which the employee has the potential to control his or her work). Karasek found that individuals in occupations with high demands and low decision latitude suffered the most severe psychosomatic complaints and the highest levels of both depression, and job and life dissatisfaction. Other studies have confirmed that employees who perceive they are subject to high demands (job responsibility), but little control over their environment (authority and/or choices) are at increased risk for stress-related illnesses such as cardiovascular disease (Karasek, Baker, Marxer, Ahlbom, & Theorell, 1981). For example, Fox, Dwyer, and Ganster (1993) found that nurses employed in a medium-sized private hospital in the Midwest who experienced high workloads/demands with perceived low controllability showed increased physiological problems and lower attitudinal outcomes (job satisfaction), with the physiological responses continuing after the nurses left work. The researchers suggested that it was not the higher levels of workload or demands, but the nurses' perception of low controllability over the situation that caused the nurses to display symptoms of job stress (i.e., low job satisfaction, high blood pressure, and high cortisol levels).

An employee's sense of loss of control is an important form of emotional stress; therefore, employers need to pay particular attention to this matter in the workplace. Middle managers are among those with the most highly stressed positions as related to the need to respond to others' demands and project deadlines, with little perceived control over their environments. Savery and Hall (1986) relate that "managers are beleaguered by demands not only from their superiors but also from government agencies, from subordinates and union representatives pushing for a greater say in the running of the enterprise, and from community and other interest groups with their many and rising expectations. Many of these demands are also mutually exclusive" (p. 160). Savery and Hall also found that a significant relationship existed between managers' perceived lack of autonomy (i.e., control) in decision making and stress-related illnesses. The researchers further found that middle managers under 30 years of age felt more stress than older managers because of less autonomy, closer supervision, and confusion over lines of authority within the organization.

However, as previously discussed in Chapter 5 with Hackman and Oldman's job design model, a perceived lack of control may not be stressful to some employees. Some employees may want minimum control in their jobs. These employees may not want the increased responsibility that is often connected with greater job autonomy. In such situations, a greater degree of job control would actually have the reverse effect on the employee's well-being.

Minorities

As discussed in Chapter 2, the nation's workforce is becoming more culturally and ethnically diverse. Surprisingly, the literature is limited about the specific impact of workplace diversity on organizations or about the stress that such diversity imposes on members of different cultural and ethnic groups (Keita & Hurrell, 1994; Quick et al., 1997). However, managers need to be attentive to the fact that employees from ethnic minority groups may be more prone to stress than majority (i.e., nonethnic minority) groups because of issues associated with prejudice and discrimination, whether perceived or real, potential language difficulties, and cultural values and attitudes.

Quick et al. (1997) point out that "blatant prejudice is the most obvious source of stress for those in minority ethnic groups" (p. 57). For example, in an early study, Kasschau (1977) found that the "overwhelming majority" of 800 minority survey respondents identified prejudice and discrimination at work. In a more recent national study, Roberts, Swanson, and Murphy (2004) found that American minorities reported perceptions of discrimination at work at greater frequencies than nonminority Americans, and that white, African-, and Hispanic-Americans, who reported that they had been discriminated against, were found to have poorer mental health outcomes than their same-race counterparts, who did not acknowledge being discriminated against.

James, Lovato, and Khoo (1994) argue that differences in cultural values and attitudes between minority workers and majority workers constitute a major source of minority worker stress. For example, Cox, Lobel, and McLeod (1991) found that Asian-American, African-American, and Hispanic-American individuals have a more collectivist orientation than European-Americans (see discussion in Chapter 2, regarding Hofstede's four dimensions of national culture). Therefore, as a minority-culture member shifts from a work role in which he or she attempts to fit in with a majority-culture orientation, increased stress levels may occur because this attempt to fit in, or assimilate, causes a departure from the societal role within his or her collectivist community. Assimilation is the process by which an individual develops a new cultural identity, whereby the individual may eventually lose identification with his or her culture of origin in order to become successful in the dominant culture. Since minority cultures may have a more collectivist orientation, minority members may experience stress as they attempt to assimilate into the majority culture dominating the workplace. As an example, Bell, as cited in Richard and Grimes (1996), found that African-American women who were career-oriented experienced more stress than their counterparts who were community-oriented or family-oriented. Since minority cultures may differ in race, attitudes, and beliefs from the majority culture within an organization, minority members would find the workplace to be more stressful. Richard and Grimes (1996) point out that this is due to the minority members' need to work harder to socialize, or assimilate, into the dominant organizational culture for a significant portion of their day.

Gender

Over the years, research has been conducted on the stress levels of women, and considering that 92 percent of the 4.3 million nurses and nursing aides in the United States are female, healthcare employers need to be sensitive to the work-related stress issues experienced by women. Statistics from Roper Starch Worldwide's Global 2000 Consumer Study of 30,000 people between the ages of 13 and 65 in 30 countries showed that increased stress is felt worldwide, with women consistently reporting being more stressed than men. The most stressed women are: (1) mothers with children under the age of 13, (2) full-time working mothers, and (3) full-time working mothers with children under 13. In addition, one-fourth of women executives and professionals say they feel "superstressed."

A second study, Creating Healthy Corporate Cultures for Both Genders, revealed that stress affects women differently from men (Peterson, 2004). The study indicated that women reported nearly 40 percent more health problems than their male counterparts and noticeably higher stress. Furthermore, Swanson (2000) found that:

- Women face gender-specific work stress, such as sex discrimination and the need to balance work and family demands, in addition to general job stressors such as work overload, lack of control over their job, or underutilization of their skills.
- Barriers to financial and career advancement based on sex discrimination have been linked to more frequent psychological and physical symptoms, such as depression and increased blood pressure.
- Half of all working women will experience on-the-job sexual harassment at some point in their lives, and women who experience sexual harassment report a range of psychological symptoms including depression, anxiety, fearfulness, and feelings of guilt and shame, as well as physical symptoms such as headaches and sleep disorders. Sexual harassment is a particularly noxious stressor for women and has a significant impact on psychological distress and absenteeism beyond that attributable to regular job stressors (77–78).

Burnout

Stress occurs when job requirements do not match the capabilities, resources, or needs of the employee. Studies show that stressful working conditions are associated with increased absenteeism, tardiness, and turnover, which affects an organization's productivity and profitability.

An extreme case of job-related stress is known as burnout. Burnout, first discovered in the 1970s, has been recognized as an occupational hazard for people-oriented professions such as health care, human services, and education (Mashlach & Goldberg, 1998). Burnout symptoms include overwhelming exhaustion, feelings of frustration, anger and cynicism, and a sense of ineffectiveness and failure. Sadly, healthcare professionals have reported substantially higher degrees of burnout than managers not employed in the healthcare industry (Golembiewski & Boudreau, 1991).

Maslach and Jackson (1981) identified three dimensions associated with burnout: emotional exhaustion, depersonalization, and diminished personal accomplishment.

- Emotional exhaustion results in apathy and loss of concern, a feeling that one has reached the "end of the rope." As emotional resources are depleted, healthcare professionals feel they cannot give of themselves at an emotional or psychological level.

- Depersonalization is characterized by the development of negative and cynical attitudes toward the workplace, as well as toward people with whom the employee interacts (patients and coworkers). Individuals distance themselves and see others as things or objects.

- Diminished personal accomplishment is characterized by the tendency to evaluate oneself negatively, including viewing oneself as performing poorly in the job—a job that is viewed as having no worth or meaning (low professional efficacy).

Golembiewski and his associates (1986; 1990; Golembiewski & Boss, 1991; Golembiewski & Boudreau, 1991) studied over 13,000 managers and healthcare professionals regarding burnout. The researchers found that varying degrees of burnout existed, with healthcare workers experiencing the most advanced phases (Golembiewski & Boudreau, 1991). As illustrated in Table 12–4, Golembiewski's phase model suggests that employees who are suffering from burnout first experience depersonalization, which induces feelings of inadequacy, followed by diminishing personal accomplishment, and ending with emotional exhaustion. Golembiewski and Boudreau relate that employ-

Table 12–4 Golembiewski's Phases of Burnout

Dimensions of Burnout	Phase I	Phase II	Phase III	Phase IV	Phase V	Phase VI	Phase VII	Phase VIII
Depersonalization	Lo	Hi	Lo	Hi	Lo	Hi	Lo	Hi
Personal Accomplishment (reversed)	Lo	Lo	Hi	Hi	Lo	Lo	Hi	Hi
Emotional Exhaustion	Lo	Lo	Lo	Lo	Hi	Hi	Hi	Hi

SOURCE: "The epidemiology of progressive burnout: A primer," by R. T. Golembiewski, 1986. *Journal of Health and Human Services Administration, 8*(1), p. 18. Reprinted with permission.

ees show growing deficits or deficiencies as they move from phase to phase, such as:

- Broad ranges of perceptions or attitudes about the worksite deteriorate; for example, satisfaction and job involvement fall and tension at work increases.
- Performance appraisals tend to decrease.
- Physical symptoms increase.
- Turnover grows.
- Self-esteem falls.
- Various clinical indicators of mental health deteriorate.
- Declining quality of social and emotional life at work; for example, group cohesiveness is down and social support falls.

In support of Golembiewski's phase model, Kalliath, O'Driscoll, Gillespie, and Bluedorn (2000) found that nurses, laboratory technicians, and managers employed by a general community hospital in an urban Midwest city who reported higher levels of burnout experienced (1) decreased job satisfaction, (2) decreased satisfaction with interpersonal relationships, and (3) lower levels of organizational commitment reflected by either job turnover or increased intentions to leave their jobs.

As previously noted, symptoms of burnout may include lower job performance and satisfaction, higher job tension and turnover, and increased absenteeism. However, increased absenteeism is not always an indicator that an employee may be suffering from burnout. A new buzzword is "presenteeism," which occurs when employees show up for work but are less productive because of illness. A study of 29,000 US employees estimated that absenteeism and presenteeism cost US industry more than $60 billion a year and that more than three-fourths of lost productivity is explained by presenteeism, not by absenteeism (Stewart, Ricci, Chee, Morganstein, & Lipton, 2003). Dow Chemical Company estimates that presenteeism is its largest health-related economic impact, ahead of absenteeism, health insurance, and workers' compensation (Berry, Mirabito & Berwick, 2004).

CAUSES OF WORKPLACE STRESS

Workplace stress can be related to: (1) individual task demands, (2) individual role demands, (3) group demands, and (4) organizational demands (Kinicki & Williams, 2003) (see Table 12–5).

- Individual task demands would include unrealistic deadlines, fear of failure, new technology, lack of necessary resources (e.g., poor physical work environment, such as noise, heat, and crowding), work overload, lack of control, and repetitive, unchallenging work (work underload).
- Individual role demands include job ambiguity, role conflict, and difficulty balancing work and family life.

Table 12–5 Job Stressors

Categories of Job Stressors	Examples
Individual Task Demands (factors unique to the job)	• Workload (overload and underload) • Pace/variety/meaningfulness of work • Autonomy (e.g., the ability to make your own decisions about your own job or about specific tasks) • Shiftwork/hours of work • Physical environment (noise, air quality, etc.) • Isolation at the workplace (emotional or working alone)
Individual Role Demands (role in the organization)	• Role conflict (conflicting job demands, multiple supervisors or managers) • Role ambiguity (lack of clarity about responsibilities, expectations, etc.) • Level of responsibility • Difficulties balancing work and personal lives
Group Demands	• Relationships at work with supervisors, coworkers, and subordinates • Threat of violence, harassment, etc. (threats to personal safety) • Lack of participation in decision making • Inappropriate leadership/management styles (autocratic vs. participatory)
Organizational Demands (including organizational structure and climate)	• Management/leadership styles • Communication patterns • Career development opportunities (under-/overpromotion) • Job security • Unplanned change • Overall job satisfaction

SOURCE: "Occupational stress management: Current status and future directions," by L. R. Murphy, 1995. In C. L. Cooper and D. M. Rousseau (Eds.), *Trends in organizational behavior* (Vol. 2, pp. 1–14). New Jersey: John Wiley & Sons. Reprinted with permission.

- Group demands include poor interpersonal relationships with coworkers and/or supervisors, inadequate support, and lack of participation in decisions.
- Organizational demands encompass politics, communication problems, excess rules and regulations, organizational structure and culture, lack of career development activities, and change without clear strategic direction.

How these various demands can affect employees' stress levels is illustrated in Case Study 12–1.

Case Study 12–1 Stress in Today's Workplace

The longer he waited, the more David worried. For weeks he had been plagued by aching muscles, loss of appetite, restless sleep, and a complete sense of exhaustion. At first he tried to ignore these problems, but eventually he became so short-tempered and irritable that his wife insisted he get a checkup. Now, sitting in his primary care physician's office and wondering what the verdict would be, he didn't even notice when Theresa took the seat beside him. They had been good friends when she worked in the billing office at the drug manufacturing facility, but he hadn't seen her since she left three years ago to take a job as a member service representative at a local health maintenance organization. Her gentle poke in the ribs brought him around, and within minutes they were talking and gossiping as if she had never left.

"You got out just in time," he told her. "Since the reorganization, nobody feels safe. It used to be that as long as you did your work, you had a job. That's not for sure anymore. They expect the same production rates even though two people are now doing the work of three. We're so backed up I'm working 12-hour shifts six days a week. I swear I hear those machines humming in my sleep. Employees are calling in sick just to get a break. Morale is so bad they're talking about bringing in some consultants to figure out a better way to get the job done."

"Well, I really miss everyone," she said. "I'm afraid I jumped from the frying pan into the fire. In my new job, the computer routes the calls and they never stop. I even have to schedule my bathroom breaks. All I hear the whole day are complaints from unhappy members. I try to be helpful and sympathetic, but I can't promise anything without getting my supervisor's approval. Most of the time I'm caught between what the member wants and company policy. I'm not sure who I'm supposed to keep happy. The other reps are so uptight and tense they don't even talk to one another. We all go to our own little cubicles and stay there until quitting time. To make matters worse, my mother's health is deteriorating. If only I could use some of my sick time to look after her. No wonder I'm in here with migraine headaches and high blood pressure. A lot of the reps are seeing the employee assistance counselor and taking stress management classes, which seems to help. But sooner or later, someone will have to make some changes in the way the place is run."

Job Conditions That May Lead to Stress

The Design of Tasks: Heavy workload, infrequent rest breaks, long work hours, and shiftwork; hectic and routine tasks that have little inherent meaning, do not utilize workers' skills, and provide little sense of control.

Example: David works to the point of exhaustion. Theresa is tied to the computer, allowing little room for flexibility, self-initiative, or rest.

Management Style: Lack of participation by workers in decision making, poor communication in the organization, lack of family-friendly policies.

Example: Theresa needs to get her supervisor's approval for everything, and her employer is insensitive to her family needs.

Interpersonal Relationship: Poor social environment and lack of support or help from coworkers and supervisors.

Example: Theresa's physical isolation reduces her opportunities to interact with her coworkers or receive help from them.

Work Roles: Conflicting or uncertain job expectations, too much responsibility, too many "hats to wear."

Example: Theresa is often caught in a difficult situation trying to satisfy both the member's needs and her employer's expectations.

Career Concerns: Job insecurity and lack of opportunity for growth, advancement, or promotion; rapid changes for which workers are unprepared.

Example: Since the reorganization at the hospital equipment manufacturing facility, everyone, including David, is worried about their future with the company and what will happen next.

Environmental Conditions: Unpleasant or dangerous physical conditions such as crowding, noise, air pollution, or ergonomic problems.

Example: David is exposed to constant noise at work.

SOURCE: Adapted from "Stress at Work,".DHHS (NIOSH) Publication No. 99-101, 1999. Washingto, DC: National Institute for Occupational Safety and Health.

COPING WITH STRESS

Coping with stress at work can be defined as "an effort by a person or an organization to manage and overcome demands and critical events that pose a challenge, threat, harm or loss to that person and that person's functioning or to the organization as a whole" (Schwarzer, 2004, p. 342). Coping is considered as one of the top skills inherent in effective managers. With population samples from business, education, health care, and state governments, Whetton and Cameron (1993) identified 402 effective managers on the basis of responses from peers and superiors. Responses from the participants revealed that coping with stress was second on a list of 10 skills attributed to effective managers.

Stress is inevitable, but the degree of experienced stress can be modified in two ways: by changing the environment and/or by changing the individual. This is referred to as stress management. Stress management can refer to a narrow set of individual-level interventions (e.g., relaxation training, biofeedback, meditation) or a broader meaning that includes any type of stress intervention (Murphy, 1995). However, for stress management interventions to be successful, they need to target characteristics of the individual worker, the job, and the organization.

Schwarzer (2004) provides managers with a model using four perspectives for assisting themselves and others to cope with job-related stress (refer to Figure 12–3). The distinction between each perspective is based on time-related stress appraisals and on the perceived certainty of critical events or demands. The four perspectives are: (1) reactive coping, (2) anticipatory coping, (3) preventive coping, and (4) proactive coping.

- Reactive coping refers to efforts to deal with a stressful encounter that is either ongoing or has already happened, such as a job loss or demotion.
- Anticipatory coping pertains to efforts to deal with an inevitable event that is certain to occur in the near future, such as public speaking, a job interview, or downsizing.
- Preventive coping refers to an effort to "build up" resistance resources, whereby the level of stress felt by an individual is reduced (minimizing severity of impact) if a critical event should occur in the future. For example, an individual returns to school to earn a master's degree in health administration or completes the requirements to become a board-certified healthcare executive in case of a possible job loss due to a merger or buyout.

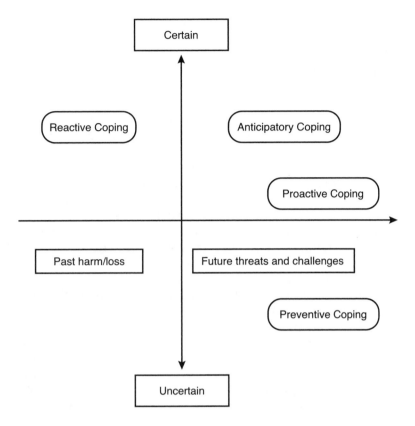

Figure 12–3 Four Coping Perspectives

- Proactive coping is defined as an effort to "build up" general resources that facilitate movement toward challenging goals and personal growth, such as hardiness training and learned optimism (Schwarzer, 2004).

Schwarzer (2004) points out, "The distinction between these four perspectives of coping is highly useful because it moves the individual's focus away from mere responses to negative events towards a broader range of risk and goal management that includes the active creation of opportunities and the positive experience of stress" (p. 349).

ORGANIZATIONAL COPING STRATEGIES

At the organizational level, when reactive or anticipatory coping occur, managers' efforts are involved with reducing the harm or loss to the organization. Managers are concerned with putting out fires as opposed to using their efforts to develop and implement preventive and proactive coping strategies, which are more beneficial for both the organization and the employee. For example, preventive coping is called for when no specific event is envisioned but a more general threat in the distance comes into view, such as an economic decline, a potential merger or downsizing, an aging workforce, or new technology (Schwarzer, 2004).

The healthcare industry is using preventive coping strategies regarding the envisioned future shortage of healthcare leaders due to an aging workforce. For example, among its 191 hospitals, HCA, Inc., anticipates that many of its baby boom–generation chief executive officers (CEOs) will retire within the next 10 years. Furthermore, given the likelihood that those vacancies will be filled by incumbent chief operating officers (COOs), HCA anticipates that it will face a hospital leadership gap at the COO level. To address this challenge proactively, HCA created an intensive COO development program. This program is a development-in-place approach whereby the program is not supplemental to the duties of a regular hospital job, but instead individuals are hired by HCA for the sole purpose of participating in the program with the goal of developing critical, advanced executive-level skills. Participants are given the title of "associate administrator" and assigned to an HCA hospital. The current CEO of the hospital serves as the associate administrator's mentor and superior over a two- to four-year period. After successfully completing the development program, the associate administrator would be promoted to COO for one of HCA's hospitals (HCA, 2004).

Preventive and proactive coping are also referred to as primary prevention or organizational prevention (Quick et al., 1997). Organizational prevention is designed to enhance an employee's health and performance at work by eliminating the stressors that lead to distress. These methods include modifying work demands and improving relationships in the workplace (Schwarzer, 2004). Anticipatory coping is related to secondary prevention; the goal is changing individual stress responses to necessary demands. Reactive coping may be referred to as tertiary prevention, which attempts to minimize the amount of individual and organizational distress that results when organizational stressors and resulting stress responses have not been adequately controlled (Quick et al., 1997) (see Figure 12–4).

To illustrate these coping concepts, consider the following: A physician displays inappropriate behavior* toward a nurse (a stressor), which leads to the nurse experiencing anxiety (a stress response), and in turn, the nurse resigns (an organizational consequence of distress). Primary prevention would attempt to eliminate the stressor by the hospital establishing a zero-tolerance policy regarding inappropriate physician behavior (preventive and/or proactive coping). Secondary prevention would address the problem by providing programs to improve interpersonal relations between physicians and nurses (anticipatory coping). These programs may include improving team building and communication skills, whereby the physician recognizes that nurses are an integral part of the patient's healthcare team and, as such, interactions are based on mutual respect and trust. Tertiary prevention might include establishing an employee assistance program designed to assist nurses to cope with confrontational behavior that may be displayed by physicians.

---

*Inappropriate physician behavior may be defined as "any inappropriate behavior, confrontation or conflict, including verbal abuse to physical and sexual harassment" (Rosenstein, 2002, p. 26).

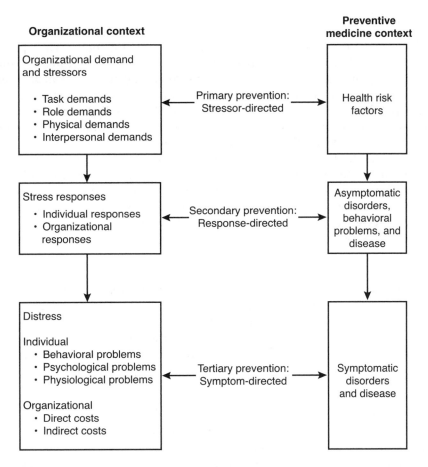

Figure 12–4 Stages of Preventive Stress Management

The preceding example is based on a recent study that linked inappropriate physician behavior with nurses leaving the nursing profession. Rosenstein (2002) surveyed 1,200 nurses, physicians, and executive administrators at several hospitals affiliated with VHA, a national network of community-owned hospitals and healthcare systems, to assess how these disparate groups viewed nurse–physician relationships, disruptive physician behavior, the institutional response to such behavior, and how such behavior affected nurse satisfaction, morale, and retention.

Rosenstein found that daily interactions between nurses and physicians strongly influence nurses' morale. All respondents indicated that they were concerned with the significance of nurse–physician relationships, and over 90 percent of all respondents reported witnessing disruptive physician behavior and that they saw a direct link between this disruptive behavior and nurse satisfaction and retention. In addition, 30 percent of the nurse respondents reported knowing at least one colleague who had resigned because of disruptive physician behavior.

Work Setting

As discussed previously, an employee's work setting may create physical stress because of noise, lack of privacy, poor lighting or ventilation, and so forth. As such, an organization should redesign employees' physical settings to minimize distressful effects (i.e., primary preventive and proactive coping). For example, Williams (2003) found that the odds of feeling stress because of fear of accident or injury were 7.2 times higher for employees working in health occupations than those in the management, business, finance, or science fields. This high source of workplace stress by healthcare workers may be caused by their constant exposure to risk of infection, long hours, and irregular shifts. Other studies have shown that the creation of pleasant and suitable work areas can elevate an employee's job satisfaction, job safety, and mental health, which indirectly may improve job performance.

Job Design

Another important component of reducing work-related stress is job design. Proper job design accommodates an employee's mental and physical abilities. According to the MFL Occupational Health Centre (2000), a Canadian community health center whose mission is to improve workplace health and safety conditions and eliminate hazards, employers can better design jobs by:

- Clearly defining jobs and responsibilities that reduce role conflict and/or role ambiguity;
- Giving workers a say in how they do their jobs;
- Giving workers opportunities to learn new skills;
- Allowing time for social interactions among workers;
- Making work schedules flexible for responsibilities outside of work;
- Clearly communicating about job security;
- Training managers to apply participative-management styles as part of a culture that emphasizes open communication, support, and mutual respect;
- Implementing effective performance-management systems with clear expectations and procedures that are understood by managers and staff;
- Ensuring that effective change management accompanies organizational change (see Chapters 17 and 18 of this text regarding change management).

INDIVIDUAL COPING STRATEGIES

At the individual level, one of the most well-documented techniques for reducing stress is through the relaxation response (see Exhibit 12–2). However, relaxation is a reactive coping strategy as a result of an individual's appraisal of a threat or harm/loss situation such as failing to meet a work goal, conflict with a colleague or supervisor, or job loss. Reactive coping strategies do very little if anything to solve the underlying problems; therefore, employees need to learn to use preventive and proactive coping strategies so

Exhibit 12–2 How To De-stress

One of the most well-documented techniques for reducing stress is through the relaxation response, a term coined by Dr. Herbert Benson of Harvard Medical School to describe a state of deep, mindful rest that offsets the physical effects of stress by lowering heart rate, blood pressure, and breathing rate. The relaxation response can be elicited at any time and in any place by sitting comfortably with your eyes closed, breathing slowly, letting your muscles relax, and repeating a certain word, sound, phrase, or prayer for 10 minutes while disregarding all other thoughts. The slow, repetitive movements and meditative thoughts involved in activities such as yoga and T'ai Chi have also been found to evoke a similar physiological response, which in turn can help you to think more rationally about your own predicament and how you can work to improve it.

SOURCE: Optimistic People Live Longer, January 2003. *Tufts University Health and Nutrition Letter, 20*(11), pp. 4–5.

---

that the fight-or-flight response is not automatically engaged at the first sign of stress (Schwarzer, 2004).

Friedman (1999) suggests training employees to cope with stressful situations by improving their abilities for problem solving and conflict resolution, and developing their leadership skills. For example, when an employee is facing a stressful episode due to increasing workload, he or she can be trained beforehand how to delegate tasks, use good time management skills, and increase his or her social support system. In addition, employees need to learn how to maintain a healthy balance between work, family, and leisure activities, although this may be a difficult process for workaholics and individuals displaying other Type A personality characteristics. It is known that healthy lifestyles (e.g., nutrition and exercise) provide a protective shield against the experience of stress (Schwarzer, 2004). In addition, the use of learned optimism and hardiness training has been shown to be successful in assisting employees to reinterpret perceived threats (i.e., stressful events) into challenges, thereby transforming distress into eustress.

Learned Optimism

From extensive research throughout his career as a psychologist, Martin Seligman (1991) developed the concept of learned optimism and applied it directly to workplace productivity. According to Seligman, when pessimistic people run into obstacles in the workplace, they give up. However, when optimistic people encounter obstacles, they try harder. Seligman's learned optimism theory suggests that people can learn optimism by undoing pessimistic thinking by recognizing and then disputing negative thoughts and beliefs.

Optimism is not the same as the popular concept of "positive thinking." Optimists and pessimists attribute the reasons for success and failure differently. Drawing on attribution theory (see Chapter 7), Seligman (1991) refers to how a person interprets events as his or her explanatory style. Seligman identified three primary elements of an individual's explanatory style: stability, globality, and locus of control.

- Stability refers to whether the event's outcomes are temporary or permanent. For example, if the outcome is negative, the optimist tends to think it's an isolated incident. If the outcomes are positive, the optimist tends to think they will reoccur in the future. On the other hand, the pessimist views positive outcomes as a "one time event" and negative outcomes as more likely to occur in the future.

- Globality refers to whether the event's outcomes are specific to this one situation or whether the outcomes apply to everything in a person's life. For example, when a positive event occurs, the optimist is more likely to extend it to his or her whole life. With a negative event, the optimist will tend to isolate the incident as specific to that situation. The opposite holds true for the pessimist: Positive events are viewed as "stroke of luck," and negative events are viewed as representative of his or her whole life.

- Locus of control refers to whether the individual believes the outcome is attributable to his or her actions or to factors in the environment. For example, when a positive event occurs, the optimist attributes his or her success to his or her efforts. With a negative event, the optimist looks to causes outside of his or her control to explain the outcome, such as bad luck, whereas the pessimist will view positive events as attributable to luck, other people's hard work, or something else outside of his or her control, and will view negative events as being caused by his or her personal deficiencies.

Pessimists tend to attribute failure and negative events to permanent, personal, and pervasive factors. Optimists tend to attribute bad events to nonpersonal, nonpermanent, and nonpervasive factors. They attribute their failures to causes that are temporary rather than stable, specific to the attainment of a particular goal rather than all their goals, and see the problem as a result of the environment or setting they are in, rather than being inherent in themselves. Optimists have high self-efficacy; as such, they view setbacks, obstacles, and a noncontingent environment as challenges that provide excitement in their life (Seligman & Csikszentmihalyi, 2000). The opposite is true for pessimists. Pessimists see no relationship between their actions and goal attainment. Their low outcome expectancy causes deficits in future learning as well as motivational disturbances such as procrastination and depression (Seligman, 1991). Thus, even when the situation changes so that they can exert control over their environment so as to make progress toward their goal, pessimists do not try to do so, because they have learned that giving up is a rational response. This is because their attribution leads to what is referred to as learned helplessness (see Exhibit 12–3) (Seligman, 1991). An individual's habitual blaming of oneself undermines self-efficacy (Bandura, 1997).

Optimism may serve as a buffer against the physiological effects of stress. Research suggests that the immune function in optimists is better than in pessimists. It is not that optimists experience fewer stressful situations than pessimists; they are just more adept at coping with such situations so they can

Exhibit 12–3 Learned Helplessness

Helplessness is a learned condition that has a negative impact on an individual's physical, emotional, mental, and spiritual well-being. As explained in Chapter 7, learned helplessness is a phenomenon in which people experience failure at a task, often numerous times. They determine that the task cannot be accomplished, at least not by them; as such they stop trying. They internalize their failures (self-blame) and develop a helpless attitude.

A study on learned helplessness looked at stress levels in two groups subjected to the same loud and unpleasant noise. One group was given a button that could turn the noise off, while the second group was not given the same option. The subjects who were denied control over the noise experienced significant stress and called the noise "unbearable." The first group that had the option of turning off the noise only considered the noise "unpleasant," but chose not to turn off the sound. Just knowing that they had the option of turning the noise off was enough.

Following the sound session, the researchers observed that the group that had been subjected to helplessness in the noise experiment tended to act helpless in subsequent situations, whereas the group that had been given control to turn off the noise in the experiment looked for and chose to exercise control over subsequent situations. Both helplessness and empowerment are learned conditions. Once learned, they are extended into other areas of life.

work through the problems and develop solutions rather than feeling helpless or like victims.

Hardiness Training

The hardiness concept has been applied frequently to prevent and alleviate stress at work (Schwarzer, 2004). The HardiTraining® program (see The Hardiness Institute, Inc. at www.hardinessinstitute.com) comprises building an employee's attitudes of commitment, control, and challenge.

- Commitment refers to an individual's belief that involving oneself in life changes is the way to deepen meaning and purpose. Individuals high in commitment immerse themselves in a proactive coping process that transforms the stressfulness of a problem so that it becomes manageable and growth promoting.

- Control refers to one's belief that if he or she tries, he or she can positively influence much of what happens in his or her life. An individual maintains that even when a personal or professional problem has unchangeable aspects to it, if he or she is resourceful, there are ways to use the stressful circumstance as an opportunity for new learning. By constructively influencing outcomes, a person strengthens his or her view of oneself as capable, hardy, and a participant in the world.

- Challenge refers to an individual's attitude that everything that happens to him or her, whether negative or positive, is an opportunity to enhance one's performance, leadership, morale, conduct, and health.

Individuals high in HardiAttitudes® engage fully in their personal and work life, use life changes to promote learning and renewal, and report greater life meaning, purpose, and satisfaction (Maddi, 1998). HardiTraining® outcome studies have demonstrated their effectiveness in strengthening one's ability to resist the stressful impact of personal and professional changes.

Stress Management Programs

Organizations are developing comprehensive health promotion strategies for their employees, which include various types of individual-level stress management programs (Schwarzer, 2004). Stress management programs often consist of breathing and stretching exercises, yoga, meditation, and/or massage. The programs' goals are to lessen the adrenaline response to minor stress. For example, St. Paul Fire and Marine Insurance Company conducted several studies on the effects of stress-prevention programs in hospital settings. Program activities included (1) employee and management education on job stress, (2) changes in hospital policies and procedures to reduce organizational sources of stress, and (3) establishment of employee-assistance programs. In one study, the frequency of medication errors declined by 50 percent after prevention activities were implemented in a 700-bed hospital. In a second study, there was a 70 percent reduction in malpractice claims in 22 hospitals that implemented stress-prevention activities. In contrast, there was no reduction in claims in a matched group of 22 hospitals that did not implement stress-prevention activities (Jones, Barge, Steffy, Fay, Kuntz, & Wuebker, 1988).

Another example is Baptist Health South Florida. Baptist Health, the largest nonprofit healthcare organization in South Florida, provides a holistic approach to the well-being of its staff. The organization sponsors a healthy lifestyle program for its employees, called the Wellness Advantage. On-site fitness coaches are available to employees at each of the system's six hospital fitness centers to provide screening and personal training. Discounts are offered to employees who choose the designated "healthy" meals in the system's cafeterias. For those facing life-threatening illnesses, the system offers flexible, reduced scheduling so that staff can maintain some level of employment during stressful times. Senior management believes that the organization's success, as measured by patient satisfaction, physician satisfaction, employee satisfaction, clinical outcomes, and operating profits, is directly owed to the "healthy" infrastructure of its employees. Baptist Health's commitment to its employees is recognized nationally. The American Association of Retired Persons has recognized Baptist Health's longtime commitment to its employees by naming the health system one of the Best Employers for Workers over 50 for the past three years (May, 2004).

Crampton and colleagues (1995) related that stress management programs need to contribute to the goals and needs of both the organization and the individual. Organizations need to believe that the benefits of stress management programs outweigh their costs. Employees need to perceive that they will benefit from stress management programs or they will not voluntarily participate. To meet both organizational and individual goals, Crampton and colleagues provide the following recommendations:

Preventive and/or Proactive Coping (primary prevention)

1. Identify the major stressors in the workplace and assess which ones are controllable. Organizations should do more than simply provide stress management techniques. If the causes of stress can be reduced or elimi-

nated, they should be. Organizational-level strategies might include redesigning employees' jobs, improving the selection, placement, and orientation of new employees, providing employees with more participation and autonomy in decision making, disseminating information, providing needed education and training, reducing workloads or the work pace, modifying work schedules to be compatible with demands and responsibilities outside of work, conducting time management programs, clearly defining work roles, providing opportunities for career development, and providing emotional and task support.

2. Communicate with employees about the benefits of stress management. Explain what stress is, along with the health implications of excess stress or distress. Employees should be encouraged to lead healthier lives by lowering their stress on the job as well as at home.

Anticipatory Coping (secondary prevention)

1. Assist employees to identify their stressors and stress-tolerance levels. Before learning how to deal with stress, employees first have to identify those stressors they react to, because not everyone responds the same way to the same stressors. To aid this process, organizations might provide health-risk appraisals that test for their employees' levels of stress.

2. Develop individualized stress management programs that meet the needs of the organization's employees. Programs should be topic-specific and implemented in stages. If all aspects of a program are implemented at one time and parts of the program fail, employees will lose faith in the program and in management. This will be another cause of anxiety and stress for the employee. Stress management programs may include learning relaxation and meditation techniques, developing a good support system, undertaking outside hobbies, learning to set realistic goals, developing time management skills, and learning when to say "no" before taking on more than they can handle.

3. Communicate with employees. Providing more information about their jobs and other factors that affect them will help employees feel more in control of their circumstances and can help build cohesion. Organizations must also communicate and describe the stress management strategies available to employees and help them develop personalized action plans.

Reactive Coping (tertiary prevention)

1. Make sure employees learn to recognize symptoms of distress. For example, symptoms may include gastrointestinal problems, rapid pulse, frequent illness, insomnia, persistent fatigue, irritability, lack of concentration, and increased use of alcohol and/or drugs. Common methods used to help identify stressors and symptoms include self-report measures (e.g., interviews and surveys), behavioral measures (e.g., observation and performance measures), and physiological stress measures (e.g., heart rate and blood pressure).

2. Exercise and maintaining a nutritious diet are two of the most agreed-upon stress management techniques. Organizations can help employees by providing information and access to physical recreation facilities or equipment by either establishing on-site facilities or providing memberships to

local health clubs. One type of organizational stress management program available is to provide employees with access to an employee assistance program, a corporate psychologist, a toll-free hotline, or some other form of counseling assistance. These programs can deal with a variety of problems that range from learning to cope to dealing with substance abuse.

3. Assist employees to keep a positive perspective on life and feel a sense of purpose. It is important for employees to feel they are making a valuable contribution to the organization.

SUMMARY

Stress has become a widely used but misunderstood term. As a result, a number of misconceptions about stress exist. The first misconception is that all stress is negative. A certain degree of stress is necessary for good mental and physical health; it can be viewed as positive or constructive stress, which compels us to act with optimum performance, whereby we achieve our goals. The second misconception is that nothing can be done to eliminate or diminish workplace distress. Organizations and individuals can use preventive or proactive coping strategies (primary prevention) to change negative events into positive experiences and growth opportunities.

In the past, the phrase "healthy organization" almost always denoted a firm's financial health. But recent studies of "healthy organizations" suggest that policies benefiting workers' health also benefit the organization's bottom line. Today, the healthy organization means not only financial soundness but also the physical and mental well-being of those who make up the organization—its employees. Healthy employees create stronger businesses and healthier profits (Berry, Mirabito, & Berwick, 2004).

END-OF-CHAPTER DISCUSSION QUESTIONS

1. Define what stress means and the difference between eustress and distress.
2. Discuss the various components of Schwarzer's Phase Model of Stress and Coping.
3. Discuss the negative effects of distress from both an organizational and individual perspective.
4. Describe the various forms of stress.
5. Describe the three stages of the General Adaptation Syndrome and positive and negative effects that occur within each stage.
6. Discuss why personalities, ethnicity, and gender may affect an individual's level of stress.
7. Discuss the symptoms of burnout using Golembiewski's phase model.
8. Discuss the four categories of causes of stress in the workplace.
9. Discuss and provide examples of the various coping strategies available to organizations and individuals.

10. Discuss the concept of learned optimism and how it relates to coping with stress by individuals.

11. Discuss the concept of hardiness training and how it relates to coping with stress by individuals.

12. Discuss what is meant by the term "stress management" and available interventions for organizations and individuals.

Case Study 12–2 Scott's Dilemma—Revisited

Scott is a licensed physical therapist who works for a national rehabilitation company. The rehabilitation facility in which Scott works is located in an urban Southwest city. He has worked at this facility for four years, and up until recently was satisfied with his working environment and the interactions he shared with his coworkers. In addition, Scott received personal fulfillment from helping his patients recover from their disabilities and seeing them return to productive lives.

Last year the health system went through reorganization with some new people being brought in and others reassigned. Scott's new boss, George, was transferred from one of the system's Midwest facilities. Almost immediately upon taking his new position, George began finding fault with Scott's care plans, patient interactions, and so on. Scott began feeling as if he couldn't do anything right. He was experiencing feelings of anxiety, stress, and self-blame. Although his previous performance evaluations had been above average, Scott was shocked by his first performance review under George's authority—it was an extremely low rating.

Scott began trying to work harder, thinking that by working harder he could exceed George's expectations. Despite Scott's working long hours and addressing George's critiques, George continued to find fault with Scott's work. Staff meetings began to be a great source of discomfort and stress because George would belittle Scott and single him out in front of his colleagues.

Scott began to feel alienated from his family, friends, and colleagues at work. His eating and sleeping habits were adversely affected as well. Scott's activities held no joy for him anymore and the career that he once loved and been respected in became a source of pain and stress. He began to call in sick more often and started visualizing himself confronting and even hurting George, which created even more guilt and anxiety for Scott.

As time went on, George encouraged Scott's coworkers to leave Scott alone to do his work. The perception of the coworkers became more sympathetic to George's point of view. Scott's coworkers mused that perhaps Scott really was a poor worker and that George knew better because of his position as the supervisor of the rehabilitation department. Eventually, Scott's coworkers began to distance themselves from him, in order to protect their own interests. They began to see Scott as an outsider, with whom it was unsafe to associate.

In an effort to resolve the situation, Scott spoke to George directly, stating his feelings and expressing an interest in how they might improve the situation. Rather than making the situation better, what George perceived as Scott's insubordination served to enrage George, and the personal attacks against Scott intensified. Feeling frustrated and helpless, Scott then decided to take his problem to the Human Resources Department (HRD). A human resources manager listened to Scott's complaints and suggested that Scott return with documentation evidence of what Scott perceived to be George's mistreatment. In an effort to help ease the situation, the HRD manager discussed the issue with George, which only stirred the flames of George's anger and his negative behavior toward Scott.

As a last resort, Scott decided to go to George's boss, Rebecca. Rebecca met with George to get his side of the story. George portrayed Scott as an unproductive employee with no respect for authority. The result was a strong letter of reprimand in Scott's file for insubordination.

Discuss the symptoms of stress that Scott is experiencing. What recommendations can you make to Scott for coping with his stress?

SOURCE: Case discussion: Workplace bully, by J. Pinto, M. Vecchione, & L. Howard, October 2004. Presented at the 12th Annual International Conference of the Association on Employment Practices and Principles, Ft. Lauderdale, FL. Reprinted with permission.

Exhibit 12–4 How Vulnerable Are You to Stress?

In modern society, most of us can't avoid stress. But we can learn to behave in ways that lessen its effects. Researchers have identified a number of factors that affect one's vulnerability to stress—among them are eating and sleeping habits, caffeine and alcohol intake, and how we express our emotions. The following questionnaire is designed to help you discover your vulnerability quotient and to pinpoint trouble spots. Rate each item from 1 (always) to 5 (never), according to how much of the time the statement is true of you. Be sure to mark each item, even if it does not apply to you; for example, if you don't smoke, circle 1 next to item six.

	Always	Sometimes	Never
1. I eat at least one hot, balanced meal a day.	① 2	3 4	5
2. I get seven to eight hours of sleep at least four nights a week.	① 2	3 4	5
3. I give and receive affection regularly.	① 2	3 4	5
4. I have at least one relative within 50 miles, on whom I can rely.	① 2	3 4	5
5. I exercise to the point of perspiration at least twice a week.	① 2	3 4	5
6. I limit myself to less than half a pack of cigarettes a day.	① 2	3 4	5
7. I take fewer than five alcohol drinks a week.	① 2	3 4	5
8. I am the appropriate weight for my height.	① 2	3 4	5
9. I have an income adequate to meet basic expenses.	1 2	3 4	⑤
10. I get strength from my religious beliefs.	1 2	3 4	5
11. I regularly attend club or social activities.	① 2	3 4	5
12. I have a network of friends and acquaintances.	① 2	3 4	5
13. I have one or more friends to confide in about personal matters.	① 2	3 4	5
14. I am in good health (including eyesight, hearing, teeth).	① 2	3 4	5
15. I am able to speak openly about my feelings when angry or worried.	① 2	3 4	5
16. I have regular conversations with the people I live with about domestic problems, for example, chores and money.	① 2	3 4	5
17. I do something for fun at least once a week.	① 2	3 4	5
18. I am able to organize my time effectively.	① 2	3 4	5
19. I drink fewer than three cups of coffee (or other caffeine-rich drinks) a day.	① 2	3 4	5
20. I take some quiet time for myself during the day.	① 2	3 4	5

To get your score, add up the figures and subtract 20. A score below 10 indicates excellent resistance to stress. A score over 30 indicates some vulnerability to stress; you are seriously vulnerable if your score is over 50. You can make yourself less vulnerable by reviewing the items on which you scored three or higher and trying to modify them. Notice that nearly all of them describe situations and behaviors over which you have a great deal of control. Concentrate first on those that are easiest to change—for example, eating a hot, balanced meal daily and having fun at least once a week—before tackling those that seem difficult.

Source: "Scale developers: Lyle Miller and Alma Dell Smith of Boston University Medical Center," August 1985, *Berkeley Wellness Letter*, Berkeley, CA: University of California at Berkeley. Reprinted with permission.

REFERENCES

American Institute of Stress. (2004). Job stress. Available at: http://www .stress.org.

Bandura, A. (1997). *Self-efficacy: The exercise of control*. New York: W. H. Freeman & Company.

Barefort, J. C., Dahlstrom, W. G., & Williams, R. B. (1983). Hostility, CHD incidence, and total mortality: A 25-year follow-up study of 255 physicians. *Psychosomatic Medicine, 45,* 59–63.

Berry, L. L., Mirabito, A. M., & Berwick, D. M. (2004). A health care agenda for business. *MIT Sloan Management Review, 45*(4), 56–64.

Cox, T. H., Lobel, S. A., & McLeod, P. L. (1991). Effects of ethnic group cultural differences on cooperative and competitive behavior on a group task. *Academy of Management Journal, 34*(4), 827–847.

Crampton, S. M., Hodge, J. W., Mishra, J. M., & Price, S. (1995). Stress and stress management. *Advanced Management Journal, 60*(3), 10–18.

Evans, G. W., & Carrere, S. (1991). Traffic congestion, perceived control, and psychophysiological stress among urban bus drivers. *Journal of Applied Psychology, 76,* 658–663.

Fox, M. L., Dwyer, D. J., & Ganster, D. C. (1993). Effects of stressful job demands and control on physiological and attitudinal outcomes in a hospital setting. *Academy of Management, 36*(2), 289–318.

Friedman, I. A. (1999). Turning over schools into a healthier workplace; bridging between professional self-efficacy and professional demands. In R. Vandenberghe & A. M. Hubermann (Eds.), *Understanding and preventing teacher burnout* (pp. 166–175). Cambridge, UK: Cambridge University Press.

Friedman, M. D., & Rosenman, R. H. (1974). *Type A behavior and your heart.* New York: A. A. Knopf.

Ganster, D. C., & Fusilier, M. R. (1989). Control in the workplace. In C. L. Cooper & T. Roberston (Eds.), *International review of industrial and organizational psychology*. Chichester, UK: John Wiley & Sons.

Golembiewski, R. T. (1986). The epidemiology of progressive burnout: A primer. *Journal of Health and Human Resources Administration, 8*(1), 16–37.

Golembiewski, R. T. (1990). Differences in burnout, by sector: Public vs. business estimates using phases. *International Journal of Public Administration, 13*(4), 545–559.

Golembiewski, R. T., & Boss, R. W. (1991). Shelving levels of burnout for individuals in organizations: A note on the stability of phases. *Journal of Health and Human Resources Administration, 13*(4), 409–420.

Golembiewski, R. T., & Boudreau, R. (1991). Healthcare professional attend thyself: The epidemiology of burnout in several settings. *International Journal of Public Administration, 14*(1), 43–57. Last accessed on January 15, 2004

Hardiness Institute, Inc. Available at: www.hardinessinstitute.com.

HCA prepares future executives. (2004, July/August). *Healthcare Executive, 19,* 4.

Homsted, L. (2003). Professional practice advocacy. *The Florida Nurse, 19,* 4–5.

Integra Realty Resources. (2001). Second annual "desk rage" survey of American workers. Available at: http://www.irr.com. Last accessed February 1, 2004.

Jacobs, G. D. (2001). The physiology of mind-body interactions: The stress response and the relation response. *The Journal of Alternative and Complementary Medicine, 7*(Suppl. 1), S83–S92.

James, K., Lovato, C., & Khoo, G. (1994). Social identity correlates of minority workers' health. *Academy of Management Journal, 37*(2), 383–396.

Jones, J. W., Barge, B. N., Steffy, B. D., Fay, L. M., Kuntz, L. K., & Wuebker, L. J. (1988). Stress and medical malpractice: Organizational risk assessment and intervention. *Journal of Applied Psychology, 73*(4), 727–735.

Kalliath, T. J., O'Driscoll, M. P., Gillespie, D. F., & Bluedorn, A. C. (2000). A test of the Maslach Burnout Inventory in three samples of healthcare professionals. *Work and Stress, 14*(1), 35–50.

Karasek, R. A. (1979). Job demands, job decision latitude, and mental strain: Implications for job redesign. *Administrative Science Quarterly, 24,* 285–310.

Karasek, R. A., Baker, D., Marxer, F., Ahlbom, A., & Theorell, T. (1981). Job decision latitude, job demands, and cardiovascular disease: A prospective study of Swedish men. American *Journal of Public Health, 71*(7), 694–705.

Kasschau, P. L. (1977). Age and race discrimination reported by middle-aged and older persons. *Social Forces, 55,* 728–742.

Keita, G. P., & Hurrell, J. J., Jr. (1994). *Job stress in a changing workforce: Investigating gender, diversity, and family issues.* Washington, DC: American Psychological Association.

Kim, J. S., Yoon, S. S., Lee, S. I., Yoo, H. J., Kim, C. Y., Choi-Kwon, S., et al. (1998). Type A behavior and stroke: High tenseness dimension may be a risk factor for cerebral infarction. *European Neurology, 39*(3), 168–173.

Kinicki, A., & Williams, B. K. (2003). *Management: A practical introduction.* New York: McGraw Hill Book Company.

Kushnir, T., & Kasan, R. (1991). Work-load, perceived control, and psychological distress in Type A/B industrial workers. *Journal of Organizational Behavior, 12,* 155–168.

Lazarus, S. R. (1991). Progress on a cognitive-motivational-relational theory of emotion. *American Psychologist, 46,* 819–834.

Lazarus, S. R., & Folkman, S. (1984). *Stress, appraisal and coping.* New York: Springer.

Lazarus, S. R., DeLongis, A., Folkman, S., & Gruen, R. (1985). Stress and adaptational outcomes: The problem of confounded measures. *American Psychologist, 40,* 770–779.

Maddi, S. R. (1998). Dispositional hardiness in health and effectiveness. In H. S. Friedman (Ed.), *Encyclopedia of mental health.* San Diego, CA: Academic Press.

Maslach, C., & Goldberg, J. (1998). Prevention of burnout: New perspectives. *Applied Preventive Psychology, 7,* 63–74.

Maslach, C., & Jackson, S. E. (1981). The measurement of experienced burnout. *Journal of Occupational Behavior, 2,* 99–113.

May, E. L. (2004). Are people your priority? How to engage your workforce. *Healthcare Executive, 19*(4), 8–16.

MFL Occupational Health Centre, Inc. (2000, March). Stress at work. Available at: http://www.mflohc.mb.ca/. Last accessed January 25, 2004.

Murphy, L. R. (1995). Occupational stress management: Current status and future directions. In C. L. Cooper & D. M. Rousseau (Eds.), *Trends in Organizational Behavior* (Vol. 2). West Sussex, England: John Wiley & Sons.

National Institute for Occupational Safety and Health. (1999). *Stress at Work. DHHS (NIOSH)* Publication No. 99-101. Cincinnati, OH: Author. Also available at: http://www.cdc.gov/niosh/stresswk.html. Last accessed January 23, 2004.

Peterson, M. (2004, June). Creating healthy corporate cultures for both genders: A national employee survey. Available at Lluminari, Inc.'s Web site at: www.lluminari.com. Last accessed February 2, 2004.

Quick, J. C., Quick, J. D., Nelson, D. L., & Hurrell, J. J. (1997). *Preventive stress management in organizations*. Washington, DC: American Psychological Association.

Richard, O. C., & Grimes, D. (1996 December). Bicultural interrole conflict: An organizational perspective. *The Mid-Atlantic Journal of Business, 32*(3), 155–170.

Roberts, R. K., Swanson, N. G., & Murphy, L. R. (2004). Discrimination and occupational mental health. *Journal of Mental Health, 13*(2), 129–142.

Roper Starch Worldwide (2000). Global 2000 consumer study. Available at: www.roper.com. Last accessed February 3, 2004.

Rosenman, R. H., Friedman, M., Wurm, M., Jenkins, C. D., Messinger, H. B., & Strauss, R. (1966). Coronary heart disease in the Western Collaborative Group Study. *Journal of the American Medical Association, 195,* 86–92.

Rosenstein, A. H. (2002). Nurse–physician relationships: Impact on nurse satisfaction and retention. *American Journal of Nursing, 102*(6), 26–34.

Rotter, J. B. (1966). Generalized expectancies for internal versus external control of reinforcement. *Psychological Monographs, 80,* 1–28.

Savery, L. K., & Hall, K. (1986). Tight rein, more stress. *Harvard Business Review, 65,* 160–164.

Schwarzer, R. (2004). Manage stress at work through preventive and proactive coping. In E. A. Locke (Ed.), *Handbook of principles of organizational behavior*. London: Blackwell Publishing.

Seligman, M. E. P. (1991). *Learned optimism*. New York: A. A. Knopf. Reissue edition; March 1, 1998, Free Press.

Seligman, M. E. P., & Csikszentmihalyi, M. (2000). Positive psychology. *American Psychologist, 55*(1), 5–14.

Selye, H. (1956). *The stress of life*. New York: McGraw Hill Book Company.

Selye, H. (1974). *Stress without distress*. London: Hodder and Stoughton.

Spector, P. E. (1986). Perceived control by employees: A meta-analysis of studies concerning autonomy and participation at work. *Human Relations, 39,* 1005–1016.

Stewart, W. F., Ricci, J. A., Chee, E., Morganstein, D., & Lipton, R. (2003). Lost productive time and cost due to common pain conditions in the U.S. workforce. *Journal of the American Medical Association, 290*(18), 2443–2454.

Swanson, N. G. (2000). Working women and stress. *Journal of the American Medical Women's Association, 55,* 76–79.

Von Onciul, J. (1996, September 21). Stress at work. *British Medical Journal, 313,* 745–748.

Weber, D. O. (2004, September/October). Poll results: Doctors' disruptive behavior disturbs physician leaders. *The Physician Executive, 30,* 6–14.

Whetton, D. A., & Cameron, K. S. (1993). *Developing managerial skills: Managing stress.* New York: HarperCollins.

Williams, C. (2003). Sources of workplace stress. Perspectives on Labour and Income, *4*(6), Statistics Canada Catalogue no. 75-001-XIE.

Yerkes, R. M., & Dodson, J. D. (1908). The relation of strength of stimulus to rapidity of habit-formation. *Journal of Comparative Neurology and Psychology, 18,* 459–482.

Young, P. (1974). Stay calm and stay alive. *Management Review, 63*(4), 37–39.

OTHER SUGGESTED READING

Golembiewski, R. T., Hilles, R., & Daly, R. (1987). Some effects of multiple OD interventions on burnout and work site features. *The Journal of Applied Behavioral Science, 23*(3), 295–313.

Hackman, J. R., & Oldham, G. R. (1980). *Work design.* Reading, MA: Addison-Wesley.

Jick, T. D., & Mitz, L. F. (1985). Sex differences in work stress. *Academy of Management Review, 10*(3), 408–420.

Keenan, A., & McBain, G. D. (1979). Effects of Type A behaviour, intolerance of ambiguity, and locus of control on the relationship between role stress and work-related outcomes. *Journal of Occupational Psychology, 52,* 277–285.

Keita, G. P., & Jones, J. M. (1990). Reducing adverse reaction to stress in the workplace. *American Psychologist, 45*(10), 1142–1145.

Kowalski, R., Harmon, J., Yorks, L., & Kowalski, D. (2003). Reducing workplace stress and aggression: An action research project at the U.S. Department of Veterans Affairs. *Human Resource Planning, 26*(2), 39–53.

Kushnir, T., & Melamed, S. (1991, March). Work-load, perceived control and psychological distress in Type A/B industrial workers. *Journal of Organizational Behavior, 12*(2), 155–168.

National Institute for Occupational Safety and Health (2002, April). The Changing Organization of Work and the Safety and Health of Working People. Available at: www.cdc.gov/niosh. Last accessed February 15, 2004.

Noblet, A. (2003). Building health promoting work settings: Identifying the relationship between work characteristics and occupational stress in Australia. *Health Promotion International, 18*(4), 351–359.

Rahe, R. H., Meyer, M., Smith, M., & Kjaer, G. (1964). Social stress and illness onset. *Journal of Psychosomatic Research, 8,* 35–44.

Savery, L. K., & Hall, K. (1986). Managers and decision making—"people" and "things." *Journal of Managerial Psychology, 1*(2), 19–24.

Sparks, K., Faragher, B., & Cooper, C. L. (2001, November). Well-being and occupational health in the 21st century workplace. *Journal of Occupational and Organizational Psychology, 74*(Pt. 4), 489–509.

CHAPTER 13

Conflict Management, Decision Making, and Negotiation Skills

Nancy Borkowski, DBA, CPA, FACHE

LEARNING OUTCOMES

After completing this chapter, the student should understand:

- ☛ The definition of conflict.
- ☛ The four basic types of conflict.
- ☛ The five levels of conflict.
- ☛ The five conflict-handling modes.
- ☛ The difference between the rational and the bounded rationality approach to decision making.
- ☛ The limitations of using intuitive decision making and the heuristics or biases approach.
- ☛ How framing heuristics affects escalation of commitment.
- ☛ The four basic styles of decision making.
- ☛ The three major negotiation models.

OVERVIEW

Conflict is inevitable and unavoidable because it is a natural part of human relationships. It is a part of our everyday professional and personal lives, and therefore, it is inherent in any type of work setting (Thomas, 1976). Although there are numerous definitions of conflict, Thomas (1992) suggests that there are three common components to most definitions: (1) perceived incompatibility of interests, (2) some interdependence of the parties, and (3) some form of interaction. For example, Rahim (1985) defined conflict as an "interactive state" manifested in disagreement or differences, or incompatibility, within or between individuals and groups. For our discussions, we will define conflict as occurring when an individual or group feels negatively affected by another individual or group.

No organization is exempt from conflict; however, the healthcare setting has been referred to as one of the highest conflictual environments because of factors such as high stress, high emotions, scarce resources, competition, downsizing, mergers, excessive regulations, diversity and cultural issues, and multiple stakeholders' demands. These factors increase conflict in organizations (Gardner, 1992; Johnson, 1994). For example, research has shown that managers, both healthcare and nonhealthcare, spend an average of 30 percent of their time dealing with conflict, and this is frequently cited as one of the least enjoyable aspects of their leadership roles (McElhaney 1996; Robbins, 1990; Shelton & Darling, 2004; Thomas & Schmidt, 1976).

It is important to note that conflict does not necessarily lead to ineffectiveness. Conflict, like stress, can either be positive or negative. Positive conflict can act as a stimulus for positive change. Positive or constructive conflict can lead to creative problem solving and alternatives, increased motivation and commitment, high-quality work, and personal satisfaction (i.e., functional outcomes) (Cosier & Dalton, 1990). However, negative or unconstructive conflict can be counterproductive for an organization by diverting efforts from goal attainment (i.e., dysfunctional outcomes). Negative conflict may also affect the psychological well-being of employees. If severe, unconstructive conflicts may result in employee resentment, tension, and anxiety, which may lead to low-quality work, personal stress, and possible sabotage. For example, it is estimated that over 65 percent of performance problems result from strained relationships and that conflict accounts for up to 50 percent of involuntary employee departures (Dana, 2000; Watson & Hoffman, 1996). Negative conflict may create an organizational culture of competition versus cooperation, thereby eliminating the sustainability of supportive and trusting relationships, which are necessary for successful organizations (Baron & Richardson, 1990). For example, Forte (1997) points out that in clinical environments, conflict among healthcare professionals can be counterproductive with respect to patients, which can result in increased mortality and morbidity rates due to medical errors.

Lewicki, Weiss, and Lewin (1992) identify six major areas in conflict research: the microlevel (psychological) approach, the macrolevel (sociological) approach, the economic-analysis approach, the labor-relations approach, the bargaining and negotiation approach, and the third-party dispute approach. The microlevel approach includes research on factors that affect intrapersonal and interpersonal conflict (i.e., within and among individuals), whereas the macrolevel approach focuses on factors affecting conflict among and within groups, departments, and organizations (i.e., intragroup, intergroup, and interorganization). Economic analysis refers to economic rationality and how it applies to individual decision making. The research areas of labor relations, bargaining and negotiation, and third-party resolution relate to studies that deal with the effects of workplace and conflict resolutions and/or conflict management.

Using this framework, we will first discuss the various types and levels of conflict. Second, we will examine the various methods to deal with conflict effectively, referred to as conflict resolution or conflict management. This discussion includes individual decision making and the negotiation skills necessary for effective conflict management.

TYPES OF CONFLICT

There are four basic types of conflict: goal, cognitive, affective, and procedural (Kolb & Bartunek, 1992). Goal conflict occurs when two or more desired or expected outcomes are incompatible. It may involve inconsistencies between the individual's or group's values and norms (e.g., standards of behavior). Cognitive conflict occurs when the ideas and thoughts within an individual or between individuals are incompatible. Affective conflict emerges when the feelings and emotions within an individual or between individuals are incompatible. Procedural conflict occurs when people differ over the process to use for resolving a particular matter. As illustrated in Case Study 13–1, the different types of conflict are not mutually exclusive.

Case Study 13–1 Who's the Boss?

"Dr. Jordan on line three for you, Mary." When Mary Jones pressed the blinking button, she knew Dr. Jordan was not calling to set up their next tee time. As Chief of Surgery, Dr. Jordan had full access to the Board of Directors and Mary, the Chairperson of the Board, noticed he took full advantage of it. Lately, Dr. Jordan's calls were mostly about Harriet Briggs, the hospital's administrator. Today was no different.

"Mary, as Chief of Surgery, I have authority over all issues that affect the quality of patient care. When something or someone is compromising that quality, it is my prerogative, not the prerogative of some layman [Dr. Jordan's word for anyone not holding an MD] to do what I deem necessary to correct the situation. Don't you agree?"

Mary mentally ran through job descriptions and the hospital's charter and she could remember no clause that explicitly gave the Chief of Surgery this authority. Implicitly though, his stance was probably correct. "I'll reserve comment on that, Alex, until you tell me the specific situation that has you this upset."

The problem that concerned Dr. Jordan involved the nursing supervisor, Judith Brady, RN. Ms. Brady scheduled the hospital's surgical nurses according to her interpretation of established hospital policy. Surgeons were frustrated with her attitude that maximum utilization must be made of the hospital's operating time for training purposes. She therefore scheduled in such a way that nurses were often assigned to procedures they had not seen before. Surgeons complained that this scheduling method often added to the time it took to perform an operation. This caused problems because the Operating Room was run at full capacity. Surgeons already felt they must hurry to complete a procedure because another procedure was scheduled directly following theirs. Having to wait because a nurse did not automatically know what instrument is needed next only exacerbated this problem and did not permit them sufficient time to complete a surgical procedure in the proper manner. The surgical staff was concerned that this scheduling system was impacting quality of care. Furthermore, some of the surgeons had complained that Ms. Brady clearly favored some physicians over others and tended to assign more experienced nurses to their procedures.

The situation came to crisis earlier in the morning when Dr. Jordan, following a confrontation with Ms. Brady, told her she was fired. Ms. Brady then made an appeal to Harriet Briggs, the hospital administrator. Harriet overturned Ms. Brady's dismissal and then instructed Dr. Jordan that discharge of nurses was the purview of the hospital administrator and only she had the authority to do so. Dr. Jordan vehemently disagreed. The conversation ended with Dr. Jordan yelling, "This is clearly a medical problem and I am sure the Board of Directors will agree with me." Dr. Jordan then called Mary.

After listening to Dr. Jordan, Mary decided to call Harriet Briggs to get her side of the story. Harriet told Mary, "I cannot be responsible for improving patient care if the board will not support me. I must be able to make decisions and develop policies and procedures without worrying whether or not the board will always side with the physicians. As you already know, Mary, I am legally responsible for the care that patients receive here at the hospital. And another thing, the next time Dr. Jordan tells me that I should restrict my activities to fund raising, maintenance, and housekeeping, I will not be responsible for my actions!"

The severity of the problem was obvious, but the answers were not. All Mary knew was she needed to fix the situation quickly.

Discuss the goal, cognitive, affective, and procedural conflicts illustrated in this case.

SOURCE: "Musical operating rooms: Mini-cases of health care disputes," by R. Friedman, 2002. *International Journal of Conflict Management, 13*(4), pp. 419–420. Reprinted with permission.

LEVELS OF CONFLICT

There are five levels of conflict: intrapersonal conflict (within a person), interpersonal conflict (between or among individuals), intragroup conflict (within a group), or intergroup conflict (between or among groups), and interorganizational conflict (between or among organizations).

Intrapersonal Conflict

Intrapersonal conflict occurs within the individual and may involve some form of goal, or cognitive or affective conflict. Intrapersonal goal conflict happens when several alternative courses of action are available and when the outcome is important to the individual, whether positive or negative (Locke, Smith, Erez, Chah, & Schaffer, 1994). Brehm and Cohen (1962) identified three types of intrapersonal conflict, which may develop involving alternative courses of action:

- *Approach / Approach:* The approach/approach type occurs when an individual must choose among two or more alternatives, each of which is expected to have a positive outcome. For example, Judy Lewis, a recent graduate of a local university's Master of Health Services Administration (MHSA) program, has been offered job positions in two different health-care organizations. The first is a managed care coordinator position with a national, publicly held laboratory company. The second is a network analyst position with a fast-growing third-party administrator. The salary levels of both positions are comparable.

- *Avoidance / Avoidance:* The avoidance/avoidance type occurs when an individual must choose among two or more alternatives, each of which is expected to be or result in a negative outcome. For example, after Judy Lewis accepted the position as the managed care coordinator with the laboratory company, management announced that because of a recent merger, the company is in the process of rightsizing. Two options were presented to Judy: to retain her position by relocating to the organization's headquarters, which is 1,000 miles away from her hometown, or be laid off.

- *Approach / Avoidance:* The approach/avoidance type occurs when an individual must choose an alternative that is expected to have both positive and negative outcomes. Judy Lewis chooses the relocation option. Although Judy realizes she will gain valuable experience working in the organization's corporate headquarters with opportunities for advancement, she is saddened by the fact that she must leave her family, friends, and familiar surroundings.

Intrapersonal conflict may also be a consequence of cognitive dissonance, which occurs when individuals recognize inconsistencies in their thoughts and behavior. As discussed in Chapter 3, individuals seek consistency among their beliefs and/or opinions (i.e., cognitions), and when an inconsistency arises between an individual's attitude or behavior (i.e., dissonance), something must change to eliminate or lessen the conflict. When there is a discrepancy between an individual's attitude and behavior, it is more likely that the individual's attitude will change to accommodate his or her behavior, thereby reducing or eliminating the intrapersonal conflict (Brehm & Cohen, 1962).

In the workplace, dissonance occurs most often within the context of role conflict. The three types of role conflict are: (1) the person and the role, (2) intrarole, and (3) interrole. Person-role conflict occurs when the expectations associated with a work role are incompatible with the individual's needs, values, or ethics—for example, a pharmaceutical representative who believes that making untested claims about a new drug is unethical, but whose work role requires him or her to do so. Intrarole conflict occurs when an individual experiences different expectations from his or her role. For example, a hospital's purchasing manager reporting administratively to the vice president of operations and functionally to the medical director may face conflicting expectations, as the former may, because of decreasing reimbursements, stress cost efficiency by restricting choices of prosthesis devices in the surgery department, whereas the latter may emphasize having available whatever prostheses the surgeons prefer to use without regard to cost. Interrole conflict occurs when there is a clash between work and nonwork role demands. For example, if an individual must travel extensively or work excessive hours, it may conflict with family needs or demands to spend time together.

Interpersonal Conflict

Interpersonal conflict is a natural outcome of human interaction. Interpersonal conflict involves two or more individuals who believe that their attitudes, behaviors, or preferred goals are in opposition. Kottler (1996) relates that there are three major sources of interpersonal conflict: (1) personal characteristics and issues, (2) interactional difficulties, and (3) differences around perspectives and perceptions of the issues. Porter-O'Grady and Epstein (2003, p. 36) summarize these components as follows:

Personal Characteristics and Issues: As a result of the diversity of today's workplace, an extensive range of differences exists between persons and cultures. These differences are embedded with a kind of emotional content related to variations in beliefs, behaviors, roles, and relationships. Individuals function in the context of these diverse characteristics, further validating differences others see in us.

Interactional Difficulties: As we mature and socialize, we learn effective communication and relational skills. A lack of communication skills, combined with our personal and cultural differences, creates powerful deficits in our ability to relate to one another. Because of this broad-based inadequacy, relational conflicts regularly emerge.

Perspective and Perceptive Differences: When combined with personal differences and communication inadequacies, dissimilarity in the way people view issues and interactions is a common source of interpersonal conflict. This source of interpersonal conflict may include erroneous perceptions based on incomplete information, disparate interpretations of meaning, or personal bias.

Many interpersonal conflicts involve goal conflict or role ambiguity. Role ambiguity involves a lack of clarity or understanding regarding expectations about an individual's work performance. Often, the misunderstanding is the result of perceptual differences regarding an issue or process. Unclear performance expectations may easily intensify interpersonal conflicts and undermine sustainability of healthy relationships. Role ambiguity may cause stress reactions, such as aggression, hostility, and withdrawal behavior (Jackson & Schuler, 1985).

Intragroup Conflict

Intragroup conflict involves clashes among some or all of a group's members, which often affect the group's processes and effectiveness (Chapters 14 and 15 provide a detailed discussion of group dynamics and the various interactions between group members.). Jehn and Mannix (2001) suggest that there are three types of intragroup conflict: (1) relationship, (2) task, and (3) process.

- Relationship conflict is an awareness of interpersonal incompatibilities. It includes affective components such as feeling tension and friction. Relationship conflict involves personal issues such as dislike among group members and feelings such as annoyance, frustration, and irritation.
- Task conflict is an awareness of differences in viewpoints and opinions pertaining to a group task. Similar to cognitive conflict, it pertains to conflict about ideas and differences of opinion about the task. Task conflicts may coincide with animated discussions and personal excitement but, by definition, are void of the intense interpersonal negative emotions that are more commonly associated with relationship conflict.
- Process conflict is an awareness of controversies about aspects of how task accomplishment will proceed. More specifically, process conflict pertains to issues of duty and resource delegation, such as who should do what and how much responsibility different people should be assigned. For example, when group members disagree about whose responsibility it is to complete a specific duty, they are experiencing process conflict.

Intergroup Conflict

Intergroup conflict involves opposition and clashes between groups. Under extreme conditions of competition and conflict, the groups develop attitudes toward one another that are characterized by a failure to communicate, distrust, and a self-interest focus (see Case Study 13–2). Nulty (1993) relates that there are four categories of intergroup conflict: (1) vertical conflict, (2) horizontal conflict, (3) line-staff conflict, and (4) diversity-based conflict.

- Vertical conflict occurs between employees at different levels in an organization. For example, when supervisors attempt to control subordinates, subordinates may resist because they believe that the controls infringe too much on their autonomy to perform their jobs. Vertical conflict may also arise because of poor communication, goal or value incompatibility, or role ambiguity (Pondy, 1967).

- Horizontal conflict occurs between groups of employees at the same hierarchical level in an organization. It occurs when each department or team strives only for its own goals, disregarding the goals of other departments and teams, especially if those goals are incompatible (see Case Study 13–3; also, Pondy, 1967).

- Line-staff conflict occurs over authority relationships. Most managers are responsible for the processes that create the organization's services or products. Staff managers often serve an advisory or control function that requires specialized technical knowledge. Line managers may feel that staff managers are imposing on their areas of legitimate authority. Staff personnel may specify the methods and partially control the resources used by line managers. Line managers often believe that staff managers reduce their authority over employees, although their responsibility for the outcomes remains unchanged (March & Simon, 1993).

- Diversity-based conflict relates to issues of race, gender, ethnicity, and religion. These conflicts may encompass all five levels of conflict—intrapersonal, interpersonal, intragroup, intergroup, and interorganizational.

Case Study 13–2 Turf Battles

Andrea Bevans, chief operating officer of Holy Name Hospital, knew it was a matter of when, not if. The memo she had just read was the first salvo in what promised to be another turf battle within the medical staff organization. In the memo, the hospital's vascular surgeons demanded that radiologists not be allowed to perform balloon angioplasty. Bevans knew that this treatment used a balloon at the end of a catheter and that after the catheter had been threaded into an artery in the peripheral vascular system, the balloon was inflated to break up deposits that narrowed the arteries.

The memo stated that vascular surgeons had the background, training, expertise, and proven outcomes using surgical skills and that they could best learn and apply the new techniques, if those techniques were appropriate at all. To allow radiologists to work inside the peripheral vascular system would violate previously tried and tested relationships and would cause other, unspecified, disruptions. The memo ended with a chilling, thinly veiled threat: "Should the hospital allow radiologists to perform balloon angioplasty, it may not be possible for members of the surgical staff to be available to treat untoward events, should they occur as the result of a procedure done by radiologists."

Bevans reread the memo and mused about the path of modern medicine. It was reaching the point where many conditions were treated without a scalpel. She thought fleetingly about "Bones," the Star Trek physician, who had only to pass a device over a patient's body to make a diagnosis. "Is this where we're headed?" she thought. "But, enough of science fiction," she said to herself. "How do I solve yet another turf battle without too many casualties, not the least of whom could be me?"

Discuss the intergroup conflicts reflected in the Turf Battle case study.

SOURCE: "The developing crisis in medical staff organization," by K. Darr, 1996. *Hospital Topics,* 74(4), pp. 4–6. Reprinted with permission.

Case Study 13-3 The Managed Care Factor

Cedars-Sinai is a 400-bed community hospital located in a major East Coast metropolitan area. The hospital has a reputation as a high-quality, low-cost provider. The medical staff at Cedars-Sinai comprises board-certified physicians who are predominantly solo practitioners or are part of two- or three-physician practices. No single- or multispecialty group practices are affiliated with Cedars-Sinai. Medical staff matters are handled cautiously and conservatively by the hospital administration.

Nine years ago a large West Coast health maintenance organization (HMO) established a presence on the East Coast and grew rapidly. Because of its fine reputation, Cedars-Sinai has become a major provider of services for the HMO, and many of the HMO's physician–employees have admitting privileges. Almost 20 percent of Cedars-Sinai's inpatient days come from the HMO.

Following a review of the HMO's utilization patterns, a West Coast consultant noted the large difference in hospital inpatient days per 1,000 enrollees between East and West Coast branches of the HMO. The HMO's clinical director was asked to assess how many days of care and, consequently, how many premium dollars could be saved with various levels of progress toward the West Coast utilization patterns.

Word of this study came to the attention of Cedars-Sinai's chief executive officer (CEO), who was immediately alarmed by the implications. He knew that if the HMO's physicians reduced the lengths of stay for their patients by moving utilization patterns toward the West Coast experience, shockwaves would run through the majority of the members of his medical staff— the voluntary, fee-for-service physicians. The consequences of such a disparity in patient-day utilization patterns could be a decision by the medical staff leadership not to reappoint the HMO's physician–employees to the medical staff because the voluntary medical staff would judge that the lengths of stay were inappropriately short and risked patient morbidity and mortality.

Discuss the horizontal conflict reflected in the Managed Care Factor case study.

SOURCE: "The developing crisis in medical staff organization," by K. Darr, 1996. *Hospital Topics, 74*(4), pp. 4–6. Reprinted with permission.

Interorganizational Conflict

Interorganizational conflict occurs between organizations as a result of interdependence on membership and divisional or system-wide success. For example, as Longest and Brooks (1998) point out, healthcare organizations participate in a variety of forms of organizational integration. The most extensively integrated organizations are integrated delivery systems (IDS). As integration levels increase, senior managers increasingly become involved in interorganizational conflict. Integration that involves extensive linking of providers at different points in the patient care continuum—and even more so when IDSs are linked with insurers or health plans and perhaps with suppliers in very highly integrated situations—brings into close interactive proximity what are often quite disparate organizations. Conflicts are unavoidable; knowledge and skills useful in managing them effectively are imperative. Interpersonal/collaborative competence is, of course, required of senior managers in all settings, but in an IDS, such competence becomes more complex overall, especially given the new dimension of managing interorganizational conflict (Longest & Brooks, 1998).

CONFLICT MANAGEMENT

Winder (2003, p. 20) points out that:

> Disagreements between people are an inherent and normal part of life. These disagreements can stem from differences in perceptions, lifestyles, values, facts, motivations or procedures. Differing goals, expectations or methods can turn disagreements into conflict, which can be damaging to both parties. Conflict may also be positive and beneficial in that it can force clarification of policy or procedures, relieve tensions, open communications and resolve problems. In its negative form, conflict can direct energy from real tasks, decrease productivity, reduce morale, prevent cooperation, produce irresponsible behavior, breakdown communication, and increase tension and stress, all resulting in loss of valuable human resources.

Understanding how conflict arises in the workplace is helpful for anticipating situations that may become conflictual. However, individuals also need to understand how they cope with or handle these conflictual situations. Thomas and Kilmann (1974), building on Blake and Mouton's (1964) work in the area of leadership, identified five conflict-handling modes (see Chapter 9 for discussion of Blake and Mouton's Managerial Grid). Thomas and Kilmann describe the five conflict-handling modes within two dimensions: (1) assertiveness (i.e., attempt to satisfy one's own concern) and (2) cooperativeness (i.e., attempt to satisfy others' concerns). The five conflict-handling modes are: (1) competition, (2) avoidance, (3) compromise, (4) accommodation, and (5) collaboration (see Figure 13–1).

Competition involves assertive and uncooperative behaviors and reflects a win–lose approach to conflict. A dominating or competing person goes all out to win his or her objective and, as a result, often ignores the needs, concerns, and expectations of the other party (Rahim, Garrett, & Buntzman, 1992). When dealing with conflict between subordinates or departments, competition-style managers use coercive powers such as demotion, dismissal, negative performance evaluations, or other punishments to gain compliance (Winder, 2003). When conflict occurs between peers, a competition-style manager will try to get his or her own way by appealing to his or her supervisor in the attempt to use the supervisor to force the decision on his or her peer (Blake & Mouton, 1984b).

However, in some situations competition-style management is appropriate. For example, when the issues involved in a conflict are trivial or when emergencies require quick action, this style may be appropriate. It is also appropriate when unpopular courses of action must be implemented for long-term organizational effectiveness and survival (e.g., cost cutting, and dismissal of employees for poor performance). This style is also appropriate for implementing the strategies and policies formulated by higher-level management (Dewine, Nicotera, & Perry, 1991; Rahim et al., 1992).

Collaboration involves highly assertive and cooperative behaviors and reflects a win–win approach to conflict. A collaborating-style manager attempts to find

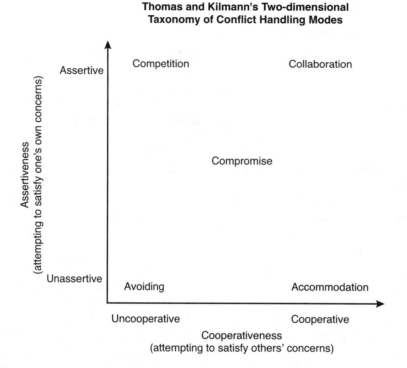

Figure 13–1 Thomas and Kilmann's Two-dimensional Taxonomy of Conflict Handling Modes

a solution that maximizes the outcomes of all parties involved. Managers who use the collaborating style see conflict as a means to a more creative solution, which would be fully acceptable to everyone involved (Winder, 2003). This involves openness, exchange of information, and examination of differences to reach an effective solution acceptable to all parties. Rahim et al. (1992) suggest that when issues are complex, the collaboration conflict-handling mode emphasizes the use of skills and information possessed by different employees to arrive at creative alternatives and solutions. This style may be appropriate for dealing with the strategic issues relating to objectives and policies, long-range planning, and so forth. However, as Winder (2003) points out, this style requires sufficient interdependence and parity in power among individuals so that they feel free to interact candidly, regardless of their formal superior/ subordinate status. In addition, this style requires expending extra time and energy; therefore, sufficient organizational support must be available to resolve disputes through collaboration (Winder, 2003).

Compromising is the "middle ground," with managers displaying both assertive and cooperative behaviors. It involves give-and-take, whereby both parties give up something to reach a mutually acceptable agreement. According to Rahim et al. (1992), it may mean splitting the difference, exchanging concessions, or seeking a middle-ground position. Compromising may be appropriate when the goals of the conflicting parties are mutually exclusive or when both parties, who are equally powerful (e.g., labor and management), have reached a deadlock in their negotiation.

According to Winder (2003), heavy reliance on this style may be dysfunctional because the compromising style may create several problems if used too early in trying to resolve conflict. First, the people involved may be encouraged to compromise on the stated issues rather than on the real issues. The first issues raised in a conflict often are not the real ones, so premature compromise may prevent full diagnosis or exploration of the real issues. Second, accepting an initial position presented is easier than searching for alternatives that are more acceptable to everyone involved. Third, compromise may be inappropriate to all or part of the situation, because it may not be the best decision available.

Compared to the collaborating style, the compromising style does not maximize optimal outcomes for all involved parties. Compromise achieves only partial satisfaction for each person. Kabanoff (1991) points out that this style is likely to be appropriate when agreement enables each person to be better off or at least not worse off than if no agreement were reached, achieving a total win–win agreement is not possible, and conflicting goals or opposing interests block agreement on one person's proposal.

Accommodating involves cooperative and unassertive behaviors and is the opposite of competing. Accommodations may represent an unselfish act, a long-term strategy to encourage cooperation by others, or a submission to the wishes of others (Winder, 2003). This style is associated with attempting to play down the differences and emphasizing commonalities to satisfy the concern of the other party. An obliging person neglects his or her own concern to satisfy the concern of the other party; as such, accommodating-style managers may be perceived as weak and submissive because these individuals try to reduce tensions and stress by reassurance and support (Rahim et al., 1992; Winder, 2003).

According to Lee (1990), accommodating is generally ineffective if used as a dominant style, but it may be effective on a short-term basis when individuals are in a potentially explosive emotional conflict situation, and smoothing is used to defuse it; when keeping harmony and avoiding disruption are especially important in the short run; and when the conflicts are based primarily on the personalities of the individuals and cannot be easily resolved. In addition, this style is useful when an individual believes that he or she may be wrong or the other party is right and the issue is much more important to him or her. It can be used as a strategy when a party is willing to give up something with the hope of getting something in exchange from the other party when needed (Rahim et al., 1992).

Avoiding involves unassertive and uncooperative behaviors and is the opposite of collaborating. It is associated with withdrawal, buck-passing, or side-stepping situations (Rahim et al., 1992). This approach often reflects a decision to let the conflict work itself out, or it may reflect an aversion to tension and frustration. Because ignoring important issues often frustrates others, consistent use of the avoidance conflict-handling mode usually results in frustration by others. When unresolved conflicts affect goal accomplishment, the avoiding style will lead to negative results for the organization (Winder, 2003).

The avoiding style is useful when the issue is trivial, where the potential dysfunctional effect of confronting the other party outweighs the benefits of the resolution of conflict; there isn't enough information available to the individual to effectively deal with the conflict at that time; the individual's power is so low relative to the other person's that there is little chance of causing change (such as disagreement with a new strategy approved by top management); or when other individuals can more effectively resolve the conflict (Baron, Fortin, Frei, Hauver, & Shack, 1990; Rahim et al.,1992).

Culture and gender play an important part in an individual's conflict-handling style. For example, Golnaz and Rahmatian (2003) examined levels of effectiveness as well as preferences in styles of resolving interpersonal conflict among the following ethnic/racial groups: Asian, Mexican American, Mexican, Chicano, and Caucasian. Golnaz and Rahmatian also examined levels of effectiveness and preferences in styles between men and women. The researchers found that Caucasians showed a greater preference for assertive modes of behavior, while Mexican-Americans, Mexicans, Chicanos, and Asians favored nonassertive modes of behavior. In addition, men demonstrated more assertive behaviors and women demonstrated more nonassertive behaviors. Likewise, Kirkbride, Tang, & Westwood (1991) found that Chinese conflict-handling behavior is influenced by Chinese values, which emphasize conflict avoidance, emotional composure, and nonconfrontation.

Regardless of an individual's conflict-handling style, successful managers need to understand how conflict originates and know its sources so that they can proactively control situations that may develop into dysfunctional outcomes.

DECISION-MAKING MODELS

Before we begin our discussion of conflict negotiation models, a review of individual decision making is necessary. Why? Because as Thompson (1990, p. 524) points out, "negotiation is a complex decision-making task in which negotiators are faced with alternative courses of action and choices." It is important for us to understand how individuals make these choices or decisions, because negotiation occurs "whenever the allocation of gains among participants to an agreement is subject to their own choice rather than predetermined by circumstances" (Cross, 1969, p. 1).

Managers face different types of problems (i.e., well-structured and poorly structured) and use different types of decision-making models. When managers confront a well-structured problem, defined as one that is straightforward, repetitive, familiar, and easily defined, they use a routine approach by relying on an organization's policies and procedures. For example, two employees request the same vacation period. Because the manager must ensure adequate coverage in the workplace, he or she follows company policy by granting the vacation request to the employee with the most seniority. However, middle and senior managers usually deal with poorly structured problems, those that are new and complex, where information is limited and incomplete.

In the context of behavioral decision making, there are various means that an individual can use to choose the optimal or most desired outcome. Individuals use the rational approach to decision making when there is sufficient time for an orderly, thoughtful process. However, because of time, resource, information constraints, and the complexity of today's healthcare organizations, managers are limited or "bounded" as to their rational decision making. The bounded rationality perspective takes into consideration that managers, because of the complexity of problems, limited time, personal bias, and other factors, will not be able to weigh all possible alternatives to a problem and, therefore, must sometimes rely on intuitive decision making or the heuristics and biases approach.

Rational Approach

The rational approach to decision making, also referred to as the economic rationality model, is a systematic analysis of the problem followed by the choice and implementation of a solution in a logical, step-by-step sequence (Daft, 2004). The rational model is considered the "ideal" method of decision making. Daft (2004, pp. 449–450) explains the rational model using an eight-step approach, as illustrated in Figure 13–2:

1. *Monitor the Decision Environment:* In the first step, a manager monitors internal (within the organization) and external (outside the organization) information that will indicate deviations from planned or acceptable behavior. The manager talks with colleagues and reviews financial statements, performance evaluations, industry indices, competitors' activities, and the like.

2. *Define the Decision Problem:* The manager responds to deviations by identifying essential details of the problems: where, when, who was involved, who was affected, and how current activities are influenced.

3. *Specify Decision Objectives:* The manager determines what performance outcomes should be achieved by a decision.

4. *Diagnose the Problem:* In this step, the manager digs below the surface to analyze the cause of the problem. Additional data might be generated to facilitate this diagnosis. Understanding the cause enables appropriate treatment.

5. *Develop Alternative Solutions:* Before a manager can move ahead with a decisive action plan, he or she must have a clear understanding of the various options available to achieve desired objectives. The manager may seek ideas and suggestions from other people.

6. *Evaluate Alternatives:* This step may involve the use of statistical techniques or personal experience to gauge the probability of success. The merits of each alternative are assessed, as is the probability that the alternative will reach the desired objectives.

7. *Choose the Best Alternative:* This step is the core of the decision process. The manager uses his or her analysis of the problem, objectives, and alternatives to select a single alternative that has the best chance for success.

8. *Implement the Chosen Alternative:* Finally, the manager uses managerial, administrative, and persuasive abilities and gives directions to ensure that the decision is carried out. The monitoring activity (step 1) begins again as soon as the solution is implemented.

Steps in the Rational Approach to Decision-making

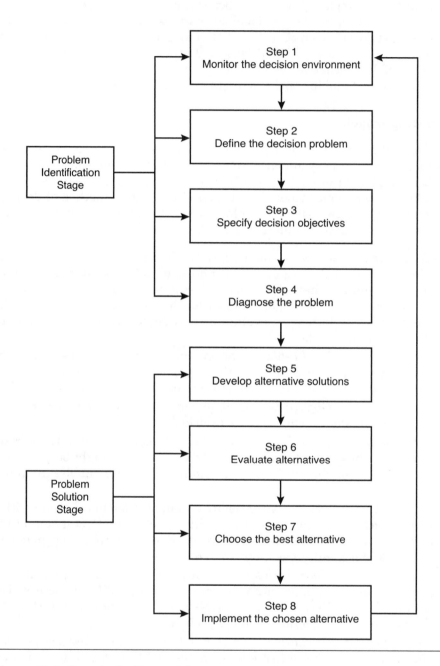

Figure 13–2 Steps in the Rational Approach to Decision Making (SOURCE: *Organization Theory and Design* (8th ed., p. 449), by R. L. Daft, 2004. Mason, OH: South-Western Used with permission.)

However, under most circumstances, managers do not possess complete information about a problem and/or all the plausible alternatives. In addition, managers are under the constraints of limited time and resources, personal bias, and other factors, which make rational decision making unrealistic. Therefore, managers are bounded or limited regarding their rational decision making. The concept of bounded rationality embraces the realism that evaluation of alternatives and decision making are constrained by human actions (Forest & Mehier, 2001).

Bounded Rationality Model

The bounded rationality model of decision making, proposed by Simon (1957), recognizes that individuals have cognitive limitations, which prohibit the processing of all the necessary or optimal information necessary for decision making; as such, an individual will limit his or her search for information prior to decision making. Dequech (2001, p. 913) explains the concept of bounded rationality in the following manner:

1. Individuals often pursue multiple objectives, which may be conflicting. The alternatives from which to choose in order to pursue these objectives are not previously given to the decision maker, who, thus, needs to adopt a process for generating alternatives.

2. The limits in the decision maker's mental capacity compared with the complexity of the decision environment usually prevent him or her from considering all the alternatives. Those limits are also present when the decision maker has to consider the consequences of the alternatives, so that the decision maker employs some heuristic procedure for that purpose.

3. Finally, the decision maker adopts a "satisfying" rather than an optimizing strategy, searching for solutions that are "good enough" or satisfactory, given some aspiration levels.

The expression "bounded rationality" is used to denote the type of rationality that managers resort to when the environment in which they operate is too complex relative to their cognitive limitations. Because of these limitations, managers may employ the use of intuitive and/or heuristic strategies for decision making.

Intuition

Intuitive decision making can be understood as a cognitive "short-circuiting," where a decision is reached even though the reason for the decision cannot be easily described (Hall, 2002). In other words, intuitive decision making involves using one's professional judgment based on past experiences rather than sequential logic or explicit reasoning (Daft, 2004). Agor (1985, 1986a, 1986b) suggests that intuition is most useful to managers in situations of uncertainty. Agor advocates reliance on intuition when a high level of uncertainty exists, when there is little precedent, when variables are not scientifically predictable and analytical data are of little use, when facts are limited and don't clearly point the way to go, when several alternatives seem plausible, and when time is limited and there is pressure to come up with the right answer.

There is some debate as to the degree to which an individual's intuitive ability can be developed and improved (Bennett, 1998). Some argue intuitive abilities are closely related to personality types (Myers, 1980). Others claim that job characteristics or situational factors encourage managers to develop and improve their intuitive abilities (Agor, 1986a, 1986b; Behling & Eckel, 1991; Wally & Baum, 1994). In top-level decision-making environments, this ability is certainly an asset and has been shown to be a benefit to senior managers (Agor, 1986a, 1986b; Eisenhardt and Bourgeois, 1988; Hayashi, 2001; Simon, 1987). For example, Agor (1985, 1986a, 1986b) conducted a series of studies and found that senior managers always score higher than middle- and lower-level managers in their abilities to use intuition to make decisions on the job. Therefore, it is not surprising that Peters and Waterman (1984) relate that the 10 best-run companies in America encouraged the use of intuitive skills, nurturing its development in their management culture, and that business schools are designing courses to help develop MBA students' intuitive skills for decision making (Agor, 1985, 1986b).

Heuristics or Biases Approach

In addition to using intuition to deal with the problems of uncertainty and complexity, managers use judgmental heuristics strategies to simplify their decision making. Heuristics are guidelines or "rules of thumb" that help make our world manageable by simplifying complex tasks (Kahneman, Slovic, & Tversky, 1982; Tversky & Kahneman, 1974). Heuristic processing strategies enable managers to cut through overwhelming data by applying simplifying assumptions to the information. Although the use of heuristics may result in accurate predictions by managers, it also can give rise to an array of errors and biases. Tversky and Kahneman (1974) describe three commonly used heuristics: (1) availability, (2) representativeness, and (3) anchoring and adjustment.

Availability bias is an intuitive technique where the perceived probability of an event is influenced by the ease of recollection. More easily recalled events are given a higher probability. More frequent events are often the most easily recalled, but the most easily recalled are not necessarily the most frequent (Hall, 2002). Ease of recall is also affected by salience (i.e., the degree to which some information is perceived as being more relevant to the decision being made) related to the emotional strength of a memory, with memories associated with strong emotions being recalled more easily. Performance appraisals of staff are affected by the use of availability heuristics by managers while evaluating them. It is common to find the most recent and vividly etched event—positive or negative—influencing the appraisal. (See "A Case of Abuse or Neglect?" in Case Study 13–4.)

Representativeness bias is an intuitive technique where probabilities are evaluated by the degree to which the given sample matches, or is representative of a class of samples or populations. In the workplace, representativeness heuristics can be traced as the reason behind many cases of employee discrimination. (See "A Case of Abuse or Neglect?" in Case Study 13–4.)

Anchoring and adjustment bias is an intuitive technique used when a series of estimates is used to obtain a "proposed" answer to a current problem. People create the preliminary solution on the basis of initial information (anchoring), and thereafter modify the answer when more information becomes available (adjustment). For example, when the salary of a new employee is being set, the anchoring and adjustment heuristic is used. The employee's starting salary is invariably set close to the last paid salary, without regard to what the new job description may entail. In other words, the initial value significantly influences the process of the adjustment toward the new value, irrespective of the rationality in the choice of the initial value. (See "A Case of Abuse or Dependency?" in Case Study 13–5.)

Case Study 13–4 A Case of Abuse or Neglect?

A significant portion of Dr. Smith's private practice comprised clients who had been referred to him from a psychiatric hospital. These included a former inpatient at the hospital, Ms. Sarah Jacobson. During the initial 20 minutes of the intake session, Sarah reported that she was 15 years old and was in her sophomore year in high school. Sarah told Dr. Smith that her parents were divorced and that her mother had custody of her and her two younger sisters. The client reported that her mother repeatedly said that she was tired of taking care of her and her sisters and that she thought that her mother wanted the children out of the home. Sarah went on to say that she had been placed in the hospital because of her aggressive and defiant behavior toward her mother. In addition, Sarah stated that she thought that her mother had become involved with another man prior to the divorce and that her mother liked him more than she liked her children. Sarah expressed considerable anger toward her mother and the belief that her mother was trying to "get rid of her."

Dr. Smith's case notes indicated that Sarah seemed agitated and felt persecuted by her mother. As he was conceptualizing the case, he recognized the similarity between this case and previous referrals from the hospital and recalled that the diagnosis in those cases had been paranoid schizophrenia. The case notes indicated that Sarah seemed to be functioning at an adequate level to be treated as an outpatient and that Dr. Smith regarded her as suffering from paranoid schizophrenia.

Sarah attended only one other session, as she failed to keep subsequent appointments. Approximately three weeks after his last meeting with Sarah, Dr. Smith received information from the Division of Family Services that Sarah's mother had been charged with neglect and abandonment of Sarah and her two younger siblings. Two weeks after Sarah had been released from the hospital, her mother had failed to pick up the younger children from day care and had left the city with her male friend.

Discussion

Dr. Smith used the availability heuristic when formulating his diagnosis. Symptoms of psychopathology were very salient and accessible to Dr. Smith, because many of his cases were referrals from the psychiatric hospital. Dr. Smith also used the representativeness heuristic by comparing Sarah to former clients. Had Dr. Smith referred to DSM-III-R (American Psychiatric Association, 1987) criteria when forming his diagnosis in addition to relying on his previous experience, he would have realized that Sarah's symptoms did not meet the criteria for schizophrenia.

Source: "Bias in the counseling process: How to recognize and avoid it," K. A. Morrow and C. T. Deidan, 1992. *Journal of Counseling and Development, 70*(5), pp. 571–577. Reprinted with permission.

Case Study 13–5 A Case of Abuse or Dependency?

Mr. Larson was a counselor employed by a community health clinic that offered both medical and psychological care. Mr. Larson made a practice of reviewing all records on file at the center before seeing each new client. Prior to the initial session with Ms. Irma Busse, Mr. Larson reviewed her file, which indicated no health problems and no previous visits for psychiatric reasons. The only remarkable entries were a broken arm sustained six months earlier and an indication that the attending physician suspected abuse. The physician's notes indicated that Irma's husband always accompanied her during examinations and that she deferred to him to answer the physician's questions.

During the initial session, Mr. Larson noticed that Irma had her collar buttoned to her neck, was slightly stooped when she walked, and did not make immediate eye contact when she spoke. She had a quiet voice and indicated that she had come to counseling because she was having marital problems. During this interview, Irma discussed how important her marriage was to her and how difficult it was for her to do things on her own, and indicated that all she wanted was to make her husband happy. After the session, Mr. Larson reviewed the interview and concluded that the client was a victim of spouse abuse and was unable at this time to recognize the need to leave her husband. He decided that the course of counseling would be to help Irma become aware of the dangerous nature of the situation, provide information about the shelter for battered women, and attempt to convince Irma that she needed to leave her husband for her own safety.

As counseling progressed, Irma made other statements such as "I'm afraid to go anywhere without my husband" and "I just don't know if I could get along without him." These seemed to support both his and the physician's earlier conclusions that Irma was a battered wife. After speaking to several family members, it became apparent that Irma had not been abused. Rather, it seems as though she was a very dependent person and that her needs were directed primarily toward her husband, although others had experienced her dependency as well.

Discussion

Mr. Larson's perceptions seem to have been skewed by the physician's notes (anchor), which suggested that Irma may have been abused. Because of the dangerous nature of abusive situations, Mr. Larson focused on assisting the client to prepare to move out of her home and into a shelter. He failed, however, to recognize that this client, through her verbal and nonverbal behavior, was reflecting strong dependency. Mr. Larson maintained his initial impression of Irma (i.e., the "battered wife" label) until much later in the counseling process when he obtained substantial contradictory information from family members (adjustment).

SOURCE: "Bias in the counseling process: How to recognize and avoid it," by K. A. Morrow and C. T. Deidan, 1992. *Journal of Counseling and Development, 70*(5), pp. 571–577. Reprinted with permission.

As illustrated by these two case studies, there are many similarities between clinical decision making and managerial decision making. Extensive literature exists regarding the use of intuition and heuristics in medical decision making because of the high degree of uncertainty within the practice of medicine. As Sox, Marshal, Higgins, and Marton (1988, p. 17) point out, "medicine is the art of making decisions without adequate information." As such, decisions made by clinicians through the use of intuition or heuristics can have a tremendous impact on healthcare managers. Clinicians make the decisions as to the commitment of scarce resources to patients and the associated care and treatment plans (Hall, 2002; Thompson, 2003). However, it is the responsibility of healthcare managers to provide the resources for clinicians to perform their work, and their health systems are "judged" on the clinical outcomes of the patient populations they serve. As such, healthcare managers need to appreciate not only how intuition and heuristics play a part in their own decision making but also how they affect the decision making of clinicians because both impact the achievement of organizational goals.

Escalation of Commitment and Framing Heuristic

In addition to Tversky and Kahneman's (1974) three commonly used heuristics, there is another area that may cause low-quality decision making—escalation of commitment. Staw (1981) defines the problem of escalation of commitment as when a manager continues to allocate more resources to a losing proposition. One reason escalation of commitment may occur is because a manager does not want to admit that he or she has made a mistake (Staw & Ross, 1987). Research finds that if a manager feels personally responsible for an initial decision that is failing, he or she is more likely to allocate additional resources than another person who was not responsible for the initial decision (Staw, 1981). For example, one of the main reasons for the bankruptcy of the Allegheny Health System in Pennsylvania was the unwillingness of the top leaders of the organization to make midcourse corrections in their grand plans on the basis of what was and was not working in hospitals and office practices in Philadelphia and Pittsburgh (Bottles, 2001).

Another reason escalation of commitment may occur is due to framing heuristic. Framing heuristic is a tendency to make a decision based on the form or manner in which information is presented. For example, Levin, Schnittjer, and Thee (1988) conducted a study where one group was given a description of an experimental cancer treatment that was shown to have a 40 percent success rate; the other group was told that the procedure had a 60 percent failure rate. Although both statements are true, the way the researchers worded the statements affected a person's opinion of its effectiveness and whether or not he or she would recommend the treatment to a family member. The participants were more optimistic about the treatment when its success rate was emphasized and less optimistic when the failure rate was emphasized.

Staw and Ross (1987) suggest that to avoid escalation of commitment, managers can: (1) recognize that they may be biased toward escalation, (2) see escalation for what it is (i.e., an overcommitment to a strategy by defining failure ambiguously, or by ignoring others' concerns), and (3) avoid overcommitment by looking at the strategy from an outsider's perspective.

Decision-style Model

Managers have different styles when it comes to making decisions and solving problems. Rowe and Boulgarides (1983, 1998) developed a decision-style model that proposes that managers differ along two dimensions in the way they approach decision making: value orientation and tolerance for ambiguity. Value orientation reflects the extent to which an individual focuses on either task and technical concerns or people and social concerns when making decisions. Tolerance for ambiguity reflects the extent to which a person has a high need for structure or control in his or her life.

As illustrated in Figure 13–3, the decision-style model encompasses four basic styles: directive, analytic, conceptual, and behavioral. Boulgarides and Cohen (2001, pp. 59–60) describe the four basic styles as follows:

1. *Directive:* Low tolerance for ambiguity and low cognitive complexity. The focus is on technical decisions, and this style is generally autocratic. The decision maker may adopt this style because of a high need for power. Because of the use of little information and few alternatives, speed and satisfactory solutions are typical. The decision makers tend to be focused and are frequently aggressive. Generally they prefer structure and specific information, which is given verbally. Their orientation is internal to the organization and short range. They tend to operate with tight controls. Although they are efficient, these decision makers have a high need for security and status. They have the drive required to achieve results, but they also want to dominate others.

2. *Analytic:* This decision maker has a much greater tolerance for ambiguity than the directive-style manager and also has a more cognitively complex personality that leads to the desire for more information and the consideration of many alternatives. Because of the focus on technical decisions and the need for control, the analytic style contains an autocratic bent. The analytic style is typified by the ability to cope with new situations (but in a structured manner) and problem solving. Position and ego are important to individuals who use an analytic decision-making style. As such, these individuals often reach top positions within an organization or start their own companies. They are not particularly quick in their decision making, and they enjoy variety and prefer written reports. They also enjoy challenges and examine every detail in a situation.

3. *Conceptual:* Including both high cognitive complexity and people orientation, this decision-making style tends to use data from multiple sources and considers many alternatives. Similar to individuals using the behavioral decision-making style, conceptual-style decision-makers share goals with subordinates in trusting and open relationships. These

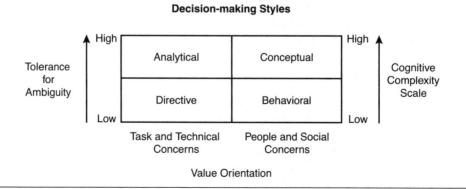

Figure 13–3 Decision-making Styles

individuals tend to be idealists who may emphasize ethics and values in their behavior. They generally are creative and can readily understand complex relationships. Their focus is long range with high organizational commitment. They are achievement-oriented and value praise, recognition, and independence. They prefer loose control over power and will frequently encourage the participation of those they lead. They may be characterized as thinkers rather than doers.

4. *Behavioral:* Although low on the cognitive complexity scale, this leader has a deep concern for the organization and the development of people. Behavioral-style managers tend to be supportive and are concerned with subordinates' well-being. They provide counseling, are receptive to suggestions, communicate easily, show warmth, are empathetic, are persuasive, and are willing to compromise and accept a looser style of control. With low data input, this style tends toward a short-range focus and uses meetings primarily for communicating. These managers avoid conflict, seek acceptance, and tend to be more people-oriented, but sometimes are insecure.

Of the four decision-making styles, individuals have a tendency to resort to a single, dominant style (i.e., default mode of decision making). However, with training, managers can use all four styles effectively as different situations are presented.

Conflict Negotiation Models

Rubin and Brown (1975) define negotiation as the process by which two or more parties decide what each will give and take in an exchange. Since the 1960s, there has been extensive research in the field of conflict resolution or conflict management. From this research, three major negotiation models have been developed: (1) distributive, (2) integrative, and (3) interactive. Each of these models is associated with different goals and indicators of success, and each may be most appropriately applied in different contexts (Winder, 2003).

Distributive Model

The distributive model originated within the field of labor negotiations (Lewicki et al., 1992; Stevens, 1963; Walton & McKersie, 1965) and can be described as a set of behaviors for dividing scarce resources. Distributive negotiation is often referred to as "hard-bargaining" or a win–lose, zero-sum approach. The negotiators are viewed as adversaries who reach agreement through a series of concessions with the goal of obtaining the greater "piece of the pie." Tactics used in the distributive negotiation model are withholding information, guarded communications, power positioning, limited expressions of trust, use of threats, and distorted statements and demands (Walton & McKersie, 1965). Brett and Shapiro (1998) referred to distributive negotiations as a tug-of-war game with each party trying to tug the other to its own side. The winner wins when the opponent's strength gives out and the opponent is pulled across the midline. The result is a one-sided agreement, where resolved issues favor one side more than the other.

Winder (2003) outlines the four win–lose strategies practiced by negotiators using the distributive approach. The first negotiating strategy is the "I want it all" tactic. This tactic involves making extreme offers and then granting concessions grudgingly, if at all. One party hopes to wear down the resolve of the other by pressuring the other to make significant concessions and forcing the other party into a position of nonreciprocation. The second negotiating strategy is "time warp." The time-warp tactic communicates an arbitrary deadline for acceptance of the offer. For example, the negotiators will relate to the other party that an offer is only good until a certain date and time. If not accepted by the arbitrarily set deadline, the offer will be withdrawn. The third negotiating strategy is the "good cop, bad cop" scenario. In this scenario, one party attempts to sway the negotiator by alternating sympathetic with threatening behavior. The fourth negotiating strategy is the "ultimatum" tactic, which is designed to try to force one party to submit to the will of the other. In this negotiation approach "take it or leave it" offers are presented, and one party overtly tries to force acceptance of demands—one party is unwilling to make any concessions, and the other party is expected to make all of the concessions (Fisher, Ury, & Patton, 1991).

Integrative Model

The integrative negotiation model, similar to the distributive model, evolved primarily within the field of labor negotiations (Follett, 1940, 1942; Lewicki et al., 1992; Walton & McKersie, 1965). It is currently one of the most frequently used models of conflict resolution because of its collaborative versus confrontational approach.

Integrative negotiation is a cooperative, interest-based, agreement-oriented approach to dealing with conflict that is viewed as a "win–win" or mutual-gain dispute. Integrative negotiation is a process by which parties attempt to explore options to achieve mutual gains versus unilateral gains. Parties recognize and define a problem, search for possible solutions to it, evaluate the solutions, and select one that maximizes joint gains (Lewicki et al., 1992).

Filley (1975), building on the work of Walton and McKersie (1965), developed an integrative decision-making model. Filley's six-step approach is as follows:

1. Create an environment that promotes equality, cooperation, communication, and information sharing
2. Review and adjust perceptions
3. Review and adjust attitudes (i.e., create processes that maximize information-sharing and "clear the air" of past hostilities and negative attitudes)
4. Define the problem
5. Search for alternatives
6. Achieve consensus

The concept of integrative negotiation is based on a value system that stresses interpersonal trust, cooperation, a willingness to share information combined with open communication, and a search for mutually acceptable outcomes (Lewicki et al., 1992). This model looks beyond the existing resources and aims to expand the alternatives and increase the available payoffs to both parties through joint problem solving (Winder, 2003).

Fisher and Ury (1981) and Fisher et al. (1991) define integrative negotiation as "principled negotiation." The researchers suggest that negotiations should be grounded in substantive concerns when the participants:

- Separate the people from the problem. In other words, separate the issues in conflict from the personal relationships. Negotiators should be hard on the issues, but to do so in a cooperative relationship with the other party.

- Focus on interest or need rather than position. In other words, do not allow individual egos to negate the negotiation process. This requires trust, respect, and open communication by both parties.

- Identify best alternative to a negotiated agreement (BATNA) for both parties. By identifying BATNAs, the parties' goal will be to achieve better outcomes than their BATNA through negotiations.

- Invent options or alternatives that provide mutual gain. Brainstorming, prior to and during meetings, will assist in developing creative alternatives.

- Insist on using only objective criteria to judge solutions. When negotiations are based on objective versus subjective criteria, discussions focus on equitable solutions, not false assumptions.

The integrative-conflict model encourages equitable solutions to problems. Negotiators are viewed as partners who cooperate in searching for a fair agreement that meets the interest of both sides and seeks to maximize the gain for all the parties involved (Winder, 2003) (see "Creating a Win–Win Situation" in Case Study 13–6).

Case Study 13–6 Creating a Win–Win Situation

A hospital anesthesiology department is deeply financially troubled. Department leaders approach senior hospital administrators seeking additional funds. Department leaders say without funding they will lose staff and be forced to close operating rooms. The administrators take the position that if they provide funding to the anesthesiology department, every department will demand it. Furthermore, the anesthesiology department has enjoyed the privilege of having an exclusive contract. If rooms are closed, the hospital may entertain looking at other anesthesiology practices. The senior vice president for medical affairs (i.e., VPMA) is called in to mediate. A meeting is set up to negotiate a solution.

Applying Fisher's principled negotiations, how should the VPMA proceed?

The first component of principled negotiation is to attack the problem over which the parties are negotiating. The further apart the positions, the more likely emotions will obscure the objective merits of the problem. Most negotiations are as much about emotion as they are money. The negotiation process will deteriorate rapidly if both sides firmly settle into their respective positions. If the anesthesiology group and hospital administration settle into their respective positions of closing rooms and denying the anesthesia group their exclusive contract, the negotiation soon will become a series of personal attacks.

The first step is for the VPMA to acknowledge that negotiation is an emotional undertaking. As mediator, he or she should encourage both parties to consider what they would be thinking if they were on the other side of the table. The point is to get both parties to address the problem and not to react immediately to emotional outbursts.

Relationship building and the "spirit of the deal" are important factors to keep in mind. The way to accomplish this relationship building is simple. Lay down the ground rules so that each party agrees to show the same degree of honesty, respect, and fairness that it would demand from others.

The ultimate objective of any negotiation is to satisfy the underlying interests of each side in the best way possible. As mediator, the VPMA must get each party to recognize the importance of each other's interests.

What are the interests of each group in this example? For the anesthesiologists, it may be increasing salaries to retain current staff and recruit new staff, while not having to work unreasonable or unsafe amounts of time to achieve this goal. For the hospital, it may be maintaining or even increasing operating room time to retain and attract high-volume surgeons.

The point is that each side has multiple interests. Positions such as "We will close down an operating room" obscure the underlying interests. Both parties must be cautioned to recognize and avoid any preconceived perceptions they may have about the other party.

For example, not all anesthesiology groups seeking stipends are greedy. Not all hospital administrators are clueless to clinical issues. No attempt should be made to discard any solutions until there has been a discussion of the problem and interests at hand.

With the interests articulated and understood, the VPMA should begin to look at options, looking first for shared or common interests. In this example, it is a common interest for both the anesthesiology group and hospital to keep the operating rooms open and running, since both derive revenue from the cases (i.e., common ground).

Unfortunately, it may be difficult or impossible to find common ground in many situations. As a result, capitalizing on differences may hold the key to developing options for achieving agreement. For example, the hospital may state that in order to provide a stipend, the anesthesiology group must be willing to expand operating room coverage in the evenings. The anesthesiology group may claim it does not have the staff to expand coverage and there is no need for expansion.

Could there be a solution in the disagreement? If both sides agree to look at both decreasing room turnover time and more accurate posting of procedure times by surgeons on the basis of historical data, the interest of the hospital in providing time for high-volume surgeons, and the anesthesiologists' interest in not expanding evening coverage, might be achieved. Remember that agreement often can be based on disagreement.

Once the parties begin looking at options, the problem can be discussed on the basis of objective criteria. The VPMA must have both parties prepare objective data to present prior to negotiating a solution. The anesthesiology group should be prepared to have benchmarks as to current salaries, workload, and operating room staffing models. The hospital should know how other institutions handle stipends, the legal implications, and objective criteria used to judge performance.

Source: "The role of the physician executive in negotiation," by D. P. Tarantino, 2004. *Physician Executive, 30*(5), pp. 71–73. Reprinted with permission.

Interactive Model

When negotiations become locked into a win–lose situation, a third party may be invited to assist in resolving the issues (Schwarz, 1994). Interactive problem solving is a form of third-party consultation or informal mediation. Third-party facilitators can be mediators, arbitrators, or consultants. Depending on the situation, a third-party facilitator may have high or low control of either the conflict-resolution process and/or the outcomes. For example, the third party in intraorganizational conflicts is most often the person in the hierarchy to whom the contesting parties report (Lewicki et al., 1992). In this situation, the mediator/supervisor would have high control of both the conflict-resolution process and the outcomes. Mediators usually have high control of the conflict-resolution process and low control of the outcomes (as demonstrated by the VPMA in Case Study 13–6); whereas, arbitrators have a low control of the conflict-resolution process and high control of the outcomes.

In general, interactive negotiation is designed to facilitate a deeper analysis of the problems and issues forcing the conflict. According to Winder (2003), interactive negotiation usually begins with an analysis of the needs of each of the parties and a discussion of the constraints faced by each side that make it difficult to reach a mutually beneficial solution to the conflict. After the analytical dialogue, the parties engage in joint problem solving versus a fight to be won. Interactive negotiation is less focused on directly helping parties reach binding agreements (excluding arbitration) and is more devoted to improving the process of communication, increasing perspectives and understanding, enabling the parties to reframe their substantive goals and priorities, and engaging in more creative problem solving. Other goals include improving the openness and accuracy of communication, improving intergroup expectancies and attitudes, reducing misperceptions and destructive patterns of interaction, inducing mutual positive motivations for creative problem solving, and ultimately, building a sustainable working relationship between the parties (Winder, 2003).

Managers need to understand and appreciate that negotiation is not a zero-sum game. Managers who demonstrate effective conflict-resolution skills are often seen as competent, effective leaders (Gross & Guerrero, 2000; Stamato, 2004). A study by Eckerd College's Management Development Institute (2003) found a significant link between a person's ability to resolve conflict effectively and his or her perceived effectiveness as a leader and suitability for promotion. The sample for the study consisted of 172 employees (90 male, 82 female) from five different types of organizations. Approximately one-half of the participants were middle-level managers or higher in their organization; all of them participated in a program focusing on workplace conflict. The study revealed a strong correlation between certain conflict-resolution behaviors and perceived effectiveness as a leader and promotion potential. Employees who were perceived as good at creating solutions, expressing emotions, and reaching out were considered more effective. Destructive behaviors, on the other hand, such as winning at all costs, displaying anger, demeaning others, and retaliating were found to be the worst career advancement and leadership behaviors. Avoidance behaviors were found to be particularly problematic for would-be negotiators because individuals who are uncomfortable with negotiating, or perceive themselves to be unskilled or ineffective in negotiating, often avoid conflict and thus fail to manage differences effectively. Of particular significance is the study's finding that negotiation skills are an important aspect of leadership.

SUMMARY

In this chapter, we have seen that conflict can have both positive and negative outcomes, that conflicts originate from a variety of sources, that conflict-handling behavior can be learned and that it is adaptive to the situation, and that collaborative behavior is strongly desired as a way to manage conflict.

END-OF-CHAPTER DISCUSSION QUESTIONS

1. Explain the definition of conflict.
2. Describe the four basic types of conflict.
3. Discuss the five levels of conflict.
4. Describe the five conflict-handling modes.
5. Explain the difference between the rational and the bounded rationality approaches to decision making.
6. Explain the limitations of using intuitive and the heuristics or biases approach to decision making.
7. Describe how framing heuristics affects a manager's escalation of commitment.
8. Discuss the four basic styles of decision making.
9. Describe the three major negotiation models.

Case Study 13–7 What Went Wrong?

Tim Hardwood, CEO of Community Health System, hung up the phone with a heavy sigh. Tim had just received the news from Mary Martin, Vice President of Human Resources, that negotiations had stalled between the health system and the service employees' union. Mary related, "As of now, the 2000 service employees at our three hospitals are without a contract and threatening to strike. But don't worry, Tim. I told the union negotiators that the health system is prepared to handle a strike." "A strike, the media will have a field day with this!" Tim wondered, "What went wrong?"

Jim Brentward, one of the union negotiators, sat across the table from Mary Martin. Jim related that his members understood that the health system was having financial difficulties because of the current state of the industry with decreasing reimbursements and increasing regulations, but the union members were not pleased with the health system's proposed offer for salary increases and benefit package over the next four years. He related that "unless the health system signed a contract by 5:00 PM Friday with acceptable salary and benefit increases, members of the union are threatening to strike." Jim continued, "The union plans to hold an informational picket on Thursday, and although the union doesn't want to strike, it's a strong possibility. After the informational picket, we will hold a strike vote and see what our members have to say about the situation."

Mary was shocked by Jim's comments. She simply could not believe that Community's service employees would threaten to strike! Because of her position as Vice President of Human Resources, Mary knew that the service employees represented by Jim's union were in the bottom-end of the health system's pay scale. These employees included patient transporters, housekeeping, and cafeteria workers. Mary also knew that union benefits paid during a strike represented only 50 percent of the employee's/member's weekly salary. Mary felt confident that because of financial restraints, the employees would never vote to strike; they had too much to lose. In addition, she knew that Community Health System was considering outsourcing its dietary departments to Thomson Healthcare Food Services. If the employees did strike, although Mary considered it very unlikely, that aspect of services would continue without interruption. Knowing this inside information, Mary decided she wasn't going to let Jim and the other union negotiators bully her. Mary responded by stating that the health system would not give in to the union's demands and it was prepared for a strike.

Explain to Tim Hardwood what went wrong. If you were hired as the mediator, how would you go about resolving the situation to achieve a win/win agreement?

Case Study 13–8 Conflict-handling Styles

For each of the five scenarios described below, determine what is the most appropriate conflict-handling style(s).

Scenario One

A radiologist on the staff of a large community hospital was stopped after a staff meeting by a colleague in internal medicine. On Monday of the previous week, the internist referred an elderly man with chronic, productive cough for chest X-ray, with a clinical diagnosis of bronchitis. Thursday morning the internist received the radiologist's written X-ray report with a diagnosis of "probable bronchogenic carcinoma." The internist expressed his dismay that the radiologist had not called him much earlier with a verbal report. Visibly upset, the internist raised his voice, but did not use abusive language.

How should the radiologist handle this conflict with the internist?

Scenario Two

The Family and Community Medicine Division of a large-staff model HMO serves a population that is ethnically diverse. The senior management team of the HMO, spurred by repeated complaints from representatives of one racial group, has encouraged the division, all of whose physicians are white, to diversify. Several black and Hispanic physicians with strong credentials apply for the open positions, but none are hired. Weeks later, a young female family physician learns from several colleagues that the division director has identified her as racist and the obstructionist to recruiting. The comments attributed to her are not only false but are also typical of discriminatory statements that she has heard the division chief utter. The rumors about her "behavior" have circulated widely in the division.

How should the young female family physician handle this conflict with the division chief?

Scenario Three

A manager who reports to the Vice President for Clinical Affairs (VPCA) of a tertiary-care hospital hired a young woman to supervise development of a large community outreach program. During the first four months of her employment, several behavioral problems came to the VPCA's attention: (1) complaints from community physicians that the coordinator criticizes other physicians in public; (2) concerns from two community leaders that the coordinator is not truthful; and (3) written reports about the project that label and blame others, sometimes in language that is disrespectful. The VPCA spoke several times to the manager about these problems. The manager reported other dissatisfactions with the coordinator's performance, but he showed no sign of dealing with the behavior. Two more complaints come in, one from an influential community leader.

How should the VPCA handle this conflict with the manager?

Scenario Four

The medical school in an academic health center recently implemented a problem-based curriculum, dramatically reducing the number of lectures given and substituting small-group learning that focuses on actual patient cases. Both clinical and basic science faculty are feeling stretched in their new roles. In the past, dental students took the basic course in microanatomy with medical students. The core lectures are still given but at different times that do not match with the dental-curriculum schedule. The anatomists insist that they don't have time to teach another course specifically for dental students. The dean has informed the chair of the Department of Anatomy and Cell Biology that some educational revenues will be redirected to the dental school if the faculty do not meet this need.

How should the dean handle this conflict with the chair of the Department of Anatomy and Cell Biology?

Scenario Five

The partners in a medical group practice are informed by the clinic manager that one physician member of the group has been repeatedly upcoding procedures for a specific diagnosis. This issue first came to light six months ago. At that time the partners met with him, clarified the Medicare guidelines, and outlined the threat to the practice for noncompliance. He argued with their view, but ultimately agreed to code appropriately. There were no infractions for several months, but now he has submitted several erroneous codes. One member of the office staff has asked whether Medicare would consider this behavior "fraudulent."

How should the partners handle the situation with the other physician partner?

SOURCE: "Managing low-to-mid intensity conflict in the health care setting," by C. A. Aschenbrener-Siders, 1999, *Physician Executive, 25*(5), pp. 44–50. Reprinted with permission.

REFERENCES

Agor, W. H. (1985). Intuition as a brain skill in management. *Public Personnel Management Journal, 14*(1), 15–24.

Agor, W. H. (1986a). How top executives use their intuition to make important decisions. *Business Horizons, 29*(1), 49–53.

Agor, W. H. (1986b). The logic of intuition: How top executives make important decisions. *Organizational Dynamics, 14*(3), 5–18.

Baron, R. A., & Richardson, D. R. (1990). *Human aggression* (2nd ed.). New York: Plenum Books.

Baron, R. A., Fortin, S. P., Frei, R. L., Hauver, L. A., & Shack, M. L. (1990). Reducing organizational conflict: The role of socially induced positive affective. *International Journal of Conflict Management, 1*, 133–152.

Behling, O., & Eckel, N. (1991). Making sense out of intuition. *Academy of Management Executive, 5*(1), 46–54.

Bennett, R. H. (1998). The importance of tacit knowledge in strategic deliberations and decisions. *Management Decision, 36*(9), 589–600.

Blake, R. R., & Mouton, J. S. (1964). *The managerial grid.* Houston, TX: Gulf Publishing.

Blake, R. R., & Mouton, J. S. (1984a). *Solving costly organizational conflicts.* San Francisco, CA: Jossey-Bass.

Blake, R. R., & Mouton, J. S. (1984b). *The managerial grid III* (3rd ed.). Houston, TX: Gulf Publishing.

Boulgarides, J. D., & Cohen, W. A. (2001). Leadership style vs. leadership tactics. *The Journal of Applied Management and Entrepreneurship, 6*(1), 59–73.

Bottles, K. (2001). The good leader—Management skills. *Physician Executive, 27*(2), 74–76.

Brehm, J., & Cohen, A. (1962). *Explorations in cognitive dissonance.* New York: John Wiley & Sons.

Brett, J. M., & Shapiro, D. L. (1998). Breaking bonds of reciprocity in negotiations. *Academy of Management Journal, 41*(4), 410–424.

Cosier, R. A., & Dalton, D. R. (1990). Positive effects of conflict: A field assessment. *International Journal of Conflict Management, 1*, 81–92.

Cross, J. (1969). *The economics of bargaining.* New York: Basic Books.

Dana, D. (2000). *Conflict resolution: Mediation tools for everyday worklife.* New York: McGraw-Hill Book Company.

Daft, R. L. (2004). *Organization theory and design* (8th ed.). Mason, OH: South-Western.

Dequech, D. (2001). Bounded rationality, institutions, and uncertainty. *Journal of Economic Issues, 35*(4), 911–929.

Dewine, S., Nicotera, A. M., & Perry, D. (1991). Argumentativeness and aggressiveness: The flip side of gentle persuasion. *Management Communication Journal, 4,* 386–411.

Eckerd College's Management Development Institute. (2003). Leadership effectiveness study—Conflict and your career. Available at: http://www.conflict dynamics.org/.

Eisenhardt, K., & Bourgeois, L. (1988). Politics of strategic decision making in high velocity environments: Towards a mid-range theory. *Academy of Management Journal, 31,* 737–770.

Filley, A. C. (1975). *Interpersonal conflict resolution.* Chicago, IL: Scott, Foresman.

Fisher, R., & Ury, W. (1981). *Getting to yes.* New York: Penguin Books.

Fisher R., Ury, W., & Patton, B. (1991). *Getting to yes: Negotiating without giving in* (2nd ed.). New York: Penguin Books.

Follett, M. P. (1940). Constructive conflict. In H. C. Metcalf & L. Urwick (Eds.), *Dynamic administration: The collected papers of Mary Parker Follet* (pp. 30–49). New York: Harper (original work published in 1926).

Follett, M. P. (1942). *Creative experience.* New York: Longmans, Green and Co.

Forest, J., & Mehier, C. (2001). John R. Commons and Herbert A. Simon on the concept of rationality. *Journal of Economics, 3*(35), 591–605.

Forte, P. S. (1997). The high cost of conflict. *Nursing Economics, 15,* 119–123.

Friedman, R. (2002). Musical operating rooms: Mini-cases of health care disputes. *International Journal of Conflict Management, 13*(4), 419–420.

Gardner, D. L. (1992). Conflict and retention of new graduate nurses. *Western Journal of Nursing Research, 14,* 76–85.

Golnaz, S., & Rahmatian, M. (2003). Resolving conflict: Examining ethnic-racial and gender differences. *Equal Opportunities International, 22*(2), 25–39.

Gross, M. A., & Guerrero, L. K. (2000). Managing conflict appropriately and effectively: An application of the competence model to Rahim's organizational conflict styles. *International Journal of Conflict Management, 11*(3), 200–226.

Hall, K. H. (2002). Reviewing intuitive decision-making and uncertainty: The implications for medical education. *Medical Education, 36,* 216–224.

Hayashi, A. M. (2001). When to trust your gut. *Harvard Business Review, 79*(2), 59–65.

Jackson, S. E., & Schuler, R. S. (1985). A meta-analysis and conceptual critique of research on role ambiguity and role conflict in work settings. *Organizational Behavior and Human Decision Process, 36,* 16–78.

Jehn, K. A., & Mannix, E. A. (2001, April). The dynamic nature of conflict: A longitudinal study of intragroup conflict and group performance. *Academy of Management Journal, 44*(2), 238–251.

Johnson, M. (1994). Conflict and nursing professionalization. In J. M. McCloskey & H. K. Grace (Eds.), *Current issues in nursing* (4th ed., pp. 643–649). St. Louis, MO: Mosby.

Kabanoff, B. (1991). Equity, equality, power, and conflict. *Academy of Management Review, 16,* 416–441.

Kahneman, D., Slovic, P., & Tversky, A. (Eds.). (1982). *Judgment under uncertainty: Heuristics and biases.* Cambridge, UK: Cambridge University Press.

Kirkbride, R. S., Tang, S. F. Y., & Westwood, R. I. (1991). Chinese conflict preferences and negotiating behavior: Cultural and psychological influences. *Organization Studies, 12,* 365–386.

Kolb, D. M., & Bartunek, J. M. (1992). *Hidden conflict in organizations: Uncovering behind-the-scenes disputes.* Newbury Park, CA: Sage.

Kottler, J. (1996). *Beyond blame: A new way of resolving conflicts in relationship.* San Francisco: Jossey-Bass Publishers.

Lee, C. (1990). Relative status of employees and styles of handling interpersonal conflict. *International Journal of Conflict Management, 1,* 327–340.

Levin, I. P., Schnittjer, S. K., & Thee, S. L. (1988). Information framing effects in social and personal decisions. *Journal of Experimental Social Psychology, 24,* 520–529.

Lewicki, R., Weiss, S., & Lewin, D. (1992). Models of conflict, negotiation and third party intervention: A review and synthesis. *Journal of Organizational Behavior, 13,* 209–252.

Locke, E. A., Smith, K. G., Erez, M., Chah, D.O., & Schaffer, A. (1994). The effects of intra-individual goal conflict on performance. *Journal of Management, 20,* 67–92.

Longest, B. B., & Brooks, D. H. (1998). Managerial competence at senior levels of integrated delivery systems. *Journal of Healthcare Management, 43*(2), 115–135.

McElhaney, R. (1996). Conflict management in nursing administration. *Nursing Management 24,* 65–66.

March, S., & Simon, H. (1993). *Organizations* (2nd ed.). Cambridge, UK: Blackwell.

Morrow, K. A., & Deidan, C. T. (1992). Bias in the counseling process: How to recognize and avoid it. *Journal of Counseling & Development, 70*(5), 571–577.

Myers, I. (1980). *Introduction to type.* Palo Alto, CA: Consulting Psychologists, Inc.

Nulty, P. (1993, February). Look at what unions want now. *Fortune,* 128–133.

Peters, T. J., & Waterman, Jr., R. H. (1984). *In search of excellence: Lessons from America's best-run companies.* New York: Warner Books.

Pondy, R. L. (1967). Organizational conflict. Concept and models. *Administrative Science Quarterly, 12,* 296–320.

Porter-O'Grady, T., & Epstein, D. G. (2003). When push comes to shove: Managers as mediators. *Nursing Management, 34*(10), 34–38.

Rahim, M. A. (1985). A strategy for managing conflict in complex organizations. *Human Relations, 38,* 81–89.

Rahim, M. A., Garrett, J. E., & Buntzman, G. F. (1992). Ethics of managing interpersonal conflict in organizations. *Journal of Business Ethics, 11*(5/6), 423–432.

Robbins, S. (1990). *Organization theory* (3rd ed.). Englewood Cliffs, NJ: Prentice Hall.

Rowe, A. J., & Boulgarides, J. D. (1983). Decision-styles: A perspective. *Leadership & Organization Development Journal, 4*(4), 3–9.

Rowe, A. J., & Boulgarides, J. D. (1998). *Managerial decision making.* New York: Macmillan Publishing Company.

Rubin, J. Z., & Brown, B. R. (1975). *The social psychology of bargaining and negotiation.* New York: Academic Press.

Schwarz, R. M. (1994). *The skilled facilitator: Practical wisdom for developing effective groups.* San Francisco, CA: Jossey-Bass.

Shelton, C. D., & Darling, J. R. (2004). From chaos to order: Exploring new frontiers in conflict management. *Organization Development Journal, 22*(3), 22–41.

Simon, H. A. (1957). *Administrative behavior* (2nd ed.). New York: Macmillan.

Simon, H. A. (1987). Making management decisions: The role of intuition and emotion. *Academy of Management Executive, 1,* 57–64.

Sox, H. C., Marshal, A. B., Higgins, M. C., & Marton, K. I. (1988). *Medical decision-making.* New York: Butterworths.

Stamato, L. (2004, July/August). The new age of negotiation. *Ivey Business Journal Online.* Available at: www.iveybusinessjournal.com/archives.

Staw, B. M., (1981). The escalation of commitment to a course of action. *Academy of Management Review, 6*(4), 577–587.

Staw, B. M., & Ross, P. (1987). Knowing when to pull the plug. *Harvard Business Review, 65*(2), 68–74.

Stevens, C. M. (1963). *Strategy and collective bargaining negotiation.* New York: McGraw-Hill Book Company.

Tarantino, D. P. (2004). The role of the physician executive in negotiation. *Physician Executive, 30*(5), 71–73.

Thomas, K. W. (1976). Conflict and conflict management. In M. Dunnette (Ed.), *Handbook of industrial and organizational psychology* (pp. 889–935). Chicago, IL: Rand McNally College Publishing Company.

Thomas, K. W. (1992). Conflict and negotiation processes in organizations. In M. Dunette (Ed.), *Handbook of industrial and organizational psychology* (2nd ed., Vol. 3, pp. 651–717). Palo Alto, CA: Consulting Psychologists Press.

Thomas, K. W., & Kilmann, R. H. (1974). *Thomas-Kilmann Conflict Mode Instrument.* Tuxedo, NY: Xicom, Inc. (Currently available through Consulting Psychologist's Press.)

Thomas, K., & Schmidt, W. (1976). A survey of managerial interests with respect to conflict. *Academy of Management Journal, 19*(2), 315–318.

Thompson, C. (2003). Clinical experience as evidence in evidence-based practice. *Journal of Advanced Nursing, 43*(3), 230–237.

Thompson, L. (1990). Negotiation behavior and outcome: Empirical evidence and theoretical issues. *Psychological Bulletin, 108,* 515–532.

Tversky, A., & Kahneman, D. (1974). Judgment under uncertainty: Heuristics and biases. *Science, 185,* 1124–1131.

Wally, S., & Baum, R. (1994). Personal and structural determinants of the pace of strategic decision making. *Academy of Management Journal, 37,* 932–956.

Walton, R. E., & McKersie, R. B. (1965). *A behavioral theory of labor negotiations: An analysis of a social interaction system.* New York: McGraw-Hill Book Company.

Watson, C., & Hoffman, L. R. (1996). Managers as negotiators. *Leadership Quarterly, 7*(1), 63–85.

Winder, R. (2003). Organizational dynamics and development. *Futurics, 27*(1/2), 5–30.

OTHER SUGGESTED READING

Agor, W. H. (1984). *Intuitive management: Integrating left and right brain management skills.* Upper Saddle River, NJ: Prentice Hall.

Ashford, B. E. (2001). *Role transitions in organizational life: An identity-based perspective.* Mahwah, NJ: Lawrence Erlbaum Associates.

Bates, B. (1975). Physician and nurse practitioners: Conflict and reward. *Annals of Internal Medicine, 82,* 702–706.

Brett, J. F., Northcraft, G. B., & Pinkley, R. L. (1999). Stairways to heaven: An interlocking self-regulation model of negotiation. *Academy of Management Review, 24*(3), 435–451.

Davis, M. H., Capobianco, S., & Kraus, L. (2004). Measuring conflict-related behaviors: Reliability and validity evidence regarding the conflict dynamics profile. *Educational and Psychological Measurement, 64*(4), 707–731.

Elangovan, A. R. (2002). Managerial intervention in disputes: The role of cognitive biases and heuristics. *Leadership & Organization Development Journal, 23*(7), 390–399.

Friedman, R. A., Tidd, S. T., Currall, S. C., & Tsai, J. C. (2002). What goes around comes around: The impact of personal conflict style on work conflict and stress. *International Journal of Conflict Management, 11*(1), 32–55.

Gigerenzer, G. (2007). *Gut feelings: the intelligence of the unconscious.* New York: Penguin Group.

Kahneman, D. (1991). Judgment and decision making: A personal view. *Psychological Science, 2*(3), 142–154.

Kilmann, R. H., & Thomas, K. W. (1977). Developing a forced-choice measure of conflict-handling behavior: The mode instrument. *Education and Psychological Development, 37,* 309–325.

Kolb, D. M., & Putman, L. L. (1992, May). The multiple faces of conflict in organizations. *Journal of Organizational Behavior, 13,* 311–324.

McWilliams, C. (2003). Healthcare decision making for dementia patients: Two problem cases. *Internet Journal of Law, Healthcare and Ethics, 2*(1), 12–19.

O'Connor, K. M., DeDreu, C. K., Schroth, H., Barry, B. Lituchy, T. R., & Bazerman, M. H. (2002). What we want to do versus what we think we should do: An empirical investigation of intrapersonal conflict. *Journal of Behavioral Decision Making, 15,* 403–418.

Shelton, C. D., & Darling, J. R. (2004). From chaos to order: Exploring new frontiers in conflict management. *Organization Development Journal, 22*(3), 22–41.

Thomas, K. W. (1992). Conflict and conflict management: Reflections and update. *Journal of Organizational Behavior, 13,* 265–274.

PART V

Groups and Teams

As we learned in Chapter 5, people are social beings and require satisfying a need for affiliation or achieving a sense of belonging. Groups help satisfy this need. In Chapter 14, we examine group dynamics. Group dynamics is a term, created by Kurt Lewin, used to describe the subfield of organizational behavior that attempts to understand the nature of groups, how they develop, and how they interact with the members, other groups, and their environments. In Chapter 15, we discuss the various types of groups and their related functions. Chapter 16 examines the use of teams in today's complex health service organizations. In health care, as in most organizations, few jobs can be performed start to finish by one person. To complete a task requires resources from many individuals. Today, we see the widespread use of multidiscipline teams to deliver effective and efficient health care.

CHAPTER 14

Overview of Group Dynamics

Nancy Borkowski, DBA, CPA, FACHE

LEARNING OUTCOMES

After completing this chapter, the student should understand:

- ☛ The importance of group dynamics.
- ☛ The characteristics that define a group.
- ☛ The meaning of group interaction and methods to measure it.
- ☛ What motivates individuals to join and remain in groups.
- ☛ The various roles members assume in groups and the importance of these roles.
- ☛ The meaning of group norms and how they are formed and sustained.
- ☛ The factors that contribute to or inhibit group cohesiveness.
- ☛ The impact of conformity to group performance.
- ☛ The impact of groupthink to group decision making.

OVERVIEW

Human beings are social animals. Although we are born into and leave the world in a singular manner, we spend the majority of our time working, worshiping, learning, and playing in groups. Because we spend so much of our time in groups, there is great interest in understanding the inner workings of groups and their members. This research is referred to as the study of group dynamics, which is the attempt to understand the behavior in which people interact with, influence, and are influenced by others within groups.

Why is understanding group dynamics important to managers? It is important to the success of an organization. More and more organizations are moving toward a stronger emphasis on their employees working in groups and/or teams. A study by Blackburn and Rosen (1993) found that Federal Express had 4,000 employee teams, Motorola used 2,200 problem-solving teams, more than 60 percent of Cadillac's workforce is a member of some type of team, and at any given time 76 percent of Xerox's employees serve on some type of task force or on advisory teams. It is estimated that, on average, managers spend 50 percent to 80 percent of their working day in one sort of group or another. In the healthcare setting, this estimate is not surprising. Healthcare managers, both clinical and administrative, participate in numerous groups on a daily basis, such as operating room teams, disease management teams, patient safety committees, biomedical ethics committees, patient care teams, trauma teams, and emergency-preparedness and disaster-management teams. Therefore, managers need to understand the variables involved in relating to groups: (1) formation and development, (2) structure, and (3) interrelationships with individuals, other groups, and the organizations within which they exist, so that they may effectively manage them (Turner, 2000).

Our discussion of groups is divided into three sections. In the present chapter we define what a group is, discuss why individuals join groups, and then examine the interactions and behavior of members within a group. In Chapter 15 we discuss the various types of groups, their formation and development, and the various group decision-making processes. In Chapter 16 we discuss teams and team building. Although many use the terms groups and teams interchangeably, there are differences. The concept of groups is broader than the concept of teams. Katzenbach and Smith (1993) point out that teams are a special form of groups that have highly defined tasks and roles and demonstrate high group commitment. Because of these characteristics, we discuss the nature of teams separately.

WHAT IS A GROUP?

Social scientists usually define a group using four characteristics: (1) two or more people in social interaction, (2) a stable structure, (3) common interests or goals, and (4) the individuals perceiving themselves as a group. For example, two patients waiting to be treated in a hospital's emergency department are not a group. This collection of two individuals is not a group because: (1) There is no interaction between the two patients, nor are they attempting to influence each other; (2) patients in an emergency department constantly change; therefore, a stable environment does not exist for future interactions; (3) although patients may share similar goals (e.g., restoring their healthy status, alleviation of pain), they are not working in a coordinated effort to achieve a common goal; and (4) they do not perceive themselves as a group, only as individuals occupying space in the same location at the same time. However, a group exists when volunteer members of the local chapter of the American Heart Association meet to plan the next fund-raising event, or when a multidisciplinary medical team convenes for the purpose of developing clinical practice guidelines for patients admitted to the hospital with congestive heart failure. These groups represent collections of individuals with a common interest or goal in a stable environment (although members may join and leave the group at various times), wherein members interact with one another with the intent of influencing the other(s). One important factor relating to group dynamics is understanding the interactions that occur between a group's members.

GROUP INTERACTION

Tubbs (2001) defines group interaction as the process by which members of a group exchange verbal and nonverbal messages in an attempt to influence one another. Therefore, interaction includes talking, listening, nonverbal gestures, and any other behavior to which people assign meaning. Can we observe these interactions to better understand the dynamics within a group? Yes, we can. On a formal level, researchers may use a sociogram to record their observations of the interactions between members of a group (see Figure 14–1).

A sociogram is a pictorial method of mapping out and recording the contributions of members to a group interaction. In the example shown in Figure 14–1, the number of inputs is recorded as lines in the circles, each of which represents a participant in the interaction. The arrows show the direction of the contributions made, and their thickness indicates the intensity of the traffic. Where an arrow points outward, that indicates a contribution made to the group as a whole, rather than to an individual member. Where a member addresses the group in general, rather than a particular member, arrows are shown pointing outward to reflect that.

However, a sociogram is limited to documenting the direction and intensity of communication, not the content of what was communicated by the members in their attempt to influence one another. Therefore, researchers can use other assessment tools, such as the Bales' Interaction Process Analysis, that can provide insight about the content of the members' communication (see Figure 14–2).

As noted by Sprott (1958), there are 12 categories of interactions with Bales' Interaction Process Analysis; these interactions are classified as relating to either emotion or task. The emotional responses are either positive (items 1 to 3) or negative (items 10 to 12). Task responses are either giving (items 4 to 6) or asking for information (items 7 to 9). The 12 categories are also grouped into pairs, as noted in Table 14–1. The interactions of these 12 categories greatly influence the roles assumed by members and group norms.

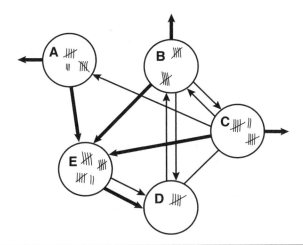

Figure 14–1 A Typical Sociogram

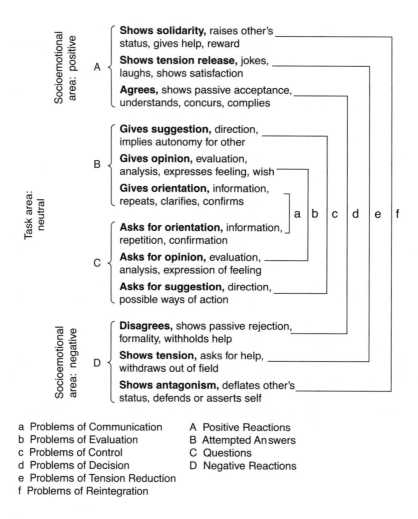

a Problems of Communication   A Positive Reactions
b Problems of Evaluation   B Attempted Answers
c Problems of Control   C Questions
d Problems of Decision   D Negative Reactions
e Problems of Tension Reduction
f Problems of Reintegration

Figure 14–2 Bales' Interaction Process Analysis

WHY DO PEOPLE JOIN GROUPS?

Individuals join groups for many reasons and many of these reasons are explained with Maslow's Hierarchy of Needs (see Chapter 5). Individuals join groups to satisfy their need for belonging (i.e., the need to have close contact with others and to be accepted by them), in addition to social and affection needs. Groups can satisfy an individual's need for safety by reducing the sense of powerlessness and anxiety, which one may experience in ambiguous or threatening situations. Members may join because group affiliation can be an important part of an individual's self-esteem as well as social identity. People need to have a positive opinion of themselves, which arises in part from acceptance by others in a group and evidence that other group members share their views and values. Furthermore, a group can help members achieve stated

Table 14–1 Bales' Interaction Process Analysis: Twelve Categories Paired

Items	Description	Example
1 and 12	Orientation	How well do the group members cohere? Bales gives the example of a man who makes an offensive remark directed at another member (item 12); however, the laughter that follows is classified under item 2.
2 and 11	Emotional response only	Bales gives the example of a member sighing heavily and examining his fingernails.
3 and 10	Acceptance or rejection	
4 and 9	Control	Asking for suggestions such as "I think we should do this" or "How do you think we ought to tackle this?" By asking for suggestions, a member is getting the others to commit themselves. By committing themselves, members limit their future choices. This is a method of bringing other members under control, which may or may not lead to resentment.
5 and 8	Opinion	"Have we done that?" "We ought to make sure that we do this." Any comments that involve summarizing the issues.
6 and 7	Orientation	Setting out the problem and giving factual information.

Source: *Interaction process analysis: A method for the study of small groups*, by R. F. Bales, 1950. Chicago: University of Chicago Press. Reprinted with permission.

goals that the member, by himself or herself, could not have achieved alone. Group membership can satisfy a number of needs for an individual, in addition to the member contributing to other members and the group achieving objectives. However, deciding whether to join a group or to continue membership with a group poses an approach/avoidance conflict for people (see Chapter 13). As such, an individual will perform a cost/benefit analysis of the relationship. Members will continue with their association as long as the rewards (satisfaction of needs) outweigh or are equal to the costs of being a member, such as required time to participate and financial commitment. This cost/benefit analysis is analogous to Adam's Equity Theory of Motivation (see Chapter 6).

ROLES OF GROUP MEMBERS

Functional Role Theory, as introduced by Benne and Sheats (1948), identified the functional roles they observed individual group members assuming in small group interactions. The three roles identified were task, maintenance, and individual (sometimes called "self-centered") roles (see Exhibit 14–1).

Exhibit 14–1 Benne and Sheats' Functional Roles of Group Members

Task Roles—Groups have members who play roles relating to job completion:

- *Initiator-contributor:* Generates new ideas.
- *Information-seeker:* Asks for information about the task.
- *Opinion-seeker:* Asks for the input from the group about its values.
- *Information-giver:* Offers facts or generalization to the group.
- *Opinion-giver:* States his or her beliefs about a group issue.
- *Elaborator:* Explains ideas within the group, offers examples to clarify ideas.
- *Coordinator:* Shows the relationships between ideas.
- *Orienter:* Shifts the direction of the group's discussion.
- *Evaluator-critic:* Measures group's actions against some objective standard.
- *Energizer:* Stimulates the group to a higher level of activity.
- *Procedural-technician:* Performs logistical functions for the group.
- *Recorder:* Keeps a record of group actions.

Maintenance Roles—Groups also have members who play certain social roles:

- *Encourager:* Praises the ideas of others.
- *Harmonizer:* Mediates differences between group members.
- *Compromiser:* Moves group to another position that is favored by all group members.
- *Gatekeeper/expediter:* Keeps communication channels open.
- *Standard setter:* Suggests standards or criteria for the group to achieve.
- *Group observer:* Keeps records of group activities and uses this information to offer feedback to the group.
- *Follower:* Goes along with the group and accepts the group's ideas.

Individual Roles—Member roles that can be counterproductive to the group accomplishing its task or goals:

- *Aggressor:* Attacks other group members, deflates the status of others, and shows other aggressive behavior.
- *Blocker:* Resists movement by the group.
- *Recognition seeker:* Calls attention to himself or herself.
- *Self-confessor:* Seeks to disclose nongroup-related feelings or opinions.
- *Dominator:* Asserts control over the group by manipulating the other group members.
- *Help seeker:* Tries to gain the sympathy of the group.

SOURCE: "Functional roles of group members," by K. Benne and P. Sheats, 1948. *Journal of Social Issues, 4,* 41–49. Reprinted with permission.

Task-oriented roles focus on goal accomplishment; maintenance roles focus on relationships; and individual roles focus on individual needs, which may in the long run be harmful to the group's overall success. Benne and Sheats' task and maintenance roles are similar to the two communication patterns, task-oriented and socioemotional, that were identified by Bales (1950, 1953, 1970, 1999) with his research of group members' interactions. Bales' task role relates to a member's activities that help the group accomplish its goals (e.g., concern for production), and his or her socioemotional role is described as the activities that a member performs to promote harmonious relations within the group (e.g., concern for people) (refer to Figure 14–2).

Members may assume different roles depending on the needs of the individual or group. However, Bales found that some members engaged in more task and socioemotional activities than others and, as a result, were offered leadership status in the group. But Bales also found that the person who engaged in the most task activities was not the same person who performed the most socioemotional activities. Therefore, two leaders emerged: the task leader, who was rated as having the best ideas, offering the most guidance, and being most influential in forming the group's opinions, and the socioemotional leader, who was the best liked. The usual explanation for the emergence of the second leader is that a task leader's sense of purpose gives rise to activities (e.g., unpopular orders, sharp criticism) that hurt group members' feelings. The second leader emerged to smooth things over and restore harmony to the group.

Belbin (1981, 1993, 2004) studied the performance of a team and how performance was directly affected by the roles that members play. Belbin developed the Team Role Theory, which proposes that for optimal operation of a management team, nine (originally eight) personality-related team roles needed to be fulfilled. The roles are: chairman/coordinator, shaper, plant, teamworker, completer/finisher, company worker/implementator, resource investigator, monitor/evaluator, and specialist. Belbin's nine roles can be categorized as either task/task-oriented, maintenance/socioemotional positive, or individual/socioemotional negative with Benne and Sheats' Functional Role Theory and Bales' Interaction Analysis (see Table 14–2). All groups need task leadership as well as attention to details and a concern for people for effectiveness. Understanding the various members' roles is important to understanding the interactions that either push toward or hinder a group from meeting its goals, including member satisfaction with the interactions. The role(s) a member assumes and the resulting interactions greatly influence the group's norms.

GROUP NORMS

Every group has a set of norms, which is an implied code of conduct about what is acceptable and unacceptable member behavior. Norms can be written or unwritten, positive, negative, or neutral and applied to all members of the group or only to certain ones. In addition, groups will apply "punishment" or sanctions to members if their behavior deviates from the group's norms. Norms can dictate the performance level of groups (e.g., high- or low-productivity work groups), the appearance of group members (e.g., bankers wear dark suits), or the social arrangement within the group (chair of the committee sits at the head of the conference table).

If written, norms become the formal rules of conduct for group members (see Exhibit 14–2). Most organizations have formal rules of conduct, which are delineated in their policies and procedures manual. For example, a hospital would have written policies as to clinical research protocols; infection-control procedures for handling blood and other body fluids; the proper attire to be worn in operating room suites; and processes to ensure that the correct surgical site is used, that the correct patient is operated on, and that procedure before surgery is performed.

Table 14–2 Comparison of Members' Roles

Benne and Sheats (1948)	Bales (1950)	Belbin (1981, 1993)	Description (Belbin)
Task	Task-oriented	Chairman	Also referred to as the coordinator—The mature and confident person who enables others to give their best, keeps the team oriented toward its goals, and is rarely the source of ideas
Task	Task-oriented	Shaper	The top-down leader, energetic, challenging, and pressurizing, who drives his or her ideas to conclusion
Task	Task-oriented	Plant	The creative and unorthodox problem solver, probably not very good with people
Maintenance	Socioemotional	Teamworker (positive)	Interpersonally perceptive and caring person who enables individuals to work together, but who may be indecisive under pressure
Task	Task-oriented	Completer/ finisher	The rules person who dots the i's and crosses the t's and will not give up until the job is satisfactorily completed and who may be a worrier
Task	Task-oriented	Company worker	Who implements, gets things done to meet goals, and who may be somewhat inflexible
Task	Task-oriented	Resource investigator	Who is out and about, seeking new ideas and exploring opportunities, and who may become bored with routine
Individual (negative)	Socioemotional	Monitor/ evaluator	Who is judgmental, looking for faults, and seeking to prevent errors, but who may not inspire others
Task	Task-oriented	Specialist	Single-minded and dedicated, who has unique knowledge but whose contributions are limited to that knowledge

Exhibit 14–2 Formal Rules of Conduct

Notice of Monthly Meeting of the
Biomedical Ethics Committee of Glen Haven Hospital

- Monthly meetings are held on the first Tuesday of each month.
- Meetings begin at 5 PM and end at 7 PM.
- If you are unable to attend the meeting, please notify the Secretary of the committee.
- No item will be discussed unless noted on the agenda. If you wish to add an item for discussion, please notify the Chair of the committee no less than two weeks prior to the scheduled meeting. The Chair must approve all agenda items.
- Issues requiring a vote of committee members will pass by a majority (hand) vote.
- New business will be discussed during the last 15 minutes of the meeting (no exceptions!).

However, in most instances group norms are unwritten and learned by members through their interactions with others. For example, Crandall (1988) studied groups of cheerleaders, dancers, and female sorority members with high rates of eating disorders and noted that these groups adopted the behaviors of binging and purging as normal methods of weight control. The most popular members of the group binged and purged at the rate established by the norms of the group, and those who did not binge and purge when they first joined the group were more likely to take up the practice the longer they were members of the group. This alignment of behavior within a group is part of an individual's socialization process. This process of socialization explains how unwritten norms become the "standards" for the group, as members begin to internalize the group's norms as their own behavior standards.

Since most group norms are unwritten, they are usually not easily identified until violated. When group norms are violated, members of the group will attempt to convince the "deviant" to conform to the group's standards of behavior. If the use of persuasion is not successful, the group may punish the member by withdrawing any "special" status that he or she may hold, or psychologically reject (e.g., ignore) the member. The final consequence for a member who refuses to conform would be dismissal from the group. Through this process, members learn the range or boundaries of acceptable behavior within a group. For example, Feldman (1984) describes the norms about productivity that frequently develop among piece-rate workers. A person produces 50 widgets and is praised by his coworkers; a person produces 60 widgets and receives a sharp teasing from them; a person produces 70 widgets and is ostracized by the group. Not all behavior deviations will be enforced, only those violations that have some significant effect on the group meeting its goals (see Table 14–3). Norms are powerful forces not only over the behavior of group members, but also in determining the degree of cohesiveness and conformity of the group.

Table 14–3 Why Norms Are Enforced

Four Conditions Under Which Group Norms Are Most Likely to Be Enforced	Example
If norms facilitate group survival	Members do not discuss internal problems with members of other organizational units
If norms simplify, or make predictable, what behavior is expected of group members	Negative comments on presentations or proposals will be made on an individual basis, not during large, formal meetings
If norms help the group avoid embarrassing interpersonal problems	Members do not discuss romantic involvement so that differences in moral values do not become salient
If norms express the central values of the group and clarify what is distinctive about the group's identity	Levels of productivity should remain relatively stable because the group is more concerned with maximizing group security than about individual profits

SOURCE: "The development and enforcement of group norms," by D. C. Feldman, 1984. *The Academy of Management Review, 9,* 47–53. Reprinted with permission.

COHESIVENESS

The degree of cohesiveness (e.g., camaraderie) of a group is determined by various factors, which may include members' dependence and physical location/proximity. The more significant factors tend to be: (1) the size of the group, (2) experience of success by the group, (3) group status, and (4) outside threats to the group.

Size of the Group

Researchers have determined that the size of the group has a direct impact on the cohesiveness of a group. When there are too many members, it becomes too difficult for members to interact. Luft (1984, p. 23) concluded that "cohesion tends to be weaker and morale tends to be lower in large groups than in comparable smaller ones." What is the acceptable size group? Kameda, Stasson, David, Parks, and Zimmerman (1992) suggest that five members appear to be the optimum group size. Five-member groups are small enough for meaningful interaction yet large enough to generate an adequate number of ideas (Tubbs, 2001). Small groups may also avoid the problem of social loafing.

Social Loafing

Social loafing refers to the decreased effort of individual members in a group when the size of the group increases (Tubbs, 2001). Ringelmann (1913) identified this social phenomenon when he noticed that as more and more people were added to a group pulling on a rope, the total force exerted by the group rose, but the average force exerted by each group member declined. The reason is that some members' performance became mediocre because they assumed that other members would pick up the slack. Karau and Williams (1993) found that social loafing occurs across work populations and tasks. However, the researchers noted that if the participants' dominant culture emphasized collectivism versus individualism, the degree of social loafing decreased (see Chapter 2 regarding Hofstede's four dimensions of national culture).

Subsequent studies revealed that when an individual's contribution is identified, and the person is held directly accountable for and rewarded for his or her behavior, social loafing may be eliminated (Kerr, 1983; Kerr & Bruun, 1981; Shepperd, 1993, Szymanski & Harkins, 1987). However, sometimes members will hold back if they believe other members of their group are not extending equal efforts toward accomplishing the task (refer to discussion of Adam's Equity Theory in Chapter 6).

Experience of Success

Prior success of a group reaching its goals has a direct impact on the degree of cohesiveness. No one wants to stay on a losing team! When a group fails to obtain its goals, members display a lack of unity by infighting, finger pointing, and, finally, disassociation.

Group Status

Cohesiveness is more prominent when admission into the group is more difficult to obtain because of various barriers or high criteria, for example, education levels. This perception of status, whether real or not, creates a feeling of being in the "in-group" for those individuals who were able to overcome the barriers for admission into the group, for example, a physicians' group.

Outside Threats to the Group

The cohesiveness of a group will increase if members perceive that an external force may prohibit the group from obtaining its goals. Members of the group will unite to display a unified front to the opposing force. In addition, cohesive groups will unite against nonconforming members who threaten the esprit de corps of the group. As such, cohesive groups exert pressure on members of the group to conform.

Managers should assist their subordinates' development into cohesive work groups because research has shown that cohesive units demonstrate a higher level of productivity when compared to less cohesive groups. However, managers need to be aware that group norms may mediate the relationship between cohesiveness and performance. On the one hand, if norms support performance-related activities, then cohesiveness is likely to improve performance. If, on the other hand, norms support limited output or engagement in irrelevant tasks, cohesiveness may undermine performance (Berkowitz, 1954).

In conclusion, group cohesiveness is a product of social identification. According to Hogg and Abrams (1990), the more positive a member feels about his or her group, the more motivated the person is to promote in-group solidarity, cooperation, and support. In turn, the more cohesive a group is, the more likely its members will socially interact and influence one another (Turner, 1987). Because of these interactions, we find that more cohesive groups have a tendency to pressure their members toward a higher degree of conformity, and a high degree of conformity may lower the performance level of the group.

CONFORMITY

Strong group norms and high degrees of group cohesiveness can hamper the performance of a group because of conformity pressures. Conformity involves the changing of an individual's perceptions or behaviors to match the attitudes or behaviors of others. This "normative social influence" is when we conform to what we believe to be the norms of the group in order to be accepted by its members.

One of the earliest studies in the conformity area was Sherif's (1936) experiment that involved the autokinetic effect. Sherif pointed a light in a dark space that, although stationary, appeared to move. Subjects were asked to estimate the amount of movement they observed both as individuals and as a member of a group. When in groups, the subjects changed their original estimates to more closely fit the answers of the other members. This experiment demonstrated the individual's urge to conform.

Asch (1952) also conducted conformity studies. In Asch's experiments, eight people were seated around a table. Of these eight people, seven were actually the experimenters or confederates. However, the eighth person was unaware of this situation. The group was shown two cards; each card contained different lengths of vertical lines (i.e., no two lines matched in length on either card). The participants were asked to say which of the lines matched the length of another. One after another, the participants announced their decisions. The confederates had been asked to give the incorrect response. The eighth subject sat in the next to last seat so that all but one participant had given their obviously incorrect answer before the subject gave his answer. Even though the correct answer was obvious (i.e., no two lines matched in length on either card), Asch found that one-third of the subjects conformed to the majority, one-third never conformed, and the remaining one-third gave conforming responses at least once. This experiment was designed to create pressure on subjects to conform to others, which in fact they did.

Although Asch's experiment has been criticized for being unrealistic (i.e., in the real world individuals would be making decisions on subjects more complex and more important than the length of a line), it did confirm that "humans have the tendency to conform to the goals and ideas of a small group and tend to be unwilling to go against the group even if they know the group is wrong" (Asch, 1960).

Not all people conform. There is evidence that those who do not conform tend to have a healthy level of self-esteem and to have mature social relationships, as well as being fairly flexible and open-minded in their thinking. For example, Crutchfield (1955) and Tuddenham (1958) found that there is a correlation between high intelligence and other personality traits and low conformity. Another important aspect of conformity is that it may lead to "groupthink."

GROUPTHINK

Strong conformity pressures reflect members' attempts to maintain harmony within the group. However, conformity may hamper a group's performance by decreasing innovation and increasing faulty decision making. Janis (1982) referred to this situation as "groupthink." Groupthink refers to conditions under which efforts to maintain group harmony undermine critical thought and lead to poor decisions (Janis, 1982; Janis & Mann, 1977). Janis, as cited in Tubbs (2001, p. 236), identified eight symptoms of groupthink:

Type I: Overestimation of the group—its power and morality

1. An illusion of invulnerability, shared by most or all of the members, which creates excessive optimism and encourages taking extreme risks.
2. An unquestioned belief in the group's inherent morality, inclining the members to ignore the ethical or moral consequences of their decisions.

Type II: Closed-mindedness

3. Collective efforts to rationalize in order to discount warnings or other information that might lead the members to reconsider their assumptions before they recommit themselves to their past policy decisions.
4. Stereotyped views of enemy leaders as too evil to warrant genuine attempts to negotiate or as too weak and stupid to counter whatever risky attempts are made to defeat their purposes.

Type III: Pressures toward uniformity

5. Self-censorship of deviation from the apparent group consensus, reflecting each member's inclination to minimize to himself the importance of his doubts and counterarguments.
6. A shared illusion of unanimity concerning judgments conforming to the majority view (partly resulting from self-censorship of deviations, augmented by the false assumption that silence means consent).
7. Direct pressure on any member who expresses strong arguments against any of the group's stereotypes, illusions, or commitments, making clear that this type of dissent is contrary to what is expected of all loyal members.
8. The emergence of self-appointed mindguards—members who protect the group from adverse information that might shatter its shared complacency about the effectiveness and morality of its decisions.

Was groupthink the downfall of HealthSouth? (See Exhibit 14–3.) Many of HealthSouth's former senior managers, including all former chief financial officers and the former chief executive officer (CEO) of HealthSouth, a nationwide provider of outpatient surgery and rehabilitative services headquartered in Birmingham, Alabama, had been indicted and/or found guilty of fraudulently and systemically inflating the company's earnings and assets by approximately $4 billion since the mid-1990s.

Exhibit 14–3 Five HealthSouth Officers Charged with Conspiracy to Commit Wire & Securities Fraud

Count 1 of the Information alleges that a conspiracy existed from in or about 1994 until the present between AYERS, EDWARDS, MORGAN, AND VALENTINE and with Owens, Smith, Harris, and others to devise a scheme to inflate artificially HealthSouth's publicly reported earnings and the value of its assets, and to falsify reports of HealthSouth's financial condition. It was part of the conspiracy that Owens, Smith, Harris, and others would provide the Chief Executive Officer (CEO) with monthly and quarterly preliminary reports showing HealthSouth's true and actual financial results. After reviewing these reports, Owens, Smith, Harris, and others would direct that HealthSouth's accounting staff find ways to ensure that HealthSouth's "earnings per share" number met or exceeded Wall Street analyst expectations. After Owens, Smith, Harris, and others issued instructions as to the desired earnings per share number, HealthSouth's accounting staff would meet to discuss ways to inflate artificially HealthSouth's earnings to meet the CEO's desired earnings numbers.

These meetings were known as "family" meetings, and attendees were known as the "family." At the meetings, they would discuss ways by which members of the accounting staff would falsify HealthSouth's books to fill the "gap" or "hole" and meet the desired earnings. The fraudulent postings used to fill the "hole" were referred to as the "dirt." Owens, Smith, Harris, and others would and did direct one or more of the defendants, also members of the accounting staff, to make false entries in HealthSouth's books and records for the purpose of artificially inflating HealthSouth's revenue and earnings. Owens, Smith, Harris, and others would direct one or more of the defendants to make corresponding false entries in HealthSouth's books and records for the purpose of artificially inflating the value of its assets, including, but not limited to, false entries made to (a) Property, Plant and Equipment ("PP&E") accounts; (b) cash accounts; (c) inventory accounts; and (d) intangible asset [goodwill]. When events required that financial records and reports related to units of HealthSouth were called for by auditors, purchasers, and others, Owens, Smith, Harris, and others would direct one or more of the defendants to generate records and reports that would black out the false entries. Owens, Smith, and one or more of the defendants would, for the purpose of deceiving auditors, manufacture false documents for the purpose of supporting false record entries. One or more of the defendants would and did change codes on accounts to deceive auditors.

SOURCE: Excerpt from the US Department of Justice's Press Release dated April 3, 2003. The complete press release is available at: www.usdoj.gov/usao/aln

Managers must be careful because sometimes we find that group members' desire to maintain their close team relationships, or in the HealthSouth case, "the family relationship," at all costs. When group members operate in a groupthink mode, they may engage in decision making. For example, a new medical procedure is proposed for joint replacements. Some team members are initially resistant because of high training demands, even though the new procedure would establish best practices. To preserve harmony in the group, other staff members go along with the resisting members. The team has succumbed to group thinking instead of critical thinking.

There are many who have studied the culture of the National Aeronautics and Space Administration (NASA) after the *Challenger* disaster and found evidence of this type of groupthink. Engineers did not voice their concerns and criticism because of the strong team spirit and camaraderie at NASA. In other words, it is when groups display a high degree of cohesiveness that you have to be on guard against groupthink.

Some suggested safeguards against groupthink include: (1) soliciting outside expert opinions during the decision-making process, (2) appointing a devil's advocate to challenge majority views, (3) hypothesizing alternative scenarios of a rival's intention, and (4) reconsidering decisions after a waiting period. Many researchers have questioned the effectiveness of these safeguards. For example, Bennis (1976) argues that a devil's advocate will be ignored if the group perceives the member as only role-playing.

SUMMARY

There are many factors that influence our behavior. Group dynamics is a complex subject that attempts to provide us with some understanding of how individuals interact with one another and how those interactions become visible in our resulting behavior. Burton and Dimbleby (1996) developed a model, using interpersonal communication as the foundation, to help us understand the complexity of group dynamics (see Figure 14–3).

The figure is titled "The Interface of Me and Them." Since group dynamics is the attempt to understand how people interact with and influence others within

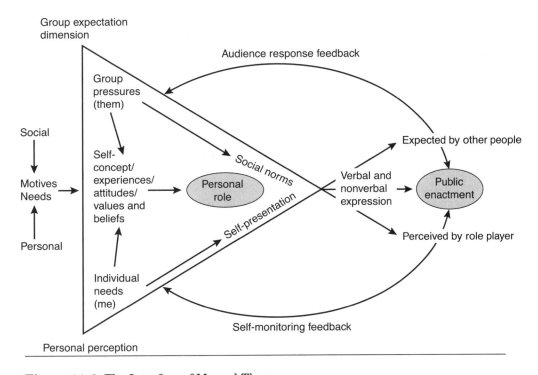

Figure 14–3 The Interface of Me and Them

groups, the title is most appropriate. When examining the model, you will notice that the bottom half is concerned with "me" and the top half represents "them." The process begins with an individual's needs or motivation, which triggers the "whole of self." The triangle represents the various interactions we have with our groups that are filtered through our self-concept, which, taken together, form our personal roles. We then communicate our role and receive feedback from both ourselves (did I play the role correctly?) and from others (did they confirm my behavior was correct?) to restart the process of redefining who we are as an individual (personal role). Although the model may appear somewhat complex, it only starts to explain the complexity of human behavior.

END-OF-CHAPTER DISCUSSION QUESTIONS

1. Define the study of group dynamics and discuss why it is important to today's managers.
2. Describe the four characteristics that define a group and provide examples of nongroups and groups.
3. Explain what is meant by "group interaction."
4. Discuss how group interactions can be measured.
5. Discuss why people join groups and what sustains their membership.
6. Explain the importance of the various roles members assume in groups.
7. Discuss how group norms are formed and sustained within groups.
8. Explain how group cohesiveness is developed and sustained.
9. Discuss why conformity can inhibit a group's performance.
10. Explain what behavior is displayed by a group operating under "groupthink."

EXERCISE 14-1

Form small groups of 4 to 5 individuals and discuss the following statement: Often employees do not act or react as individuals but as members of groups.

When discussing this statement, the members should share experiences of working in groups. Can you recall an instance in which you gave in because of the pressure to conform? Have you experienced a nonconformist in one of your groups? How did you or other members of your group react to "deviant" behavior in your group?

EXERCISE 14-2

Analyze the level of group cohesiveness in one of the groups to which you belong.

REFERENCES

Asch, S. (1952). Effects of group pressure on the modification and distortion of judgments. Reprinted in G. E. Swanson, T. M. Newcomb, & E. L. Hartley (Eds.) (1965), *Readings in social psychology* (2nd ed.). New York: Holt, Rinehart & Winston.

Asch, S. (1960). *Social psychology.* Englewood Cliffs, NJ: Prentice Hall.

Bales, R. F. (1950). *Interaction process analysis: A method for the study of small groups.* Chicago: University of Chicago Press.

Bales, R. F. (1953). The equilibrium problem in small groups. In T. Parsons, R. F. Bales, & E. A. Shils (Eds.), *Working papers in the theory of action* (pp. 111–167). Glencoe, IL: Free Press.

Bales, R. F. (1970). *Personality and interpersonal behavior.* New York: Holt, Rinehart & Winston.

Bales, R. F. (1999). *Social interaction systems: Theory and measurement.* New Brunswick, NJ: Transaction.

Belbin R. M. (1981). *Management teams: Why they succeed or fail.* London: Elsevier/Butterworth-Heinemann.

Belbin, R. M. (1993). *Team roles at work.* London: Elsevier/Butterworth-Heinemann.

Belbin, R. M. (2004). *Management teams: Why they succeed or fail* (2nd ed.). London: Elsevier/Butterworth-Heinemann.

Benne, K., & Sheats, P. (1948). Functional roles of group members. *Journal of Social Issues, 4,* 41–49.

Bennis, W. (1976). *The unconscious conspiracy: Why leaders can't lead.* New York: AMACOM.

Berkowitz, L. (1954). Group standards, cohesiveness, and productivity. *Human Relations, 7,* 509–519.

Blackburn, R., & Rosen, B. (1993). Total quality and human resources management: Lessons learned from Baldrige Award-winning companies. *The Academy of Management Executive, 7*(3), 49–66.

Burton, G., & Dimbleby, R. (1996). *Between ourselves: An introduction to interpersonal communications* (2nd ed.). London: Edward Arnold.

Crandall, C. S. (1988). Social contagion of binge eating. *Journal of Personality and Social Psychology, 55,* 588–598.

Crutchfield, R. (1955). Conformity and character. *American Psychologist, 10,* 191–198.

Feldman, D. C. (1984). The development and enforcement of group norms. *The Academy of Management Review, 9,* 47–53.

Hogg, M., & Abrams, D. (1990). Social motivation, self-esteem and social identity. In D. Abrams and M. Hogg (Eds.), *Social identity theory: Constructive and critical advances* (pp 28–47). New York: Harvester Wheatsheaf.

Janis, I. L. (1982). *Groupthink: Psychological studies of foreign policy decisions and fiascoes* (2nd ed.). Boston, MA: Houghton-Mifflin.

Janis, I. L., & Mann, L. (1977). *Decision making.* New York: Free Press.

Kameda, T., Stasson, M. F., David, J. H., Parks, C., & Zimmerman, S. (1992). Social dilemmas, subgroups, and motivational loss in task-oriented groups. In search of an "optimal" team size. *Social Psychology Quarterly, 55,* 47–56.

Karau, S. J., & Williams, K. D. (1993). Social loafing: A meta-analytic review and theoretical integration. *Journal of Personality and Social Psychology, 65,* 681–706.

Katzenbach, J. R., & Smith, D. K. (1993). *The wisdom of teams: Creating the high performance organization.* Boston, MA: Harvard Business School Press.

Kerr, N. L. (1983). Motivation losses in small groups: A paradigm for social dilemma analysis. *Journal of Personality and Social Psychology, 45,* 819–828.

Kerr, N. L., & Bruun, S. E. (1981). Ringelmann revisited: Alternative explanations for the social loafing effect. *Social Psychology Bulletin, 7,* 224–231.

Luft, J. (1984). *Group processes: An introduction to group dynamics* (3rd ed.). Palo Alto, CA: National Press.

Ringelmann, M. (1913). Recherches sur les moteurs animes: Travail de l'homme [Research on animate sources of power: The work of man]. *Annales de l'Institut National Agronomique,* 2e serie-tome XIL 1–40.

Sherif, M. (1936). *The psychology of social norms.* New York: Octagon Books.

Shepperd, J. A. (1993). Productivity loss in performance groups: A motivation analysis. *Psychological Bulletin, 113,* 67–81.

Sprott W. J. H. (1958). *Human groups.* Harmondsworth, England: Penguin Books.

Szymanski, K., & Harkins, S. G. (1987). Social loafing and self-evaluation with a social standard. *Journal of Personality and Social Psychology, 53,* 891–987.

Tubbs, S. L. (2001). *A systems approach to small group interaction.* New York: McGraw Hill Book Company.

Tuddenham, R. (1958). The influences of a distorted norm upon individual judgments. *The Journal of Psychology, 46,* 227–241.

Turner, J. (1987). *Rediscovering the social group.* New York: Basil Blackwell.

Turner, M. E. (2000). *Groups at work: Theory and research.* Mahwah, NJ: Lawrence Erlbaum Associates.

US Department of Justice, Northern District of Alabama. (April 3, 2003). Five HealthSouth Officers Charged with Conspiracy to Commit Wire & Securities Fraud. Press Release, available at www.usdoj:gov/usao/aln.

CHAPTER 15

Groups

Judith Bachay, PhD

LEARNING OUTCOMES

After completing this chapter, the student should understand the:

- ☛ Importance of a group's size.
- ☛ Three broad categories of groups.
- ☛ Difference between informal and formal groups.
- ☛ Different types of task groups.
- ☛ Five stages of group development.
- ☛ Seven stages of group decision making.
- ☛ Different methods for gathering information.

OVERVIEW

In Chapter 14, we defined what is meant by a group, why people join groups, and interactions that occur between members during their association. In this chapter, we will discuss the composition, structure, formation, and decision-making processes of groups. In Chapter 16, our focus will be on teams and the various team-building techniques available to managers.

As discussed in Chapter 14, the optimum size for a group is five members. However, we will find groups with fewer than five members and those with more. When groups have fewer than five members, problems may arise relating to an inability to make decisions and lower levels of creativity (Tubbs, 2001). If the group size becomes too large, subgroups may form, distracting from the main group's purpose, and a majority of the group's time is used for functioning purposes (e.g., organizing members, assigning roles) versus the required task (Tubbs, 2001). All these situations can cause frustration among the members and stifle the group's ability to reach its goal.

TYPES OF GROUPS

Groups can be categorized into three broad groups: primary, secondary, and reference. Within each of these categories, groups operate under an informal or formal structure. Within the definition of formal or informal groups, there are many types, such as social groups and educational groups.

Primary Groups

Primary groups usually include one's family and closest friends and/or peers. Social psychologists tend to see primary groups as those that: (1) involve regular contact between members of the group, whether through direct face-to-face interaction, technology, or other means, and (2) are fairly small (i.e., 20 members or less) (Blackler & Shimmin, 1984). In addition, primary groups: (1) involve cooperation, (2) share common goals, (3) know who all the members of the group are, and (4) have an understanding of the role(s) of each member.

Primary groups have a powerful influence on both a member's self-concept, as well as the development of an individual's perceptions and attitudes. During an individual's childhood and adolescent years, the family unit has a strong impact on the development of an individual's personality and future behaviors, both socially and in the workplace. During an individual's adult years, associations with work and professional groups will influence his or her attitudes and perceptions through various interactions with different groups.

Secondary Groups

Secondary groups comprise the larger circle of people we associate with. For example, Jane Kerry, RN, is a member of a family group, a member of a group of close-knit friends that meet for dinner once a month (friends Jane has known from high school), the president of her local bridge club, and a member of Glen Haven Hospital's neonatal intensive care unit nursing staff and quality improvement committee. After this, Jane's groups become larger. She is a member of the hospital's pediatric department, a member of the hospital's nursing staff, and a member of the hospital's overall community. In addition, she is a member of the American Nurses Association. Some of these group memberships may be short-term and others long-term. No matter what the time frame, each group will influence Jane's behavior.

Reference Groups

Reference groups are those that we compare ourselves to for developing our personal behavior and social attitudes. We may or may not be a member of one or more reference groups. For example, people will often compare themselves with and identify with supermodels, rock stars, or sports persons, though they are neither models, rock stars, nor sports persons themselves. Reference groups can be either positive or negative.

INFORMAL OR FORMAL GROUP STRUCTURE

In the workplace, two types of groups can be found: informal groups and formal groups.

Informal Groups

The informal group is organized on the basis of the members' common interests or goals. Membership is voluntary and not part of the official structure of the organization. Although informal groups usually have a short life cycle, they can have a significant effect on the organization's current and future operations.

For example, as discussed in Chapter 9, a small group of nurses, employed at a large community hospital, were unhappy about their work environment and would meet daily during lunch to discuss the situation. There had been a recent change in the hospital's senior management, which caused a high level of uncertainty among the clinical staff. The nurses also felt overworked as a result of the well-recognized nursing shortage. Their wages and benefits had been stagnant with no salary market adjustments for the past three years. Furthermore, whenever they approached management with their concerns, they perceived that these concerns were falling on deaf ears since no changes had been made. This informal group of nurses decided to contact a labor union. The labor union began an organizing effort in the hospital shortly thereafter, holding an aggressive campaign over a six-week period. There was tremendous peer pressure, as some of the well-respected nursing staff became active leaders for unionization, although they were not part of the initial organizing group. The election was held and the union was voted in by two-thirds of the nursing staff. In the weeks that followed, the clinical nursing staff remarked that they were surprised by the union's victory; they had only wanted to "scare" management into making changes to their work environment.

Managers need to be aware that informal groups can be a powerful force within their organization. With an understanding of their influence, managers can also use informal groups to initiate positive changes. For example, the administrator for a free-standing outpatient surgical center wanted to begin a cross-training program of the clinical staff to improve the organization's performance. She knew that staff would resist this "new" concept because of her past failures to implement change. Learning from her past mistakes, she enlisted the support of a group of nurses that had developed into a closely knit group. This was also the nursing group that other clinical staff looked to for guidance on patient care issues. The administrator secured the support of the informal group by showing how the change would increase the quality of care for the patients (e.g., a more knowledgeable workforce), patient satisfaction (e.g., shorter wait time for procedures to be performed), and job security (e.g., increase in the organization's financial stability). Because of the nursing group's support, the change was successfully implemented with minimum resistance from staff. Furthermore, the outcomes that the administrator predicted would occur did happen. These outcomes positively reinforced the relationship between the informal nursing group and management.

Informal groups meet the needs of individuals and, therefore, have a strong influence on the members' behaviors. If managers are aware of these groups, these groups can be enlisted to assist the organization in achieving its goals (see Case Study 15–1).

Case Study 15–1 Using Informal Groups to Promote Organizational Goals

The clinic's chief executive officer (CEO) was known for consistently seeking, listening to, and incorporating the views of others. While she worked effectively through the formal hierarchy, she also regularly sought the views of both physician and employee influence leaders. These influence leaders were part of a group that met to provide input, shape ideas, and take accurate information forth to those who looked to them for the inside scoop. Their role in helping to sell others on new directions was clearly recognized.

For example, when it came time to consider affiliating the clinic with another healthcare organization, influence leaders made site visits and came back to share their feelings with a broad cross section of the organization. Many who listened to them would have been more skeptical if the information presented had come from the lips of the CEO.

SOURCE: "Informal leadership support: An often overlooked competitive advantage," by L. H. Peters and E. J. O'Connor, 2001. *Physician Executives, 27*(3), 35–39. Reprinted with permission.

Formal Groups

Formal groups are created by the organization; therefore, they are part of the organization's formal structure. These groups can be a long-term team (e.g., functional or command) or short-term team (e.g., ad hoc committees).

A functional or command group is specified and outlined in an entity's organizational chart. For functional groups, members are grouped by similar tasks, such as financial and administrative services, ancillary services, human resources and organizational development, and nursing services (see Figure 15–1 and Chapter 21).

For command groups, members are formed into subgroups under the leader's legitimate power position within the organization. For example, all laboratory technicians report to the manager of laboratory services. The manager forms a group of laboratory technicians to discuss the implementation issues of providing clinical support for the hospital's new outpatient clinic.

Task groups include two (a dyad) or more people who are focused on an identified target, a project, or a specific issue or goal. Task groups may be either short- or long-term and may be evaluated on the basis of their identified objectives. Unlike in the functional or command groups, members can be from various functional areas and levels of organizational authority, depending on the specialized knowledge, experience, or authority that may be required by the group. For example, the CEO of a local hospital forms a task force to address the organization's disaster preparedness procedures. Members of this group would include all functional areas of the hospital, including administration, patient care, information technology, and physical plant. Task groups can be permanent groups, which may be used for policymaking or coordination of activities. Permanent groups can exist from one year to indefinitely. Ad hoc groups are generally established to deal with a specific issue or problem. These latter groups may exist for a very short period, such as from one month up to one year, depending upon resolution of problems, tasks, and issues.

A common formal group found in the healthcare industry is a psychoeducation group. Psychoeducation groups are an important source of support for patients and family members.

These groups are short-term and have as their basis both learning and psychological cognitive therapy theoretical orientations. These groups vary according to the expressed need of the community or specialized medical services specific to the healthcare institution. For example, an oncology unit may offer a psychoeducation group for women diagnosed with breast cancer. The group can help patients become involved in, and therefore become informed participants, regarding their medical care. Groups can provide information related

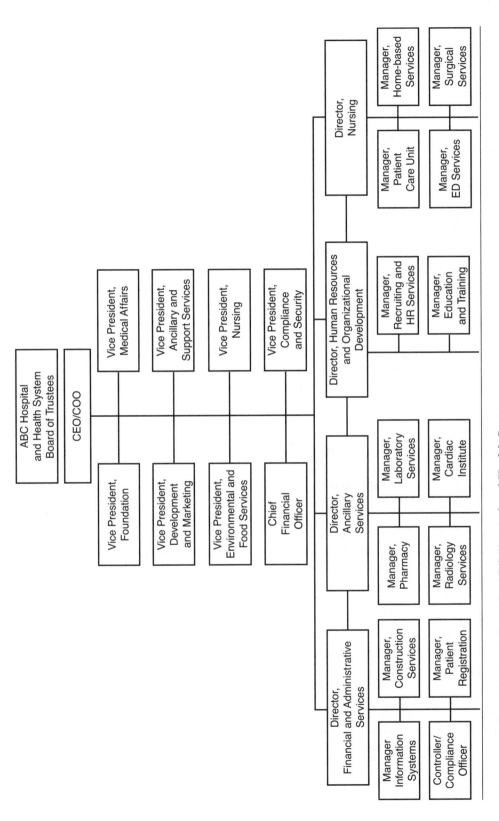

Figure 15–1 Organizational Chart for ABC Hospital and Health System

315

to the most recent research and treatment options, as well as connecting the patient with needed services, such as patient advocacy groups on community, state, and federal levels.

GROUP DEVELOPMENT

Groups go through five sequential stages of development. Some groups, on the basis of their leadership or members' prior experiences, can move through these stages more quickly than others. Because of the same factors, some groups may never experience all five stages. The five stages of development are:

1. *Forming:* During the forming stage, members try to determine what the appropriate behaviors and core values of the group are. They focus on exchanging functional information, task definition, and boundary development. They begin to establish tasks and determine how they might meet objectives. During this initial stage, members must gain an understanding about the reason or purpose for joining and find a social niche in the group.

2. *Storming:* The second stage of group development, storming, is characterized by high levels of emotion, because members are trying to find their group identity and exert their individuality. At this stage, members are claiming their social power within the group and a hierarchy is established as people question authority, react to what is supposed to be accomplished, and jockey for power within the group. Intermember criticism, scapegoating, and judgments may accompany this struggle for control.

3. *Norming:* Within the third stage, the development of cohesion and structure occurs when the group's standards, key values, and roles are accepted. The gradual development of cohesion occurs after the conflict in stage two. In this third stage, the rules for behavior are explicitly and implicitly defined. There is a greater degree of order and a strong sense of group membership.

4. *Performing:* In the fourth stage, performing, we find that members have found their role(s) within the group and that their energy is focused on the task. The group works through the problems confronting it and, when the task is almost near completion, the group moves to the final phase.

5. *Adjourning:* Adjourning is the final stage of group development, which represents the dissolution or termination of the group membership.

GROUP DECISION MAKING

Group decision making is the process of arriving at a judgment based on the feedback of multiple individuals. Such decision making is a key component to the functioning of an organization because organizational performance involves more than just individual action. Therefore, managers need to understand the ways in which the group process affects group decision making.

Group decision making usually takes longer than an individual decision (Nour & Yen, 1992); however, research confirms that groups produce more and better solutions to problems than do average individuals working alone, and the choices groups make will be more accurate and creative (Robbins, 2003). This is due to the higher levels of communication, coordination, and collaboration that occur within groups during the decision-making process (Nour & Yen, 1992).

There are four factors that play an important part regarding the quality of a group's decision. First, the group should be diverse (i.e., members should have differences in experiences, individual knowledge, talents, skills, culture, and age) (Butterfield & Bailey, 1996). Second, the members need to feel that they are in a safe environment so their ideas can be expressed freely (i.e., avoidance of conformity and groupthink). Third, the degree of task interdependence must be high (i.e., if the task is simple, members can solve the problem individually with no assistance from other members). Fourth, the group must have the potency for success (i.e., the members believe that the group can be effective) (Shea & Guzzo, 1987).

Peterson (1997) and Burn (2004) provide a model that illustrates the process by which groups make decisions (see Figure 15–2).

- *Stage 1—Problem Definition:* The better informed members are, the better they are at formulating the problem or issue at hand. Clarity about the problem is necessary for a quality decision.

- *Stage 2—Identify Alternatives:* Groups sometimes limit and restrict options on the basis of the ideas and perceptions of only a few members. Inclusivity and careful review of all available options expands problem-solving alternatives. Sometimes members believe that they have to choose the first alternative for the sake of time or that they do not have access to all of the relevant information.

- *Stage 3—Gather Information:* Information needs to be gathered about all possible consequences on the basis of the identified alternatives. Groups often neglect to take the time to gather all of the relevant information and do not develop a process by which all members can contribute to gathering information.

- *Stage 4—Evaluate Alternatives:* The group must objectively analyze all of the available alternatives and potential consequences. The challenges that emerge during this stage range from developing processes that ensure that all information is reviewed, that higher status members do not dominate, and that decisions are not made for a member's personal gain. Group members could choose the first available alternative that meets minimal standards and convince themselves and others that it is the most appropriate. Therefore, rational and objective criteria are needed to prevent flawed decisions.

- *Stage 5—Make the Decision:* The method by which the group chooses to make the decision is extremely important. Some members may try to control and bolster their own ideas without supportive evidence. Lower status members might vote with higher status members when the vote is by a show of hands; the vote might totally change if there is a secret ballot.

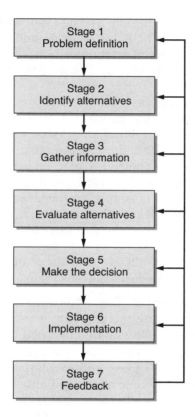

Figure 15–2 Group Decision Process Model

- *Stage 6—Implementation:* The challenges at this stage involve the resolution of all of the tasks necessary to fully implement the decision, including the identification of all of the needed resources.
- *Stage 7—Evaluate the Outcome:* After implementation, a step that is often disregarded is the attempt to evaluate the outcome. Are processes developed so that the decision group can actually measure the success or relevance of the outcome? Did the decision meet the goals and objectives? What would the group do differently? This critical inquiry is essential to learning from the experience.

The collective information processing of a group takes time to develop. This may be due to members not being aware of the information resources of the group or members being hesitant to provide information to the group. Some groups provide structured techniques so that every member participates equally and positive interaction is encouraged. These strategies include brainstorming, the nominal group, and Delphi techniques.

Brainstorming

Brainstorming requires a designated amount of time (usually five to seven minutes) to generate as many ideas as possible without discussion about feasibility or practicality. The originator of this technique (Osborn, 1957) believed that members' tendencies to judge and criticize others' offerings would deter members from freely expressing creative ideas. Osborn hypothesized that the more ideas a group developed, the greater the chance the ideas would be of higher quality. However, research does not support Osborn's hypothesis. Brainstorming groups do not produce more or higher-quality ideas than those that are generated individually (Mullen, Johnson, & Salas, 1991). Some factors that may reduce the performance of brainstorming groups include social loafing, apprehension about being judged by others, or the tendency for introverted people to withdraw when in the company of extroverted members who may compete and try to dominate the brainstorming process. People also have a difficult time thinking and listening to others at the same time. Dennis (1996) contends that computer-based brainstorming, a technique in which group members interact electronically, often anonymously, and at the same time, eradicates the interpersonal pressure. The advantages are that they are less likely to forget what they are sharing as they type; the written record of all contributions can be made available for all and at any time; and because of the anonymity, lower status members do not feel the pressure of the evaluation of their contribution by other members. In addition, computerized group support systems may also reduce the potential for groupthink.

Nominal Group Technique

The nominal group technique is a brainstorming technique that is implemented on an individual and nonverbal basis. The information obtained is then pooled. This technique is efficient because it does not require a great deal of leadership training and the group can communicate without the risks involved in verbal communication. A typical five-step process begins with a period of silence when group members write down their ideas independently. This is followed by a round-robin recording of ideas. The leader calls on each member to share one idea at a time and writes each idea down in view of the total group. There is group discussion of each idea on the list and all ideas are clarified and evaluated. The participants identify and privately rank their ideas in order of preference, and then they vote, the vote is recorded, the voting pattern discussed, and the highest ranked idea is discussed. The nominal group technique has been used extensively in business and government because of its efficiency and its capacity to limit emotional arguments.

The Delphi Technique

The Delphi technique is intended to help with the challenge faced by group members who may lack the experience to understand that the information they hold is needed to generate and evaluate options or alternatives. This technique uses a series of written communications to collect and synthesize the opinions of a group of experts into a decision. A carefully devised letter is sent to several experts that defines the problem and asks the experts for advice toward a solution. The leader collects and collates the responses for each of the experts and sends them back to the experts for commentary and additional solutions. The leader collects the letters and analyzes them for consensus. If clear consensus emerges, a decision can be made. If not, the process is repeated until consensus is achieved. This process can be time-consuming and the same result may be achieved through a face-to-face meeting of experts.

Garbage Can Decision-making Process

The "garbage can" process of group decision making is defined as many types of independently generated problems and solutions being dropped "on the table" for discussion by group members (Cohen, March, & Olsen, 1972; Lovata, 1987; Schmid, Dodd, & Tropman, 1987). This process is appropriate for group decision making in organizations where technologies are not clear, involvement of participants fluctuates in the amount of time and effort given, and choices are inconsistent and not well defined (Cohen, March, & Olsen, 1972; Lovata, 1987; Schmid, Dodd, & Tropman, 1987).

Unlike the traditional rational decision-making model described earlier, the garbage can model disconnects problems, solutions, and decision makers from one another. Specific decisions do not follow an orderly process from problem to solution but are outcomes of several relatively independent stream of events within the organization (Cohen, March, & Olsen, 1972). An illustration of the garbage can model is a hospital department, consisting of five employees, that has unallocated funds in its budget that must be "used" by the end of the fiscal year or it will be reallocated to the hospital's general funds. The employees do not want to lose the departmental money. So, they create a fictitious allocation in order to protect it, but really have no use for it. Two weeks after the end of the fiscal year, the department's computer system goes down. Fortunately, the solution (the money from the budget to replace the computer system), the problem (broken computer system), and the individuals involved (the employees) are in alignment. In other words, the timing is perfect for the combination of components to solve this problem: The employees protected budget money that could be used at a later time, the computer system went down, and the protected money could be used to buy a new computer system (Lahti, 1996).

The garbage can model provides a real-world representation of the nonrational manner in which decisions are often made within an organization. In a broad sense, the model provides some clue to understand "how organizations survive when they do not know what they are doing" (Cohen, March, & Olsen, 1972). As such, the garbage can decision-making process is not very efficient because choices are made only when the combination of problems, solutions, and individuals allow the decision to happen (i.e., are in alignment). Consequently, the alignment of the problems, solutions, and individuals often occurs after the opportunity to make a decision regarding a problem has passed or occurs even before the problem has been discovered (Cohen, March, & Olsen, 1972).

SUMMARY

Groups remain the context for most of our social and work activities. The powerful impact that groups have on people and the powerful influence that people have on groups merit our ongoing attention. In Chapter 16, we will discuss teams and team-building techniques.

END-OF-CHAPTER DISCUSSION QUESTIONS

1. Discuss why the size of a group is important to performance.
2. Explain the different broad categories of groups.
3. Describe the difference between informal and formal groups.
4. Discuss the various task groups within an organization and their purposes.
5. Explain the five stages of group development.
6. Discuss the factors that may hinder the effectiveness of a group decision-making process.
7. Explain the seven stages of group decision making.
8. Describe the various information-gathering methods a group may use.

EXERCISE 15–1

Analyze the last poor decision made by a group of which you were a member. What do you think contributed to the group's poor decision? Did the group think of alternative possibilities? Did the group move too quickly through any of the development stages? If yes, did this cause lack of cooperation or poor communication?

EXERCISE 15–2

Form small groups of 4 to 5 individuals and, within 10 minutes, brainstorm as many solutions as possible that address the following situation:

A small nonprofit organization for which you serve as a member of the Board of Directors needs to raise $500,000 in order to support its programming needs.

After the exercise is completed, personally reflect on the group interactions. Did you notice any factors that may have reduced the performance of the group (i.e., social loafing, apprehension of being criticized by others, dominate behavior by one or more members)?

REFERENCES

Blackler, F., & Shimmin, S. (1984). *Applying psychology in organizations.* London: Methuen.

Burn, S. B. (2004). *Groups: Theory and practice.* Belmont, CA: Thompson and Wadsworth.

Butterfield, J., & Bailey, J. J. (1996). Socially engineered groups in business curricula: An investigation of the effects of team composition on group output. *Journal of Business Education, 72*(2), 103–106.

Cohen, M. D., March, J. G., & Olsen, J. P. (1972). A garbage can model of organizational choice. *Administrative Science Quarterly, 17*, 1–25.

Dennis, A. R. (1996). Information exchange and use in small group decision making. *Small Group Research, 27*, 532–551.

Lahti, R. K. (1996). Group decision making within the organization: can models help? Center for Collaborative Organizations, University of North Texas, Denton. Available at: http://www.workteams.unt.edu/literature/paper-rlahti.html

Lovata, L. M. (1987). Behavioral theories relating to the design of information systems. *MIS Quarterly, 11*(2), 147–149.

Mullen, B., Johnson, C., & Salas, E. (1991). Productivity loss in brainstorming groups: A meta-analytic integration. *Basic and Applied Social Psychology, 12*, 3–23.

Nour, M. A., & Yen, D. C. (1992). Group decision support systems, toward a conceptual foundation. *Information and Management, 23*(1), 55–64.

Osborn, A. F. (1957). *Applied imagination.* New York: Scribner.

Peterson, R. S. (1997). A directive leadership style in group decision making can be both virtue and vice: Evidence from elite and experimental groups. *Journal of Personality and Social Psychology, 72*(5), 1107–1121.

Robbins, S. P. (2003). Organizational behavior (10th ed.). Upper Saddle River, NJ: Prentice Hall.

Schmid, H., Dodd, P., & Tropman, J. E. (1987). Board decision making in human service organizations. *Human Systems Management, 7*(2), 155–161.

Shea, G. P., & Guzzo, R. A. (1987). Group effectiveness: What really matters? *Sloane Management Review, 8*(3), 25–31.

Tubbs, S. L. (2001). *A systems approach to small group interaction.* New York: McGraw Hill Book Company.

CHAPTER 16

Teams and Team Building

Nancy Borkowski, DBA, CPA, FACHE

LEARNING OUTCOMES

After completing this chapter, the student should understand the:

- ☛ Various types of teams.
- ☛ Difference of a virtual team as compared to conventional types of teams.
- ☛ Various approaches for building team performance.
- ☛ Various organizational barriers to effective team building.
- ☛ Common characteristics of successful teams.

OVERVIEW

Case Study 16–1 Dr. R's Office

Dr. R works in a private practice that includes herself and one other general internist. She begins her 20-minute visit with Mr. H by thumbing through the chart to find the dates and results from his most recent hemoglobin (HbA1c), low-density lipoprotein cholesterol, eye examination, and prostate-specific antigen tests. The office has a medical records clerk who is not trained to perform these tasks. Dr. R then spends 5 minutes comparing the medication bottles brought by Mr. H with her chronic medication list. After reviewing the health maintenance form, she leaves the room to ask a medical assistant to draw up pneumonia and influenza immunizations and finds the medical assistant sitting at her desk waiting for instructions about what to do next. Returning to the examination room, Dr. R learns that Mr. H has been unable to obtain an appointment with the urologist for a prostate biopsy; she promises to arrange the appointment herself. As Mr. H leaves, Dr. R realizes that she did not need a medical degree to accomplish any of the tasks performed during the medical visit.

SOURCE: "Can health care teams improve primary care practice?" by K. Grumbach, and T. Bodenheimer, 2004. *JAMA, 291*(10), p. 1246. Reprinted with permission.

The question posed is, "Does a group of people who happen to be thrown together in a surgical suite or primary care office truly constitute a team?" The answer is obviously, "No." Not all groups are teams.

Groups are much broader than teams. Teams are special forms of groups because they have highly defined tasks and roles and demonstrate high group commitment (Katzenbach & Smith, 1993). Because of teams' distinctiveness, we begin our discussion with the definition of teams. We then examine the various types of teams, their characteristics, and the factors that either assist or hinder the effectiveness of teams in the workplace.

TEAMS

A team can be defined as a small group of people who are committed to a common purpose, who possess complementary skills, and who have agreed on specific performance goals for which the team members hold themselves mutually accountable (Katzenbach & Smith, 1993; also, see Case Study 16–2 and Case Study 16–3). On the basis of this definition, a team (1) should be composed of a small number (preferably an odd number, i.e., 5 or 7) of members to ensure consensus without discord; (2) must have specific goals; and (3) must contain members with mutual accountability, requiring interdependence and collaboration of efforts (Gordon, 2002).

Case Study 16–2 Dr. Charles Burger

A Well-functioning Primary Care Team in a Small Private Office

Charles Burger is a private practitioner in Bangor, Maine. From a distance, this remarkable primary care practice resembles thousands of physician offices throughout the country. Upon entering the office door, it is clear that—within a traditional practice setting—Dr. Burger has created a smoothly functioning primary care team. The entire office functions as one team— two physicians and two nurse practitioners are the clinicians, complemented by medical assistants, greeters, receptionists, and schedulers. The practice is financially stable and is busy, with each clinician seeing 23 to 30 patients per day. The following case typifies how the team model works.

Ms. P called Dr. Burger's office complaining of recurrent abdominal discomfort after eating. The receptionist consulted her computerized triage protocol and provided Ms. P with a same-day appointment. When she arrived, the greeter, already aware of the patient's problem, gave her a medical history questionnaire specifically related to abdominal pain, which Ms. P filled out in the waiting room. Ms. P met with the medical assistant who checked her vital signs and quickly entered her questionnaire responses into the computer. Ms. P then saw the physician, who reviewed the history, performed a relevant physical examination, and consulted a diagnostic software program. Discussing the options with Ms. P, the physician and patient decided on a diagnostic and treatment plan. Ms. P then met with the scheduler, who arranged laboratory and ultrasound studies.

Dr. Burger's staff members were all trained at a 15-week course in quality management at a nearby college. Greeters, receptionists, and schedulers (who are cross-trained) also received six weeks of in-office training.

All clinical processes in Dr. Burger's office are guided by a system. The practice has adopted advanced-access scheduling, offering patients same-day appointments. For years, the office has tracked demand and can predict how each day will unfold. On Mondays, heavy with telephone calls, more staff act as receptionists and few scheduled appointments are made.

Whereas in most offices, receptionists are not trained to properly triage patients into emergency, urgent, and routine categories, Dr. Burger designed a triage system that receptionists consult on every telephone call. When Ms. P called with abdominal complaints, the receptionist pulled up the gastrointestinal screen on the triage protocol, which prompted a series of questions including pain severity and presence of vomiting, diarrhea, black and/or bloody stools, or fever. In the case of positive answers, the protocol tells the receptionist to send Ms. P to the emergency department. For milder symptoms, an appointment is made, perhaps with previsit laboratory studies. The interaction is routed to Ms. P's medical record and a clinician's e-mail in-box.

Most communication is routinized by the office's clinical systems. Team members do not attend endless meetings. Incoming calls are routed to the e-mail inbox of the appropriate team member. Urgent messages are delivered in person. Diagnostic studies go to the appropriate e-mail inbox and the medical record. The well-trained medical assistants order clinical preventive studies on the basis of the patient's age and sex. Clinic goals and performance measures are communicated to all staff by posters prominently displayed in the office.

SOURCE: "Can health care teams improve primary care practice?" by K. Grumbach, and T. Bodenheimer, 2004. *JAMA, 291*(10), p. 1247. Reprinted with permission.

Case Study 16–3 Kaiser Permanente in Georgia

A Well-functioning Primary Care Team in a Large Group Practice

In 1997, Kaiser Permanente's Georgia region (KP/Georgia) developed primary care teams with several goals: increased patient satisfaction, improved Health Employer Data and Information Set scores, and lowered costs.

This group practice model currently consists of nine primary care offices with 25 teams. Each team has three to five clinicians (physicians, nurse practitioners, or physician assistants), two registered nurses, one to two receptionists or clerks, and six to seven licensed practical nurses or medical assistants providing care to a panel of 8,000 to 15,000 patients. Prior to the rollout of the team structure, clinicians and staff received training in team-oriented care.

Patients view their clinician, not the team, as their primary caregiver, but are aware that a nonphysician clinician may provide care for acute problems or if the physician is not available. Eighty-five percent of visits are handled by a clinician on the patient's team.

The KP/Georgia team has well-defined systems and protocols for all clinical processes, including triaging telephone calls, reviewing and informing patients of laboratory and X-ray results, making referrals, and renewing prescriptions. One registered nurse is the advice nurse, answering patient questions and triaging patients who telephone or drop in. The other registered nurse is the team co-leader, working with the physician co-leader to solve day-to-day problems, ensure that clinical systems are functioning well, and supervise team members.

Each team receives a budget based on the number of patients on the team's panel with risk adjustment according to age and disease severity. Initially given limited decision-making autonomy, teams demonstrating effective self-management are allowed flexibility in staffing mix and division of labor. Teams can decide whether they want more physicians, more nonphysician clinicians, or more support staff in their personnel mix. Some teams delegate chronic-care management functions to licensed practical nurses and medical assistants; others are less successful in this redesign. Each team decides how chronic disease registries are used to improve its panel's outcome measures. Some use the registries extensively, others minimally.

Each team receives a quarterly report on team functioning, patient satisfaction, staff satisfaction, and clinical quality measures, enabling KP/Georgia's central leadership to assess each team's functioning and allowing each team to compare itself with other teams.

SOURCE: "Can health care teams improve primary care practice?" by K. Grumbach, and T. Bodenheimer, 2004. *JAMA, 291*(10), p. 1248. Reprinted with permission.

Teams are very popular in the workplace. According to Lawler (1999), almost every organization uses some form of problem-solving team, the most common being the self-managing work teams that are used in a high majority of the Fortune 1000 companies. As teams become more of the norm in our workplace, managers need to understand the complexity of teams, whether in their work design, the composition of the members, or the factors that enable them to achieve high levels of performance and effectiveness.

TYPES OF TEAMS

On the basis of Cohen and Bailey's (1997) extensive literature review, teams can be organized into the following four categories: (1) work teams, (2) parallel teams, (3) project teams, and (4) management teams. On the basis of their work, the following descriptions of the four types of teams were developed.

- Work teams are continuing work units responsible for producing goods or providing services. Traditional work teams are directed by managers who make most of the decisions about what is done, how it is done, and who does it. However, more recently an alternative form of work team with a variety of labels—self-managing, autonomous, semiautonomous, self-directing, empowered—is gaining favor. Self-managing work teams involve employees, not managers, deciding how to carry out tasks, allocating the work within the team, and making decisions. Typically, the members of self-managing work teams are cross-trained in a variety of skills relevant to the tasks they perform.

- Parallel teams draw members from different work units or jobs to perform functions that the regular organization is not equipped to perform well. They literally exist in parallel with the formal organizational structure. They generally have limited authority and can make recommendations only to individuals higher up in the organizational hierarchy. Parallel teams are used for problem-solving and improvement-oriented activities. Examples include quality improvement teams, employee involvement groups, quality circles, and task forces.

- Project teams are time-limited. They produce one-time outputs, such as a new product or service to be marketed by the company, a new information system, or a new plant. Typically, project team tasks are nonrepetitive in nature and involve considerable application of knowledge, judgment, and expertise. The work that a project team performs may represent either an incremental improvement over an existing concept or a radically different new idea. Frequently, project teams draw their members from different disciplines and functional units so that specialized expertise can be applied to the project at hand. For example, a new drug-development team of a pharmaceutical company would draw its members from research and development, marketing, finance, and manufacturing. When a project is completed, the members either return to their functional units or move on to the next project. Cross-functional project teams were found to enhance project success as a result of their capacity to handle multiple activities simultaneously, rather than sequentially. This saves time and is important to those organizations concerned with rapid development of new services and/or products due to competition.

- Management teams coordinate and provide direction to the subunits under their responsibility, laterally integrating interdependent subunits across key business processes. The management team is responsible for the overall performance of a business unit. Its authority stems from the hierarchical rank of its members. It is composed of the managers responsible for each subunit, such as vice presidents of nursing, compliance and security, finance, and medical affairs. At the top of the organization, the executive management team establishes and manages the organization's strategic direction and performance. The use of top management teams is expanding in response to the turbulence and complexity of the healthcare environment. Management teams can help organizations achieve competitive advantage by applying collective expertise, integrating disparate efforts, and sharing responsibility for the success of the organization.

VIRTUAL TEAMS

Because of recent advances in communication technologies, a new kind of team, the virtual team, has emerged. Unlike conventional teams, a virtual team works across space, time, and organizational boundaries through various communication technologies (Lipnack & Stamps, 1997). Roebuck and Britt (2002) note that the primary difference between a conventional team and a virtual team is the dimension of physical space or distance between team members. Virtual teams allow employees to be located anywhere in the world. Virtual teams rarely meet face-to-face and are supported by technology to collaborate (Lurey, 1998). Often, these teams are set up as temporary structures existing to accomplish a particular task, or they may be more permanent teams that address ongoing organizational issues (Roebuck & Britt, 2002).

Organizations benefit from virtual teams through access to previously unavailable expertise enhanced through cross-functional interaction and the use of systems that improve the quality of the virtual team's work (Lipnack & Stamps, 1997). By using virtual teams, organizations can assign the right person to the job, regardless of where he or she lives. However, the dimension of physical distance between members does affect the way team members interact. Roebuck and Britts (2002) advise that for a virtual team to be successful, members must be firmly committed to the team's purpose and to each team member. They must want their collaborative work to be successful and be willing to go the extra mile to make sure it is successful. Team members must be persistent in overcoming the technical challenges that will occur. For example, members must be patient with other team members who may not be as comfortable communicating with new technology.

BUILDING TEAM PERFORMANCE

Katzenbach and Smith (1993) developed the team performance curve to illustrate how small groups may develop into high-performing teams (see Figure 16–1).

Katzenbach and Smith (1993, p. 85) relate that, "unlike teams, working groups rely on the sum of 'individual bests' for their performance. They pursue no collective work products requiring joint efforts. By choosing the team path instead of the working group, people commit to take the risks of conflict, joint work-products, and collective action necessary to build a common purpose, set goals, approach, and mutual accountability. People who call themselves teams but take no such risks are at best pseudoteams."

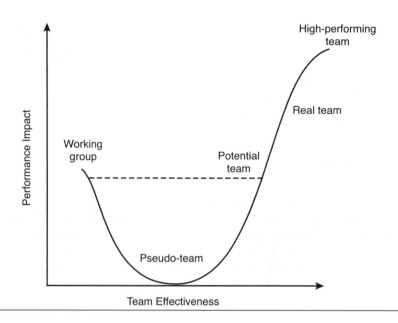

Figure 16–1 The Team Performance Curve (SOURCE: *The wisdom of teams: Creating the high-performance organization*, by J. R. Katzenbach and D. K. Smith, 1993. Boston, MA: Harvard Business School Press, p. 84. McKinsey & Company. Used with permission.)

Although there is no guaranteed how-to recipe, Katzenbach and Smith (1993, pp. 119–127) list eight approaches to building team performance:

1. *Establish Urgency and Direction:* All team members need to believe the team has urgent and worthwhile purposes, and they want to know what the expectations are. The best team charters are clear enough to indicate performance expectations, but flexible enough to allow teams to shape their own purpose, goals, and approach.

2. *Select Members on the Basis of Skills and Skill Potential, not Personality:* Teams must have the complementary skills needed to do their job. Three categories of skills are relevant: (1) technical and functional, (2) problem-solving, and (3) interpersonal. The key issue for potential teams is striking the right balance between members who already possess the needed skill levels versus developing the skill levels after the team gets started.

    Margerison and McCann (1989) have performed extensive research on the "people" side of successful team-building. On the basis of studies incorporating over 5,000 managers, they developed the Team Management Wheel, which assists managers in selecting the right "balance" for their teams regarding roles (advisers, explorers, organizers, and controllers) and "linking" skills (e.g., main role of the team leader) (see Exhibit 16–1 and Figure 16–2).

Exhibit 16–1 The Team Management Wheel

The Margerison–McCann Team Management Wheel defines members' roles and is based on the following eight characteristics:

1. *Reporter–Advisors:* Those who prefer work involving gathering and sharing of information. Supporter, helper, collector of information, knowledgeable, flexible.
2. *Creator–Inventors:* Those who prefer work that generates and experiments with new ideas. Imaginative, creative, enjoy complexity, future-oriented.
3. *Explorer–Promoters:* Those who prefer work that involves investigation and presentation of new opportunities. Persuader, influential and outgoing, easily bored.
4. *Assessor–Developers:* Those who prefer work that involves planning to ensure that ideas and opportunities are feasible in practice. Analytical and objective, idea developer, experimenter.
5. *Thruster–Organizers:* Those who prefer work that allows them to arrange and organize the way work is done. Results-oriented, analytical, organizer, and implementer.
6. *Concluder–Producers:* Those who prefer work that can be implemented systematically to produce regular outputs. Practical, production-oriented, likes schedules and plans, values effective efficiency.
7. *Controller–Inspectors:* Those who prefer work involving controlling and auditing procedures and systems. Controller, detail-oriented, inspector of standards and procedures, low need for personal interaction.
8. *Upholder–Maintainers:* Those who prefer work that involves upholding and conserving processes and procedures. Conservative, loyal, supportive, strong sense of right and wrong, motivation based on purpose.

The hub of the Team Management Wheel is the "Linker," and that is often the main role of the team leader, although all team members need to contribute to this activity. The Linker circle can be expanded into a full-range team leadership model that describes three levels of Linking that should be practiced, to varying degrees, by everyone in an organization.

At the first level of Linking are the skills arranged around the outside of the model. These skills are the People Linking Skills. They create the atmosphere in which the team works, by promoting harmony and trust. As such, everyone in a team has a responsibility to implement this level of leadership.

- Active Listening
- Communication
- Team Relationships
- Problem Solving and Counseling
- Participative Decision Making
- Interface Management

Inside the People Linking Skills are the Task Linking Skills. These skills create a solid core or foundation on which the work of the team relies. They promote confidence and stability.

- Work Allocation
- Team Development
- Delegation
- Objectives Setting
- Quality Standards

These skills tend to apply more to people on the second rung of the leadership ladder— those in more senior positions within a team, responsible for guiding others. This guiding may be done in either a supportive or directive way, but should not violate the first level of People Linking Skills. The challenge is to find the balance where the six People Linking Skills and five Task Linking skills can coexist.

At the core of the Linking Skills Wheel are the two Leadership Linking Skills of Motivation and Strategy. Leadership Linking is the third step on the leadership ladder and applies to leaders who have organizational responsibility for strategy. They need to implement these two skills along with those of the People and Task Linking Skills to achieve the status of the Linker Leader, a term used to describe someone who is effective at implementing all three levels described in the Linking Skills Wheel.

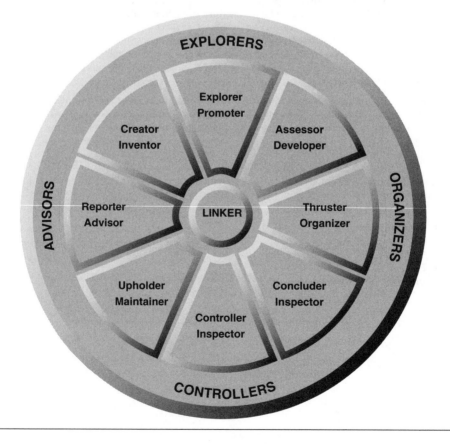

Figure 16–2 The Linking Skills Wheel (SOURCE: Team Management Systems (TMS) by Charles Margerison and Dick McCann. Reprinted with permission.)

4. *Set Some Clear Rules of Behavior:* All real teams develop rules of conduct to help them achieve their purpose and performance goals. The most critical early rules pertain to attendance ("no interruptions to take phone calls"), discussion ("no sacred cows"), confidentiality ("the only things to leave this room are what we agree will leave this room"), analytic approach ("facts are friendly"), end-product orientation ("everyone gets assignments and does them"), constructive confrontation ("no finger pointing"), and often the most important, contributions ("everyone does real work").

5. *Set and Seize upon a Few Immediate Performance-oriented Tasks and Goals:* Most teams trace their advancement to key performance-oriented events that forge them together. Potential teams can set such events in motion by immediately establishing a few challenging yet achievable goals that can be reached early on.

6. *Challenge the Group Regularly with Fresh Facts and Information:* New information causes a potential team to redefine and enrich its understanding of the performance challenge, thereby helping the team shape a common purpose, set clearer goals, and improve on its common approach.

7. *Spend Lots of Time Together:* Common sense tells us that teams must spend a lot of time together, especially at the beginning. The time spent together must be both scheduled and unscheduled. Creative insights as well as personal bonding require impromptu and casual interactions just as much as analyzing spreadsheets, interviewing customers, and so on. These meetings or interactions need not be always face-to-face. Use of technology is encouraged!

8. *Exploit the Power of Positive Feedback, Recognition, and Reward:* Positive reinforcement works well in a team context. There are many ways to recognize and reward team performance, of which direct compensation is only one. Ultimately, the satisfaction in the team's performance becomes the most cherished reward. Until then, however, potential teams must find other ways to recognize and reinforce their individual and team contributions and commitment.

BARRIERS TO EFFECTIVE TEAMWORK

The barriers to effective teamwork fall within four categories: (1) lack of management support, (2) lack of resources, (3) lack of leadership, and (4) lack of training (see Table 16–1). If these barriers exist within an organization, the likelihood that groups would be provided the opportunity to develop into high-performing teams is limited. Teams need management support, proper leadership, adequate resources, and training to reach their full potential.

Dunphy's (1996) research supports the fact that teams contribute significantly to the productivity and efficiency of organizations. In today's environment, hospitals and other healthcare providers are seeking innovative ways to reduce medical errors and costs while increasing quality of care and customer/employee satisfaction. Effective and high-performing teams

Table 16–1 Barriers to Effective Teamwork

Category	Description
Management	Lack of sufficient support and commitment from senior management
Management	Pressure for short-term results
Management and Leadership	Political meddling and power politics
Management and Leadership	Lack of trust among team members and with leadership (i.e., communication is closed and risk-taking is not encouraged or rewarded)
Leadership	Lack of clear vision, goals, and objectives
Leadership	Unwillingness to allow teams the necessary autonomy and decision-making powers
Leadership	Poor communication and interpersonal skills
Leadership and Resources	Failure to recognize and reward group efforts
Resources	Insufficient release time from other duties for team members
Training	Inadequate training and skills development
Training	Lack of project management skills

SOURCE: "Transformation through teamwork: The path to the new organization?" by S. Drew and C. Coulson-Thomas, 1996. *Management Decision, 34*(1), p. 7. Reprinted with permission.

can help accomplish these goals. However, team building is a process that takes time and resources. Management needs to invest today to reach tomorrow's goals.

COMMON CHARACTERISTICS OF SUCCESSFUL TEAMS

Elaine Biech, as cited in Gordon (2002, p. 184), outlines the 10 most commonly mentioned characteristics of successful teams:

- *Clear Goals:* Clear goals allow everyone to understand the function and purpose of the team.
- *Defined Roles:* Defined roles allow team members to understand why they are on the team and enable clear individual- and team-based goal setting.
- *Open and Clear Communication:* Effective communication is considered the most important aspect of team building. It hinges on effective listening.

- *Effective Decision Making:* Effective decision making is critical, and for a decision to be effective, the team must be in agreement with the decision and must have reached agreement through a consensus-finding process.

- *Balanced Participation:* Balanced participation ensures that all members are fully engaged in the efforts of the team. Participation is also directly linked to leader behaviors. Effective team leaders should not see their role as authoritarian and should strive to be seen as the team's mentor or coach.

- *Valued Diversity:* The team must recognize each member's expertise and value variety of knowledge, skills, and abilities. In the world of teams, diversity is larger than just race or gender.

- *Managed Conflict:* Managed conflict requires that all team members feel safe to freely state their points of view without fear of reprisal. For teams, managed conflict is almost akin to brainstorming, in that conflict allows the team to openly discuss ideas and decide on common goals.

- *Positive Atmosphere:* Postive atmosphere requires that a climate of trust be developed. One way of developing trust is to allow team members to come together in a positive atmosphere. Allowing team members to become comfortable with one another will generate a positive atmosphere, leading to enhanced creativity and problem solving.

- *Cooperative Relationships:* Cooperative relationships are a must and team members should recognize that they need one another's knowledge and skill to complete the given task(s).

- *Participative Leadership:* Participative leadership includes having good leadership role models, as well as leaders who are willing to share responsibility and recognition with the team.

I would also add *reflection* and *appreciation inquiry* to Biech's list of successful team characteristics. Teams should be encouraged to allocate time for reflection and debriefing on the results of their actions and decisions. Appreciative inquiry can help with this process by encouraging honest communication and analysis by the group (Drew & Coulson-Thomas, 1996). Appreciative inquiry encourages members to identify and reflect on periods of excellence and achievement. By looking at the past, members can develop a vision of what they want to accomplish in the future. They build on what worked best to reach their goal.

SUMMARY

In conclusion, Messmer (2004, pp. 13–14) provides an excellent guide to assist managers in the coordination of activities for building an effective team (see Exhibit 16–2).

Exhibit 16–2 Building Effective Teams: A Checklist for Managers

1. Begin by creating an action plan that specifies the group's mission, the types of expertise required to achieve this objective, and how team members will work together. Critical questions to answer include:
   - How long will the group need to be active?
   - What are the different components of the project and the deadlines for completing them?
   - Is the team responsible for generating and implementing its suggestions?
   - Will the group operate independently, or will any of its activities overlap with those managed by full-time employees currently not on the team?

2. Be sure you have researched how the project impacts the department or company so you can convey its importance at the first team meeting. Also, create a handout (e.g., a time line) and gather supporting materials that can be used for reference.

3. When selecting the team members, be sure to evaluate their interpersonal and communication skills as well as their individual professional abilities and expertise. A hospital's accountant with solid analytical skills may have the knowledge you need to assess the organization's operations, but if he or she lacks the ability to explain his or her analysis effectively to colleagues outside accounting or finance, you'll need to either help him or her develop those skills or appoint someone with a persuasive communication style to copresent.

4. Ask others in your company for recommendations of people who would be appropriate for the project. Always check with each individual's manager before making a final selection to ensure that a potential team member can commit the necessary time and effort to the initiative.

5. In addition to identifying employees who meet specific project needs, you may also want to select a coordinator. This person would periodically collect, organize, and distribute status reports to everyone in the group.

6. After team members have been identified, plan an initial meeting to review the action plan you drafted. Encourage feedback from participants so they feel more connected to the project and upcoming assignments. You may also want to establish protocols for certain practices such as conflict resolution and expenditure approvals to help prevent misunderstandings and encourage more effective collaboration. Once final guidelines and expectations have been agreed upon, distribute a revised action plan to everyone involved.

7. As team leader, you must walk a fine line between coaching and micromanaging. When participants come to you with problems or challenges, encourage them to develop their own solutions, and reward those who take reasonable risks to make improvements. Sometimes the difficulties encountered during a project can spur innovative ideas that are transferable to other groups or the company as a whole.

8. Evaluate the team's progress periodically to make sure everyone is contributing. If an individual's regular work demands are affecting his or her ability to complete project requirements, you may need to select a substitute participant who has the necessary time. Also pay attention to the level of interaction during group meetings. Sometimes a few people will speak up more than others. While you want to avoid discouraging their input, make sure that quieter team members don't feel intimidated. An administrative professional should be just as comfortable as a financial executive when sharing ideas that might help the team. You may need to solicit comments from certain employees to prompt their participation.

Exhibit 16–2 *(Continued)*

9. Providing motivation should be an ongoing priority. Even when things aren't going smoothly, do your best to keep the mood upbeat and positive. Try to begin each meeting with a summary of accomplishments before you address problems. Also take time to acknowledge and celebrate project milestones. You will help to maintain productivity and generate ongoing enthusiasm for the initiative.

10. In your role as leader, you play a pivotal role in helping the team get results. Your strategy should include careful consideration of potential participants and sufficient direction and motivation once the team is formed. The right approach will encourage more effective collaboration among participants while maximizing the team's contribution to the organization.

SOURCE: "Project teams that get results," M. Messmer, 2004. *Strategic Finance, 85*(8), pp. 13–14. Reprinted with permission.

END-OF-CHAPTER DISCUSSION QUESTIONS

1. Explain why teams and groups are not the same.
2. Describe the various types of teams used in today's organizations.
3. Explain the difference between a traditional work team and a self-managing work team.
4. Discuss the positive and negative issues of using a virtual team versus a conventional-type team.
5. Explain the difference between a working group and a high-performing team.
6. Explain the various approaches managers can use to build team performance.
7. Discuss the various organizational barriers to team effectiveness.
8. Are there other characteristics of a successful team that can be added to Biech's list?

EXERCISE 16–1

List and describe the types of teams most commonly used in your organization. Why?

EXERCISE 16–2

List the teams of which you are a member. Select one of these teams to analyze. Is this a high-performing team? If yes, why is it? If no, why isn't it?

REFERENCES

Cohen, S. G., & Bailey, D. E. (1997). What makes team work: Group effectiveness research from the shop floor to the executive suite. *Journal of Management, 23*(3), 239–390.

Drew, S., & Coulson-Thomas, C. (1996). Transformation through teamwork: The path to the new organization? *Management Decision, 34*(1), 7.

Dunphy, D. (1996). Organizational change in corporate settings. *Human Relations, 49*(5), 541–552.

Gordon, J. (2002). A perspective on team building. *Journal of American Academy of Business, Cambridge, 2*(1), 185–188.

Katzenbach, J. R., & Smith, D. K. (1993). *The wisdom of teams: Creating the high-performance organization.* Boston, MA: Harvard Business School Press/McKinsey & Co.

Lawler III, E. E. (1999). Employee involvement makes a difference. *Journal of Quality & Participation, 22*(5), 18–20.

Lipnack, J., & Stamps, J. (1997). *Virtual teams reaching across space, time and organizations with technology.* New York: John Wiley & Sons.

Lurey, J. (1998). *A study of best practices in designing and supporting effective virtual teams.* Los Angeles: California School of Professional Psychology.

Margerison, C., & McCann, D. (1989). Managing high-performance teams. *Training & Development Journal, 43*(11), 52–60.

Messmer, M. (2004). Project teams that get results. *Strategic Finance, 85*(8), 13–14.

Roebuck, D. B., & Britt, A. C. (2002). Virtual teaming has come to stay—Guidelines and strategies for success. *Southern Business Review, 28*(1), 29–39.

OTHER SUGGESTED READING

Beich, E. (Ed.) (2001). *The Pfeiffer book of successful team building: Best of the annuals.* San Francisco: Jossey-Bass/Pfeiffer.

Wise, H., Beckhard, R., Rubin, I., & Kyte, A. L. (1974). *Making health teams work.* Cambridge, MA: Ballinger Publishing Co.

Managing Organizational Change

In Part VI, we discuss organizational change and how to mange it. To manage organizational change, a leader needs to apply all the theories and concepts discussed in this textbook. The leader, or change agent, must use his or her knowledge of motivation, leadership, group dynamics, team building, and conflict management, in addition to communication and negotiation skills, to be successful. In Chapter 17, we explain the role of organization development in planned change management. In Chapter 18, we describe the strategies used for successful implementation of change within organizations.

Organization Development

Lorrie Jones, PhD

LEARNING OUTCOMES:

After completing this chapter, the student should be able to:

- ☛ Understand the role organization development (OD) plays in an organization's planned changes.
- ☛ Appreciate the function and responsibilities of the OD professional.
- ☛ Understand the components of the Action Research Model.
- ☛ Identify and understand the OD process.
- ☛ Understand the interventions used in the OD process.

OVERVIEW

Health care has been a dynamic industry in recent history. Escalating costs and various mechanisms implemented to attempt to control these costs have resulted in an environment fraught with survival struggles. In addition to the financial struggles, real and projected staffing shortages have also resulted in retention issues as well as the infiltration of labor unions into the healthcare industry. These issues have caused health systems to be in constant change. As such, health systems need the necessary strategies to successfully implement required changes. In recent years, many health systems have been turning to experts in the field of organization management (OD) to assist with change initiatives and to help ensure the long-term viability of the organization.

OD has extensive roots dating back to the early 1900s. As discussed in Chapter 1, Frederick Taylor and his theory of Scientific Management were extremely influential because it advocates exploring ways to increase the productivity of workers. The Hawthorne studies also played a predominant role in paving the way for understanding organizational behavior-oriented change processes (Ott, 1996). As the nation progressed through the Industrial Age and through the Depression and two World Wars, the emphasis on the way employees were viewed changed as the nation developed a better understanding of employee motivation. In addition, the popularity of labor unions contributed to the organization's motivation for designing a better working environment. The end result of a century of history has been organizations that understand the need to change in order to remain competitive, yet that also recognize that an emphasis on employee satisfaction is critical in meeting organizational goals. The marriage of needing change and striving for an understanding of how employees will react to change has further opened the door to the field of OD.

ORGANIZATION DEVELOPMENT

OD is a field that incorporates a number of characteristics. Most agree that OD is a planned process of change (Beckhard, 1969; Burke, 1982) using behavioral science (Beckhard, 1969; Beer, 1980; Burke, 1982; French & Bell, 1990) in an organization-wide process (Beckhard, 1969) utilizing a systematic approach (Beer, 1980; McLagan, 1989) to problem solving with the goal of improving the effectiveness of the organization. On the basis of these characteristics, OD is not a one-time training program, a quick fix change, or a "flavor of the month" initiative. Rather, OD is designed to be a planned initiative, which may be based on a needs analysis, and utilizes a strategic approach to implement the change. However, many things that occur in an organization deal with some type of change, but not all are necessarily an OD initiative. For example, expanding a service, such as an emergency department (ED), requires long-term planning, a needs assessment determined by escalating volumes or changing market conditions, a thorough cost–benefit analysis, and a strategic plan. However, this type of change may be successfully implemented without any regard for the need of OD. Why? Although the expansion of the service directly impacts the functioning of the ED staff, the overall culture of the organization may not be affected by this initiative. It is likely that most employees will be able to understand and probably welcome the expansion; therefore, the need for behavioral science intervention is not needed. One of the components of OD that is fundamental to the definition of OD is the behavioral science application. If the ED expansion were also going to require a change in the culture of the ED, then the interrelationship between the expansion and the culture shift might require the expertise of an OD professional.

Cummings and Worley (1997) describe three features of OD that differentiate it from other change initiatives: (1) it applies to an entire system; (2) it involves the impact of behavioral science on the change process; and (3) it includes planned change based on diagnosis, intervention, and redirecting, if necessary.

First, OD applies to an entire system that may include the entire organization or a division, but OD does not involve change directed at a single person or a single unit. For example, the introduction of a new computed tomography (CT) scanner into the new ED may require training for the employees utilizing this new machine, but the training in this example is targeted to new technology and to those specific individuals who will be working with the new equipment.

The second feature of OD, outlined by Cummings and Worley (1997), is the impact of behavioral science on the change process. Practitioners in the field of OD recognize the interrelationship of group dynamics, group processes, and culture on the change initiative, and great strides are taken to ensure that this relationship is cultivated throughout the change process to ensure the success of the initiative. In addition, OD practitioners understand the psychological and sociological components of change and work to assist the organization to develop a greater understanding of these dynamics. The importance of the behavioral science approach cannot be understated. Since OD involves change within an organization, the members of that organization will be directly affected by any changes. If a change initiative is implemented without an understanding of how the people within the organization will react and respond to this change, the change is likely to be difficult at best, and completely unsuccessful at worst. The behavioral science component will help the leadership of the organization understand the psychology of change, key phases in a successful change, and the importance of critical mass, as well as barriers to be prepared to overcome any anticipated time frames.

The third feature of OD is that planned change is based on diagnosis, intervention, and redirecting if the change efforts are not progressing as planned. Cummings and Worley (1997) state that OD is focused on improving organizational effectiveness and utilizes a variety of process change techniques. To achieve the goals of improving organizational effectiveness through process change techniques, OD is composed of five components: (1) OD is supported by multidisciplinary theories; (2) OD views organizations as open systems; (3) OD recognizes that if one part of the organization is impacted by change, an effect will be felt in another part of the organization; (4) OD is based on action research, which is a continuous examination of the progress of the interventions; and (5) OD is based on data (see Case Study 17–1).

Case Study 17–1 Doctor's Hospital's Organizational Change

Doctor's Hospital was facing a serious financial hardship as healthcare costs continued to spiral out of control and reimbursement plummeted. A new chief executive officer (CEO) was hired to turn things around in an effort to salvage the hospital. The CEO was determined to change the company culture, which he identified as apathetic and accustomed to mediocrity. He noted that the financial performance was suffering and attributed much of this to a variety of process issues as well as a lack of focus on the core business of patient care.

The CEO immediately took action to look at financial issues and cut costs. A drastic cost and labor reduction strategy was implemented with an aggressive timeline to turn the financial bottom line around. Within a few months, the hospital started to show less of a financial loss and things seemed to stabilize financially. However, the morale of the staff had taken a significant hit. Turnover increased as a sense of job security decreased, and the impact on the patients began to be seen in an increase in patient complaints and lowered patient satisfaction scores. A training program was introduced to remind employees about customer service with no impact on results. Finally, the CEO hired a consultant who performed an assessment. A multilevel program was implemented that incorporated all levels and all aspects of the business. This assisted leaders in understanding the link between finances, employee morale, and patient satisfaction. A culture of accountability began to emerge and began to shift the culture to one of service after two years. Finally, all business metrics began to move in the same direction.

Questions:

1. What were the key components of changing the organizational culture?
2. Why wasn't the training effective?
3. Why do you think a culture change was necessary?
4. What steps do you think the consultant recommended in order to effect this change?

THE ORGANIZATION DEVELOPMENT PROFESSIONAL

The behavioral science nature of OD requires that individuals practicing OD have a particular skill set in order to ensure success. The role of the OD practitioner consists of a variety of activities, depending on the relationship between the practitioner and the organization. Gottlieb (2001) suggests that the primary role of the practitioner is of assisting clients in achieving clarity and understanding, whereas other roles consist of assisting with diagnosis, process, providing information, or providing training activities. Ultimately, the OD practitioner is one who primarily facilitates an organization through a change initiative. The OD practitioner is similar to a therapist who guides someone through a difficult time, recommending strategies and facilitating the change process. However, just as a good therapist recognizes that ultimately the client must pave his or her own way to success, so does the OD practitioner. The OD practitioner provides the foundation for change, but it is the organization that must pave its own way. Consequently, the relationship between the organization and the OD practitioner is one that requires a delicate balance. The leaders and members of the organization must ultimately work through the process and are responsible for ensuring the success or failure of the initiative. It is critical that OD practitioners establish a psychological distance and define boundaries to clearly define roles in order to ensure a successful relationship (Browne, Cotton, & Golembiewski, 1977) (see Case Study 17–2).

Case Study 17–2 What Went Wrong?

Joan was asked to consult with a hospital that was attempting to enhance organizational effectiveness. She was able to meet briefly with the CEO before she embarked on a series of meetings with front-line managers. The managers were quite informative about the issues they observed in their departments and provided Joan with what she thought was an honest assessment of the issues. After two weeks of meetings, she met again with the CEO to review the data and recommend a course of action. The CEO seemed genuinely interested in what she had to say, but disagreed with many of her conclusions and her plan of action. He determined the problem to be poor team dynamics, whereas Joan had suggested that the team issues were a result of problem processes resulting in role ambiguity and apathy. The CEO decided that the easier course of action was to work on the team dynamics and directed Joan to pursue that course of action.

Against Joan's better judgment, she embarked on a team-building initiative involving many months and over 500 employees. As a result of the initiative, there seemed to be some better camaraderie, yet the role ambiguity and other problems persisted. Six months after the completion of the project, the CEO was commenting on the waste of time and lack of outcomes from this team-building initiative and vowed to never hire a consultant again.

Questions:

1. What went wrong?
2. What should have been done differently?
3. How effective was Joan in her role?

There are many skills that make an OD practitioner successful, including a combination of technical, interpersonal, and consulting skills (Block, 1981). Technical skills include specific education or training in some area. An example might be specific training in statistical process control whereby a particular process improvement was initiated or a Total Quality Management or Six Sigma Program implemented. Specific expertise in the psychology of change management would be another example of an appropriate expertise.

Another skill set of OD practitioners is interpersonal skills. Listening skills are as critical as is the ability to maintain a psychological distance. Marginality has also been identified as a key characteristic of an effective OD practitioner (Browne et al, 1977; Burke, 1982; Gottlieb, 2001), which involves the ability to be involved in an organization without being unduly influenced (Church, Hurley, & Burke, 1992). The ability to be collaborative is another key characteristic (Argyris, 1970) and involves the ability to facilitate rather than direct activities. In a qualitative analysis conducted by Gottlieb (2001, p. 45), clusters of roles were identified for an OD professional. These roles include:

1. Assisting in clarification, such as by asking questions, challenging, and confronting,
2. Diagnosing, which includes data gathering and the analyzing and interpreting of data,
3. Designing or assisting with the design and implementation of interventions,
4. Providing expert information on organization theory, change, or business issues,
5. Process identification, which includes assisting clients with understanding process options,
6. Facilitating interventions by guiding and directing groups through process changes or strategies to ensure effective communication during the implementation and intervention;
7. Training activities, which may run the gamut from the training needs assessment through the training design and delivery of training programs.

Overall, depending on the type of initiative, the skill level and role of the OD practitioner will vary. However, one key characteristic is the ability to apply theory to practical application.

OD practitioners are professionals who are employed by the organization, thus serving as an ongoing internal consultant, or organizations may contract for the services of an external consultant. There are pros and cons of each, and the leaders of an organization must be able to identify which type of consultant would be best suited for their organization for the issue at hand. The internal consultant has an advantage over the external consultant because the individual has a working knowledge of the organization, knows the key players, understands what interventions have been attempted previously, and may have access to data without the need to start from scratch. The downside of utilizing an internal consultant is that in some cases the consultant is too close to the individuals working in the organization and may not be able, in the eyes of the leadership of the organization, to separate the relationships. Additionally, the internal consultant, if it is someone who has been employed by the organization for a length of time, may be blind to the issues that are creating the organizational symptoms, and thus may suffer a loss of objectivity.

In contrast, an external consultant does not have an established psychological connection with the organization, so he or she may bring the objectivity that might be lacking with the internal consultant. In addition, an external consultant is often skilled at a particular intervention or set of interventions that have been used in other organizations, so the consultant brings experiences in the implementation of the intervention. Another advantage of an external consultant is that a particular skill set may exist with the external consultant that the internal consultant may not possess. For example, if an organization wants to implement Six Sigma, the internal consultant may not have the training or skill set to assist with implementation of this complex process. One disadvantage of an external consultant is that there is not a prior relationship with the organization in many cases, so the external OD practitioner must begin with rapport and trust-buildings steps. This lack of a relationship may, in some cases, hamper the data-collection steps, especially if employees are mistrusting of an outside person. It is interesting, however, that this may also be an advantage to the data-collection initiatives, as often the employees are mistrustful of providing information to an internal person for fear of retaliation.

ACTION RESEARCH

As mentioned earlier, OD is a systematic process. "What makes it systematic?" one might ask. Most OD practitioners use a model of planned change known as the Action Research Model (Cummings and Worley, 1997). According to Rothwell, Sullivan, and McLean (1995), action research can be used as a model to represent the complex activities that occur in a change process. As illustrated in Figure 17–1, the Action Research Model contains eight main steps. This model may, in fact, serve as a road map for change agents to follow as they implement change in an organization (Rothwell et al., 1995). Ultimately, the goal of action research is to base the intervention on initial research, then to follow up the process with feedback through further data analysis to determine the effectiveness or impact, make adjustments as necessary, and ultimately use the results to feed additional research (Rothwell et al., 1995).

STEPS IN THE ORGANIZATION DEVELOPMENT PROCESS

As illustrated in Figure 17–1, traditional OD theorists have identified eight steps to the Action Research Model (Burke, 1982; McLean & Sullivan as cited in Rothwell et al., 1995), which has served as the template for OD practitioners to follow. However, other practitioners have recommended that the model be consolidated into a smaller number of identified steps. The two models are

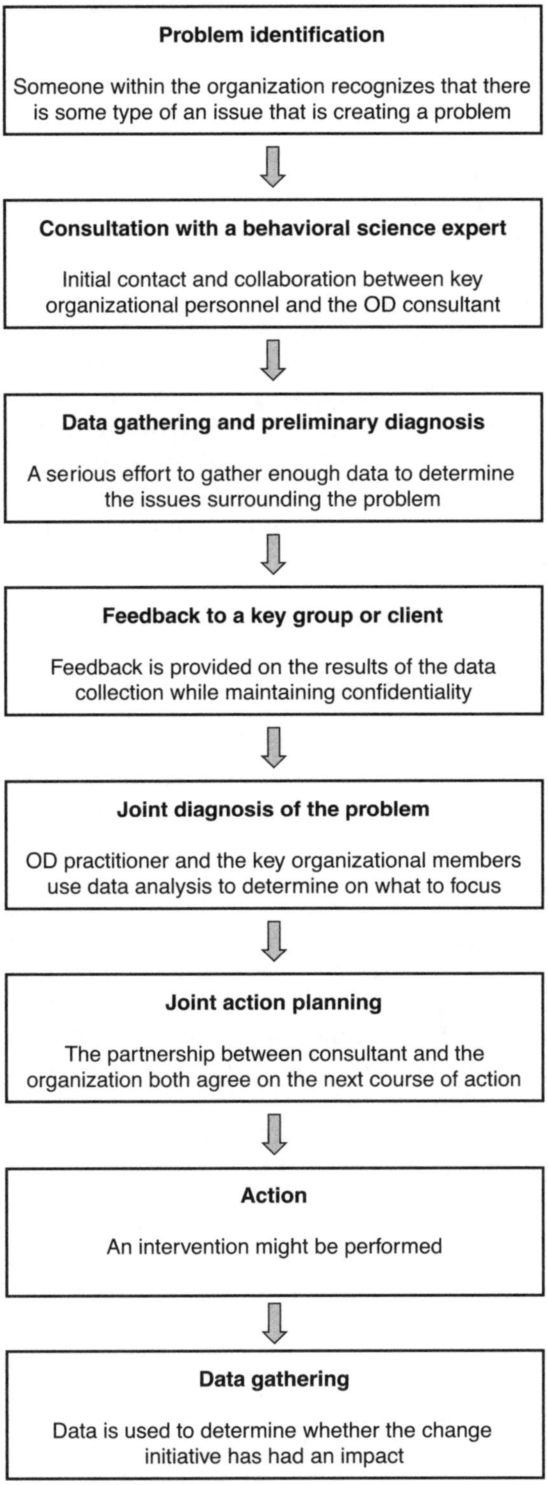

Problem identification

Someone within the organization recognizes that there is some type of an issue that is creating a problem

Consultation with a behavioral science expert

Initial contact and collaboration between key organizational personnel and the OD consultant

Data gathering and preliminary diagnosis

A serious effort to gather enough data to determine the issues surrounding the problem

Feedback to a key group or client

Feedback is provided on the results of the data collection while maintaining confidentiality

Joint diagnosis of the problem

OD practitioner and the key organizational members use data analysis to determine on what to focus

Joint action planning

The partnership between consultant and the organization both agree on the next course of action

Action

An intervention might be performed

Data gathering

Data is used to determine whether the change initiative has had an impact

Figure 17–1 Action Research Model

compared in Table 17–1. A few additional points about each of the major steps are worth noting.

Entering and Contracting

The entering and contracting phase is a critical step in this process. During this stage a contract is developed between the organization and OD practitioner, during which mutual expectations are identified. These expectations should include everything from outcomes expected—such as greater employee satisfaction, increased revenues, lower turnover; length of the engagement; and communication and reporting expectations, for example, who is the primary contact at the organization for the OD practitioner and how frequently are reports or updates, and so on, expected. In addition, ground rules need to be established that outline how to handle sensitive issues such as feedback of difficult information, maintaining employee confidentiality (whether that is an expectation), and how to terminate the engagement if there are concerns or issues from either party (Cummings & Worley, 1997; Rothwell et al., 1995).

Diagnosis

The diagnosing phase involves a strategic collection and analysis of data from the organization. There are various methods of collecting data within the organization. Cummings and Worley (1997) outline the most typically utilized methods. Usually, a variety of methods may be used, with the choice being largely determined by efficiency, sample size, and type of information that is needed. The most commonly used methods include questionnaires, interviews, observations, and unobtrusive methods.

Questionnaires are often the first method used for collecting information from an organization (Cummings & Worley, 1997). Questionnaires are often utilized because of their relative ease of administration and ability to collect information from large groups of people and to provide some response anonymity. Additionally, questionnaires, if developed correctly, enable an efficient means to quantify and analyze information. A good OD practitioner understands how to construct an effective tool for capturing the information that would be relevant for performing an organizational analysis. Such expertise is needed because it is important to understand the statistical properties of sample size, the power of results, and scale construction, as well as how to create a nonbiased instrument. Additionally, in the current litigious world, one must work to ensure that there is some validity to any questionnaire that is used in an organization and that it does not seemingly target any particular group of individuals with a biased result.

The construction of a questionnaire with an appropriate scoring scale is critical to the ability to effectively analyze the data. All too often new OD practitioners create an open-ended questionnaire and send it out to 300 employees in the hopes of collecting a variety of responses, only to discover that there is no easy way to analyze the results since every individual has written something different. One difficulty in using a questionnaire method is that it is

Table 17–1 Comparison of the Two Models for Action Research

Burke, 1982; McLean and Sullivan, 1989	Cummings and Worley, 1997	Description
1. Entry 2. Start Up	1. Entry and contracting	Key leaders identify a need and work to begin the OD process. An OD practitioner is identified and the key components of the working relationship between the organization and practitioner are established. Ground rules, mutual expectations, and deliverables are identified.
3. Assessment and feedback	2. Diagnosing	Data-collection techniques are employed to determine the extent of issues identified by the organization. A diagnosis of relevant organizational processes, interpersonal relationships, or group analysis may be employed.
4. Action planning		Steps are taken to work with the organization to ensure long-term success of any intervention. Key relationships are established and mutual plans are developed. The impact of change on any change initiative is reviewed, and steps put into place to assist the organization through the change process.
5. Intervention	3. Planning and implementing change	The planning phase is similar to the action planning phase just listed. The plan is implemented and carried out. The process of managing change is implemented, and steps taken to ensure the success of the intervention.
6. Evaluation 7. Adoption	4. Evaluating and institutionalizing change	The change process is evaluated through data analysis and comparison to previous data. The change becomes part of the organization, and the members of the organization begin to adopt these strategies and take ownership for their success.
8. Separation		The OD practitioner begins the disengagement process from the organization if it is an external consultant or the disengagement of the project if it is an internal consultant.

rare that everyone who receives a questionnaire is going to complete it. It is likely that you have received many satisfaction surveys at home, only to throw them in the trash or forget to complete them. The reality is that there is typically a relatively low response rate for questionnaires, and the missing data mean that a piece of the puzzle is missing. This nonresponse bias is impossible to interpret but exists and makes an impact on analysis. Therefore, it is common for OD practitioners to attempt to send questionnaires to as many employees as possible to ensure a sample with enough respondents to reduce statistical error of the results.

A second type of data-collection tool is the use of interviews (Cummings & Worley, 1997). Occasionally, the interview is used as a follow-up to results obtained in the questionnaire, but this method is also used to capture data that cannot be readily obtained in the questionnaire. Through a two-way communication approach, an effective interviewer can delve into issues identified by the employee and attempt to get to the heart of any issue identified. Coding of responses is a hurdle for analyzing the results of the interview. Additionally, the interviewer may hear the responses that the interviewee wants to be heard. This response bias may make it difficult to obtain valid results, but this can be overcome to some degree through effective rapport building and reassurance of confidentiality from the interviewer. The final disadvantage for this approach is that it is very difficult to conduct a large number of interviews, so the sample size tends to be small.

Another method for data collection is that of observation (Cummings & Worley, 1997). An observation is designed to allow the OD practitioner to see first-hand what is occurring with either a particular group of people or a process. For example, one organization might be concerned with the lack of teamwork among a group of employees, and the questionnaire data collection revealed a variety of potential reasons for these issues. Because the results were somewhat ambiguous, the OD practitioner might decide to go in and actually observe the interpersonal dynamics occurring between the team members. This might reveal communication patterns, leadership issues, or ineffective conflict resolution strategies within the team that might not otherwise be discovered through traditional data-collection strategies. In another example, a process might be observed in order to determine whether there are inherent inefficiencies that might not be recognized by the employees performing the various tasks within the process because they become so accustomed to performing those tasks regularly. Therefore, it is obvious that there are some distinct advantages to the observation method of data collection. However, as with all data-collection techniques, there are also some pitfalls. The most apparent is that of the "Hawthorne Effect" (as explained in Chapter 1), which is when employees behave differently simply because they are being observed. Many employees become concerned that they will face some outcome if, during the observation, some negative data are collected regarding their work performance. Since ultimately the goal for many employees is job security, it is probable that in some cases the employee may in fact alter their behavior simply to "look good." Additionally, the observers face considerable difficulty in coding observed behavior into some type of aggregate result. Observers must also guard against their preconceived ideas of what should occur, so that they are in fact recording actual behavior rather than either an ideal or a judged version of what actually occurred.

Finally, one additional type of data collection frequently utilized by OD practitioners is that of the unobtrusive method (Cummings & Worley, 1997). The interesting component in this type of data collection is that the data are obtained directly from preexisting information. This type of data exists in various formats throughout every organization. Examples of this include financial reports; human resources information such as turnover, vacancy rates, performance appraisals, and exit interviews; safety reports; and customer satisfaction information, to name a few. The advantage of this type of data is that they are relatively easy to utilize once they are obtained, although in some organizations the information systems or mechanisms by which organizations collect information are either cumbersome or in some cases nonexistent. A second advantage of these data is that they are typically free of biases that may be introduced as a result of other data-collection strategies.

Planning and Implementing Change

There is an enormous variety of interventions that are utilized by OD practitioners. According to Cummings and Worley (1997, p. 141), there are three major criteria needed for an effective intervention: "(1) the extent to which it fits the organization; (2) the degree to which it is based on casual knowledge of intended outcomes, and (3) the extent to which it transfers competence to manage change to organization members." Essentially, the types of OD interventions that are typically utilized fall into several broad categories (Cummings & Worley, 1997).

A brief overview of these interventions is outlined below, although some will be discussed in greater detail later in the chapter. These interventions include the following:

1. *Strategic Interventions:* Strategic interventions deal with large-scale organizational strategic issues, such as ensuring the organization maintains a competitive advantage, and marketing strategies, as well as other organizational performance issues. Assessing the organizational environment and external factors impacting performance may identify an intervention whereby a diversification in products or change in geographic location may be identified as the key to long-term organizational success (see Chapter 20).

2. *Technostructural Interventions:* Technostructural interventions deal with structural issues within an organization, such as organizational design issues or work design issues. An example of this might be the recognition through data collection that an organization with a functional structure is no longer efficient in its business strategy. The structure is providing some limitations that are ultimately impacting on coordination between products and services and resulting in customer service or quality issues. As a result, the recommended OD intervention is to move from a functional structure to a matrix organization (see Chapter 21).

3. *Human Process Interventions:* Human process interventions deal primarily with issues between people within an organization. Often there are distinct communication barriers, a history between employees, or perhaps ineffective leadership. In these interventions the data might point to a problem involving fundamental communication processes, and, therefore, the recommended intervention might be a strategy to assist the group with improving interpersonal relationships. An intervention such as communication training involving the Johari Window (as explained in Chapter 4) or a team-building strategy might be appropriate in these cases.

4. *Human Resource Management Interventions:* Human resource management interventions deal with larger-scale typical human resource issues. Interventions in this arena might be based on data suggesting that there is an exodus of good employees from the organization. Exit interviews might reveal that employees are disenchanted with reward programs or with organizational succession planning. Interventions such as a career planning system might be a way to address such concerns.

Evaluating and Institutionalizing Change

The true test of the effectiveness of an OD intervention is the outcome. In order to truly know whether there is an effective outcome, there has to be some sort of follow-up evaluation and measurement. The follow-up evaluation should be predetermined at the outset and agreed upon by both parties as part of the original contract.

It is critical that the OD practitioner be viewed solely as the facilitator of the new process rather than as the owner. It is therefore extremely important that the impact of the intervention be transferred back to the organization. In other words, the organization must transfer responsibility and accountability from the OD practitioner to the organization and with that ensure that the proper steps have been taken to implant the new strategy into the fabric of the organization.

ORGANIZATION DEVELOPMENT INTERVENTIONS

Listed below are some typical OD interventions suggested by Rothwell and colleagues (1995) that might be utilized by OD practitioners:

1. *Team Building:* Team building can be done in a variety of ways, from providing assessments to team members, team-building workshops, or in-depth group analysis. Regardless of the strategy utilized, the goal is to increase the effectiveness and cohesiveness of either an intact work group or a project team.

2. *Process Improvement:* The process improvement intervention is designed to look at work processes and the way an individual may work within the process. The goal is to improve efficiency.

3. *Total Quality Management:* The total quality management intervention is designed to enable groups of people to work together on a single problem and through a regimented process utilizing specific problem-solving tools, work to solve the issue at hand. Some of the tools that the team is

trained to use are Pareto diagrams, cause-and-effect diagrams, brain-storming, and flowcharts, as well as a host of other tools. Team members are trained on these techniques. Teams typically meet regularly over a long period of time in an effort to solve the problem or mission that they have been given. This intervention not only is an effective intervention for problem solving or process improvement, but also impacts on team dynamics as well as provides opportunities for employee involvement.

4. *Work Redesign:* As noted in Chapter 5, the work of Hackman and Old-man (1980) suggests that there is a significant relationship between core job dimensions (skill variety, task identity, task significance, autonomy, and feedback) and critical psychological states (experienced meaningfulness of work, experienced responsibility for outcomes of work, and knowledge of actual results of work activities). The relationships between these produce personal and work outcomes (internal motivation, high-quality work performance, high satisfaction, and low absenteeism and turnover). On the basis of this model, OD practitioners may opt to look at the design of the job to determine what core job dimensions are inherent in the work. Depending on the outcome of the analysis, a redesign of the job may be recommended so that specific psychological states are addressed in the core job.

5. *Structural Change:* As mentioned earlier and fully described in Chapter 21, it is possible to change the organizational structure if it is determined that the current structure is ineffective. Changing the structure essentially changes reporting relationships, which is designed to streamline and improve quality outcomes.

6. *Training:* Training is often seen as the only intervention needed. Often organizations fall into the trap that a training program will be the panacea that addresses and solves all of its organizational issues. This is clearly not the case; however, training is considered to be a very effective intervention when conducted with the right goal in mind or as an adjunct to an additional initiative. The goal of training should be to improve a skill base.

7. *Performance-management Systems:* Performance-management systems intervention is one of the Human Resource Management Interventions. A performance-management system is composed of goal setting, appraisal, and reward systems. Some organizations have none of the components in place; some have one or two components, or all. This intervention may involve designing a performance-management system within an organization where none exists or the redesign of one in an organization with an ineffective system in place. The goal of this strategy is to identify the appropriate mechanisms, specific to an individual, for measuring employee performance.

In addition to the preceding OD interventions, there are a variety of other techniques that may be used. One relatively new intervention is Appreciative Inquiry. Appreciative Inquiry is designed to be a paradigm shift away from the traditional Action Research Model (Cooperrider & Srivastva, 1987) and in essence suggests that for organizational change to take place, the organization needs to begin with the recognition of its positive attributes and then ask the questions that will take it along the path toward the organization it visualizes itself becoming. Similar to an athlete using visualization to prepare for an upcoming competition, whereby the athlete mentally reviews every step of the competition and visualizes success, so does Appreciative Inquiry challenge the organization to capitalize on its strengths. Appreciative Inquiry is a guided change process by an OD practitioner adept at maneuvering through the maze of possibilities that might be exposed through the positive issues identified. The OD practitioner essentially helps the organization see the future and then sets the organization off on a path to make that visualization a reality (Cummings & Worley, 2001).

SUMMARY

Organization Development (OD) is a systematic process of addressing organizational issues or implementing change strategies. There are many types of interventions available and at the disposal of a good OD practitioner. The key to a successful OD initiative is one that is based on a thorough analysis of any symptoms of problems, with this analysis based on a thorough analysis of data. The partnership with the organization is critical, and the OD practitioner must work to ensure that ultimately the organization understands and accepts that the responsibility for the success of any intervention lies with the organization.

END-OF-CHAPTER DISCUSSION QUESTIONS

1. Identify and discuss the various characteristics of OD.
2. Describe the unique features of OD that differentiate it from other change initiatives.
3. How would you describe the role of the OD professional? What skills are necessary for an OD practitioner?
4. Explain the various components of the Action Research Model.
5. Identify and explain the steps necessary in the OD process.
6. Why is data collection so important to the OD process?
7. Identify and explain the various interventions used in the OD process.
8. What is Appreciative Inquiry and how is it used in the OD process?

Case Study 17–3 Gateway Hospital

Gateway Hospital is a 500-bed tertiary-care hospital located in a busy metropolitan area. A recent employee satisfaction survey scored well below the national norms on most scales. The hospital has been facing higher than average turnover and vacancy rates. Recruitment of professional positions is very difficult because the hospital has gained a reputation as a bad place to work, especially if one is new; the term "eat their young" seems to be a prevalent description. Salaries are below the local market, as are annual pay increases. In many departments there seems to be a critical shortage of staff, and closing services has been a recent topic of discussion.

Additionally, the financial picture of the organization is bleak. The payor mix has changed; Medicare cutbacks are impacting the bottom line, as are changes in private insurance funding. Key physicians are beginning to take their services elsewhere, as they sense the inefficiency of the hospital processes.

The various stresses appear to be having a significant impact on the overall morale of employees. Poor teamwork is rampant, and communication breakdowns seem to be a normal occurrence. Several leaders have been let go in an effort to address issues.

The leadership of Gateway Hospital is extremely concerned about the organizational prognosis and has decided to begin to address the issues by enlisting the assistance of a consulting team. One member of the team is a financial expert who has been hired to address the significant financial issues affecting the hospital. The time frame on fixing the financial issues is one of a critical need; since the environment is rapidly changing, the consultant must get a handle on how to help the hospital operate successfully, given the current financial downslide.

A second member of the team is hired to address the morale and employee issues. A review of the employee opinion survey is conducted, and trends are identified in exit interviews. Employee interviews and focus groups are held in an attempt to determine the root cause of the morale issues, as well as the breakdown in teamwork and communication.

The data collection is discussed with leadership; after a series of discussions, leadership admits that many of the financial pressures have created a "knee jerk" reaction to staffing issues, often cutting back dramatically on employee hours. This would create a crisis mode and the need to ask employees to work harder. This cycle has created a significant lack of trust from the employee's perspective, coupled with the fact that employees have not felt that they have been apprised of the reasons for the roller coaster changes and have not been offered any words of appreciation when they have either reduced their hours or worked in a crisis.

The consultant and the leadership agree that in order to fix the "people" issues of the organization, there will need to be a culture shift of leadership and employee interactions so that a trust can be rebuilt.

Questions

1. On the basis of these issues, what OD interventions do you think should be utilized to address the problems this hospital is facing?
2. How would you proceed if you were the consultant in this case?
3. What skill set do you think the practitioner will need in order to be effective in this organization?
4. What type of a time line would you establish if you were this consultant?

Case Study 17–4 City Hospital

City Hospital is a growing hospital in a large metropolitan city. The hospital is currently experiencing issues that many other organizations are also facing, that of the multigenerational workforce. The senior leadership of this hospital is the typical "baby boom" generation, but the population of employees is slowly growing into one of a younger workforce. The leadership is struggling to deal with issues such as iPods at work, cell phone use, Internet use, tattoos, body piercing, and so on. Equally troublesome is a different perceived commitment to the job and breakdowns in communication. Leadership has decided to hire an outside consultant to help the organization understand the impact of the multigenerational workforce and to try to help become a more cohesive organization.

1. Which OD type of OD intervention is the leadership using in this situation?
2. What obstacles do you see in this situation that may make this intervention more difficult than other types?
3. What recommendations do you have for this situation?
4. What other interpersonal issues exist in organizations besides generational that may create a need for an OD intervention?

REFERENCES

Argyris, C. (1970). *Intervention theory and method.* Reading, MA: Addison-Wesley.

Beckhard, R. (1969). *Organization development: Strategies and models.* Reading, MA: Addison-Wesley.

Beer, M. (1980). *Organization change and development: A systems view.* Santa Monica, CA: Goodyear Publishing.

Block, P. (1981). *Flawless consulting.* San Diego, CA: University Associates.

Browne, P. J., Cotton, C. C., & Golembiewski, R. T. (1977). Marginality and the OD practitioner. *Journal of Applied Behavioral Science, 13*(4), 493–506.

Burke, W. W. (1982). *Organization development principles and practices.* Glenview, IL: Scott, Foresman.

Church, A. H., Hurley, R. F., & Burke, W. W. (1992). Evolution or revolution in the values of organization development: Commentary on the state of the field. *Journal of Organization Change Management, 5*(4), 6–23.

Cooperrider, D., & Srivastva, S. (1987). Appreciative inquiry in organizational life. In W. A. Pasmore & R. W. Woodman (Eds.), *Research in organizational change and development* (pp. 129–169). Greenwich, CT: JAI Press.

Cummings, T. G., & Worley, C. G. (1997). *Organization development and change* (6th ed.). Cincinnati, OH: South-Western College Publishing.

Cummings, T. G., & Worley, C. G. (2001). *Organization development and change* (7th ed.). Cincinnati, OH: South-Western College Publishing.

French, W., & Bell, C. Jr. (1990). *Organization development* (4th ed.). Englewood Cliffs, NJ: Prentice Hall.

Gottlieb, J. Z. (2001). An exploration of organization development practitioners' role concept. *Consulting Psychology Journal: Practice and Research, 53*(1), 35–51.

Hackman, J., & Oldman, G. (1980). *Work redesign.* Reading, MA: Addison-Wesley.

McLagan, P. (1989). *Models for HRD Practice.* Alexandria,VA: American Society for Training and Development.

Ott, J. S. (1996). *Classic readings in organizational behavior* (2nd ed.). Belmont, CA: Wadsworth Publishing Company.

Rothwell, W. J., Sullivan, R., & McLean, G. N. (1995). *Practicing organization development, a guide for consultants.* San Diego, CA: Pfeiffer and Company.

CHAPTER 18

Resistance to Change and Change Management

Paul D. Maxwell, EdD

LEARNING OUTCOMES

After completing this chapter, the student should be able to:

☞ Identify the drivers of change.
☞ Understand the various change models.
☞ Identify the organizational and individual barriers to change.
☞ Understand the step-by-step change process.
☞ Understand the costs and benefits of organizational change.

OVERVIEW

As we discussed in Chapter 17, planned change arises from a single or series of changes in organizational goals and objectives (e.g., increased patient satisfaction). These changes may originate from an organization revising its mission, creating a vision, or responding to other internal or external forces.

Unplanned change arises from the unexpected, which impinge on the well-being of the organization. Unplanned changes seldom surface from known sources. Unplanned changes occur because of, for example, sudden shifts in the marketplace accompanied by reduced product/service demand, emergence of superior competitive products/services, changes in information technology, depressive economic events, natural disasters, or the death or impairment of a senior manager.

Whether planned or unplanned, changes within an organization will meet with resistance because, as Lippitt (1973, p. 3) noted, "change is a very complex phenomenon involving the multiplicity of man's motivations in both micro and macro systems and that a man gets satisfied with his equilibrium and is resistant to changing his status quo." Resistance to change is not limited to staff. Resistance may also be encountered at the entry, middle, and senior levels of management. As such, it is a top priority for managers to understand the factors involved, thereby reducing individuals' resistance to change through change management.

DRIVERS OF CHANGE

Organizations function within three identifiable environments: external/social, industry/task, and internal (see Figure 18–1).

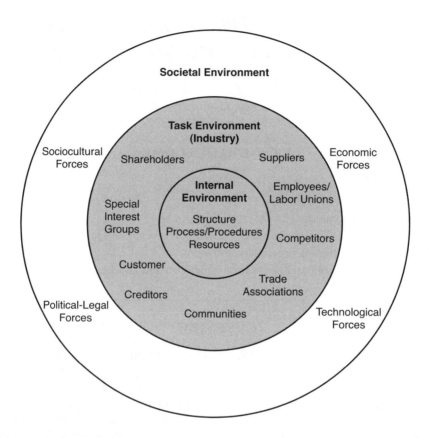

Figure 18–1 Environments (SOURCE: *Strategic management and business policy* (6th ed., p. 10), by T. L. Wheelan and J. D. Hunger, 1997. Upper Saddle River, NJ: Addison-Wesley. Used with permission.)

The primary forces creating the need for change originate in an organization's external and industry environments. Change becomes the organization's attempt to respond and adapt to new operating requirements generated by demands from these environments.

Today's organizations are facing many challenges. For example, war and terrorism are viewed as powerful political/legal forces impacting organizations worldwide. Economic forces include other countries' economic threats of inflation, deflation, and recession and the resulting general weakening of the US dollar. Technology is a major force affecting today's businesses with the increased use of and availability of the Internet. Although these external forces affect all organizations, they have had a direct impact on changes within the healthcare industry. For example, patients have become informed consumers of healthcare services, partially because of the Internet; stem-cell research and cloning capabilities have challenged an organization's ethical practices; special-interest groups such as managed care organizations and employer-sponsored health consortiums have directly impacted the way health services organizations do business; and the increase in union representation of not only nonlicensed employees but also professional groups, such as nurses and physicians, has had a direct impact on the healthcare industry. The government with its changing health policies has had a direct and major impact on the industry with the implementation of the Prospective Payment System in the 1980s, the Balanced Budget Act and the Health Insurance Portability and Accountability Act (HIPAA) in the 1990s, and the Medicare Prescription Drug, Improvement and Modernization Act of 2003.

In addition to external forces, internal forces are influencing change within health services organizations. Internal forces are related to an organization's structure, processes, and resources. Because of the many external factors cited, health services organizations are experiencing decreasing reimbursements/revenues and increasing costs, resulting in smaller profit margins, if any. Furthermore, fragmented processes do not ensure that patients are receiving appropriate and effective services. For example, the now famous Institute of Medicine (1999) study reported that between 44,000 and 98,000 patients die each year as a result of preventable medical errors. Whatever the reasons that create a need for change, a planned response must be developed and implemented by management to ensure future organizational effectiveness.

RESISTANCE TO CHANGE

Managers need to be aware that most organizational change efforts will be met with resistance. Resistance to change may arise from two sources: organizational barriers and individual barriers. Organizational barriers may include: (1) lack of change agent, (2) inadequate financial and/or capacity, (3) poor leadership and resistance to change by senior management, (4) lack of the necessary technology, (5) time restraints, or (6) poor market conditions. Overcoming organizational barriers to change may be beyond the control of the manager and is usually a topic within a strategic management course. Since our concern is to understand the behavior-oriented change process, our focus will center on understanding the individual's barriers or resistance to change.

Individual's Barriers to Change

Individuals may resist change as a result of many issues. Some of the most widely cited barriers are:

- Feelings of uncertainty based on the unknown
- Reduction in personal need fulfillment
- Real or perceived stress
- Loss of status or "personal comfort zones"
- Loss of equilibrium and personal power

Fear of the Unknown

Employees require a stable psychological condition in the workplace. In instances where changes occur, issues of professional and personal insecurity are kindled primarily by a lack of knowledge and understanding of what changes are taking place and the official causes for internal adjustments. Management's failure to furnish realistic information in a timely fashion further adds to an employee's uncertainty. This uncertainty often results in lower morale, increased absenteeism, and reductions in both quality and quantity of output.

Reductions in Personal Need Fulfillment

Lacking an understanding of management's intentions often leads to a disruption of employee expectations. Nonverbalized, mutual expectations are disrupted. In effect, the psychological contract becomes unbalanced; historical feelings of trust and perceptions of honest relationships become questionable, particularly to the "informal organization."

Real or Perceived Stress

Psychological stress will certainly be increased on the basis of real or imagined consequences of change. In many instances, stress will create a physical as well as a psychological response in the work force.

Loss of Status or "Personal Comfort Zones"

Accepting that status is a strong motivator for the work force, subsequent loss will create an immediate impact upon morale and feelings of self-worth. Increased absenteeism and reductions in both the quality and quantity of productivity may occur. Many employees view their individual areas of operation in terms of personal influence and unique contributions. Any changes in the current status of worker relationships may very well upset the individual's fiefdom or silo of interest. Change will then be viewed in personal terms, as both a loss of power and a loss of prestige.

Loss of Equilibrium and Personal Power

When current working and communication interactions are modified, a series of new employment conditions must be established. Workers who have performed comparable tasks and carried commensurate responsibilities for any period of time will quickly resent any disruptions. Responsibilities are often viewed in power or ownership terms. Therefore, any change may be perceived as a loss of two primary motivators: power and prestige.

On the basis of the Hawthorne studies (see Chapter 1), Roethlisberger (1941) proposed that an individual's attitudes affect his or her response to change. In other words, how a person feels toward a change determines his or her response. Feelings are not random. As discussed in Chapter 3, feelings and/or attitudes toward an object are based on the collective experience of one's life; thus, each employee may well be affected in a different fashion when changes are introduced in the workplace.

As illustrated in Figure 18–2, Roethlisberger's X model suggests, on the basis of his work at the Hawthorne Plant, that two primary forces are influ-

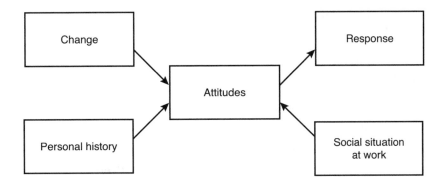

Figure 18–2 Roethlisberger's X Chart (Model for Change) (SOURCE: *Management and morale* (p. 21) by F. J. Roethlisberger, 1941. Cambridge, MA: Harvard University Press.)

encing an individual's perception, attitude, and response toward change. The first force consists of the worker's cumulative life experiences. The second, which functions within the formal organizational setting, is the influence of the social forces or informal groups. The identification of these social forces subsequently led to considerable research efforts in the area of group dynamics (see Chapter 14). These studies revealed the great potential for social forces to directly influence an individual's behavior and beliefs, which in turn serve as the foundations for establishing or changing an attitude.

LEWIN'S CHANGE MODEL

To fully understand the influence of group dynamics on an individual's attitude toward change, one would be wise to briefly review the work of Kurt Lewin (1947) and his model of Force Field Analysis. Lewin's model permits us to view change as a series of forces working in different directions. In effect, some forces and interests within an organization desiring change may well be offset by forces and interests striving to maintain the status quo.

For implementation of change, there must be an increase in the strength of the force for change (i.e., driving forces); the strength and position of opposing forces (i.e., restraining forces) must be reduced or removed. Employing this model requires an improved managerial understanding of the external and internal environments. By identifying each force, it becomes possible to distinguish between forces and issues that may be changed and those that cannot be changed.

According to Lewin (1947), change can be enacted in one or two ways: by increasing the force for change in the desired direction or by reducing the strength of any opposing forces. Borkowski and Allen's (2002) research regarding physicians' nonacceptance of clinical practice guidelines (CPGs) into their medical practice illustrates the application of Lewin's Force Field Analysis in the change process. CPGs are viewed as important tools to reduce variances of medical services received by patients and to improve quality of care by establishing "best practices." As such, there is great concern as to why CPGs have been remarkably unsuccessful in influencing physician practice patterns. Borkowski and Allen suggested that the driving forces for acceptance and implementation of CPGs represented knowledge and attitudinal change and were viewed positively by physicians, whereas the restraining forces represented changes being imposed by some external force that were viewed by physicians with resentment and negativity (see Table 18–1).

By understanding these forces or variances, a realistic approach to planning change can be undertaken. Lewin provides us with a three-step process for implementing planned change:

1. *Unfreeze:* Workers involved in perpetuating resistance acquire an understanding of variances that exist between current practices and behavior and desired activities and behavior. Using the CPG example, unfreezing may occur when managers effectively communicate the need for change (driving forces), such as mortality and/or morbidity rates, hospital readmission data, and best practices benchmarks.

2. *Change:* On the basis of new objectives, a series of revised policies, procedures, and operating practices is implemented. It is important that members of the affected work force understand the reasons for change and participate in the design of new approaches. Participating in the change design, followed by appropriate training and reorientation, presents each worker with the opportunity to buy into the new approaches. Again, using the CPG example, Borkowski and Allen (2002) found that physician participation (whether directly or indirectly) in the development of a CPG does increase the acceptance of a CPG, as measured by hospitals' reduced length of stays and inpatient costs.

3. *Refreezing:* Changes are implemented and monitored, adjusted where necessary. New organizational goals are reinforced by subsequent changes in daily activities. Continuous monitoring ensures successful operating practices. Regarding the implementation of CPGs, Borkowski and Allen (2002) found that audit and feedback of physicians' practice patterns were the most common reinforcements used by managers.

Table 18–1 Suggested Driving and Restraining Forces Regarding Physicians' Acceptance of Clinical Practice Guidelines

Driving Forces	Restraining Forces
Quality patient care (e.g., professional competence)	Administrative edicts (e.g., cost control)
Best practices (e.g., evidence-based findings)	Legislative mandates (e.g., laws and regulations)
Effective use of limited resources	Financial penalties/incentives
Good educational tools	Licensing and accreditation mechanisms
Convenient sources of advice	Utilization review

Kotter (1995, 1996), building on Lewin's Change Model, identified eight steps for managers to follow for successful organizational change. The first four steps change the status quo (i.e., unfreezing), steps five through seven introduce new policies (i.e., change), and step eight institutionalizes the changes (i.e., refreezing). The eight steps are as follows:

1. *Establish a Sense of Urgency:* Management often fails to establish a sense of urgency about the need for change. The first step should be to "unfreeze" the organization by examining market and competitive realities and discussing crises, potential crises, or major opportunities.

2. *Create a Powerful Guiding Coalition:* Management needs to create a powerful guiding coalition, a group that spans both the functions and levels of the organization (i.e., include members who are not part of senior management).

3. *Develop a Vision:* Management must create a vision to direct the change effort and develop strategies for achieving that vision.

4. *Communicate the Vision:* Management must use every vehicle possible to communicate the new vision and strategies, including teaching new behaviors by the example of the guiding coalition.

5. *Empower Others to Act on the Vision:* Management must eliminate barriers to change, and they must encourage risk taking and creative problem solving. They must change systems or structures that undermine the vision.

6. *Plan for and Create Short-term Wins:* Management must plan for visible performance improvements. In addition, employees who are involved in the improvements must be recognized and rewarded.

7. *Consolidate Improvements and Produce More Change:* Management should use the credibility achieved by short-term wins to create more change. This may include hiring, promoting, and developing employees who can implement the vision and reinvigorate the process with new projects, themes, and change agents.

8. *Institutionalize New Approaches:* Management must reinforce changes by highlighting connections between new behaviors and organizational success. Managers must also develop the means to ensure leadership development and succession.

Implementing and Monitoring the Change Process

The management of change is a systematic process involving 12 steps (see Figure 18–3). The design and implementation of planned change have three basic requirements:

1. Ample time exists for planning and implementing change.

2. Employees involved have the necessary skills and knowledge to design and implement the changes.

3. The resources required for implementation and operation of the changes are in place.

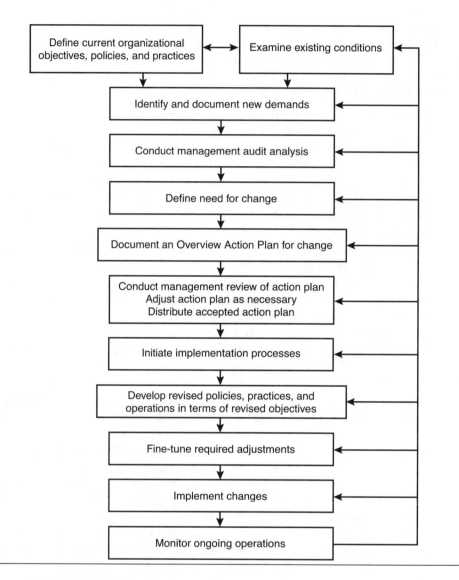

Figure 18–3 A Model for Responding to Change

Define Current Organizational Objectives, Policies, and Practices

Implementing any type of change should be based on a clear understanding of the organization's current objectives, policies, and practices. A review of considerations such as the organization's mission, structure, and responsiveness to customers may be determined by employing analytical techniques such as internal strengths and weaknesses, value-chain and financial ratio analyses.

Examine Existing Conditions (Internal and External)

An analysis of the organization's industry and its competitive relative position will result in an updated picture of growth opportunities. Reviewing external opportunities and threats will aid in acquiring an understanding of possible new strategies. As the Cheshire Cat said to Alice in Carroll's *Alice's Adventures in Wonderland*, "If you don't know where you want to go. . . . any road will do" (Carroll, 1865). A systematic and planned approach here should create an opportunity to prepare a proactive response to the need for future action.

Identify and Document New Demands

Information gathered through the two previous steps should now serve as the basis for assessing two organizational issues: (1) the need to change and (2) the ability to change.

Conduct a Management Audit Analysis

This is the first step in defining the specific needs for change. Reviewed objectives should be documented; an analysis of the resources required to reach those objectives may then be conducted and, in most instances, specific resource needs will be defined. An important aspect of this analysis is to determine who will foster change. Three possibilities exist: (1) current members of management, (2) internal organizational development specialist(s), or (3) an outside consultant.

Define Need for Change

Previous analyses will demonstrate a clear picture and documented justification for organizational change. Senior management must decide whether new objectives are to be pursued. An important strength of this approach lies in the fact that management, at all levels, has been involved in all exploration activities. The final decision should not come as a surprise, but rather as the result of consensus.

Document an Overview Action Plan and Review Process

Objectives have defined the what; attention must now be directed at the who, how, and when. Senior management may now assign the details of design to middle and functional members of management. Managers now have the opportunity to involve all employees. Participative practices will hopefully serve as mechanisms to reduce future resistance. Specific action steps, timetables, responsibilities, and preliminary budgetary considerations are now addressed. Implementation target dates should be set and communicated.

Review Action Plan, Adjust as Necessary, and Distribute

Specifics of schedules, activities, and timelines will be reviewed by senior management to ensure that the planned implementation of change is consistent with new objectives. Input received represents the cooperative effort of all middle and functional managers, who in turn have consulted with their own workforce. One would not expect any significant changes to the plan; tinkering probably will be held to a minimum. At this point in the process, management has become energized for change, and members of the organization understand that change is now necessary. Copies of the final action plan will be distributed to all members of management for implementation.

Initiate Implementation Processes

The importance of individual manager/leader skills now comes to the front. Each manager now carries the responsibility of championing change to his or her individual work force. Emphasis is now placed on both the need for change and actual changes to be designed and implemented. This step requires a great deal of communication.

Develop Revisions

Focusing on the specifics of how new practices will be developed and their specifics may now be undertaken by all members of the workforce. Individual inputs and participation should be earnestly solicited. Each idea should be discussed and explored, rather than simply being ruled out. When employees' work procedures are to be modified, gathering their input should lead to their support, to their buy-in to change. Employees who are involved in designing changes to their workplace are more apt to accept the need for change as well as the changes. Decisions may now be made with respect to the need for additional training and acquisition of resources.

Fine-tune Adjustments

The collective input of all impacted employees, at each level, will determine whether there is a need for any fine-tuning to any aspect of the planned change approach, including timetables and anticipated costs.

Implement Changes

Organization-wide knowledge of the need to change, the timetable for change, and the specifics of functional change should result in the successful implementation of the planned changes. Employing solid communications and participative practices should go a long way in reducing any of the previously identified forces that resist change. Each functional unit should carefully monitor employee response and subsequent levels of productivity.

Monitor Ongoing Operations

Change has been implemented. The organization is functioning in new directions and employing new practices. Monitoring activities and practices must be followed to ensure that, indeed, new objectives are met. A series of follow-up meetings and reviews will greatly assist the monitoring process.

THE COSTS AND BENEFITS OF ORGANIZATIONAL CHANGE

The expense of planned changes within an organization is often difficult to measure from a pure cost standpoint. Similarly, the advantages acquired from revised operations may not be readily measured. Where possible, however, every attempt should be made to evaluate the real savings obtained from a planned change by creating measurable goals. Proposed changes in products, processes, and service activities should be quantified, if possible, before the desired modifications are implemented. Questions to be addressed include such issues as:

- Have we added to the utilization of the service or product?
- Have process expenses been reduced through improved methodology and/or reduced time requirements?
- Can patients or customers be served in a more effective and efficient fashion?
- Have patient or consumer complaints been reduced?

Revising organizational structures requires addressing such issues as:

- Has the fluidity of work processes been improved?
- Have communication and coordination demands been reduced?
- Has the creation, elimination, or combining of functions resulted in more effective work flows, improved communication practices, and management monitoring?
- Have we best served the needs for expanding, retracting, or downsizing current operations?
- Have working conditions been improved and stressful conditions been reduced for our employees?
- Have we successfully implemented the use of new technology?
- Have we ensured that requirements for new operating practices and skills have been addressed and resolved?
- Has the organization become more flexible and proactive in generating responses to meeting competition?

SUMMARY

The primary objective of change is to ensure the future competitive sustainability of an organization. The rationale and need for change rise from both external and internal forces. For successful implementation, managers need to recognize and appreciate employees' attitudes, taking into consideration the various organizational and individual barriers that will create resistance to the required change. In addition, management should use a documented, step-by-step process that includes specific opportunities for feedback, evaluation, and adjustments. As Peter Senge (1990) advocates, success requires the creation of a learning organization. Organizations must develop the capacity to adapt and change continuously. Senge (1990) relates that organizations must learn to create attributes and implement practices that: (1) dismiss old ways of thinking, (2) share ideas freely, (3) create an organizational vision, and (4) establish a collective effort to design a plan to achieve the vision. To become a continuously learning organization requires management to establish a commitment to change, adopt an informal organizational structure, and develop an open organizational culture (see Chapter 19).

END-OF-CHAPTER DISCUSSION QUESTIONS

1. Identify and describe the drivers of change.
2. Explain the components of Roethlisberger's X model.
3. Explain the concept of Lewin's Change Model.
4. Identify and explain the various barriers to change.
5. Explain the components of a step-by-step approach for implementing change.
6. Why is it important for an organization to perform a cost–benefits analysis of a proposed change?

Case Study 18–1 Organizational and Cultural Change for Providing Safe Patient Care

The chairperson of the Department of Medicine (DoM) in an urban academic medical center was concerned. During the last two years, events had occurred in which patients had suffered serious harm needlessly. Although the events were few and far between, the chairperson's view of patient care safety had no place for them.

After all, the medical center had a quality-improvement department, a process-improvement oversight committee, and a risk management department. Nevertheless, despite the considerable efforts of all of these well-intentioned groups, medical errors were still occurring. This could be attributable to the constant competitive pressure to do more with less, but everyone still understood that improvements in efficiency had to be made within the boundaries of safe patient care delivery. Didn't they?

Since the physicians in the DoM were at the center of decision making in the patient care process, the chairperson felt the responsibility not only to continue his support of the medical center's efforts to improve patient safety, but also to address the issue more directly. His perception was that the medical center's current mechanisms for dealing with patient safety matters focused more on broad policy issues, as in the institutional patient safety committee (PSC). The organization's culture did not allow for an open exchange of ideas, which was needed to improve patient care in such a complex environment. Actual and potential patient safety problems were reported to risk managers, who determined the root causes and assigned blame. In addition, the medical center was in a high medical malpractice award area, which also promoted a closed, defensive attitude toward patient safety issues.

Although the DoM already had its own quality-assurance committee, the chairperson wanted to emphasize safe patient care, so he created a PSC. The PSC was going to have to deal with a number of barriers before reaching its goals. First, physicians resist changing their practice patterns unless they are supplied with hard evidence that the change will be beneficial to their patients; second, many of the solutions to patient safety problems would cross departmental boundaries; and third, many of the solutions to patient safety problems would involve the medical center's patient care information systems.

Recognizing that resident practice patterns might have to change to solve patient safety problems, the DoM chairperson appointed the associate director of the medical resident education program as a co-chairperson of the PSC. Furthermore, he appointed the associate chief of the section of medical informatics, an outgoing medical researcher and educator with a positive attitude, the second co-chairperson of the PSC.

The DoM chairperson and the PSC co-chairpersons felt strongly that safer patient care would not be readily achieved within a culture of blame. They wanted to promote a culture of collaboration, group learning, and prevention. The PSC co-chairpersons decided that the PSC meetings would be relatively informal and open to all interested parties. This would provide an atmosphere conducive to discussion and a forum for anyone who wanted to talk about patient care safety issues. PSC committee members were recruited from the chief residents, medical informatics, nursing, pharmacy, and utilization management to ensure that all aspects of patient care safety issues could be addressed in the PSC discussions.

In examining the balance of the forces that would facilitate or hinder these changes, the DoM chairperson concluded that the driving forces were adequate. Caregivers want to be effective and do well by the patient, take pride in their work, avoid the waste of scarce medical resources by providing efficient care, compete successfully in the local healthcare marketplace on the basis of effective and efficient care, and avoid malpractice (i.e., another waste of scarce medical resources). However, the DoM chairperson also knew that there were restraining forces that had to be dealt with, such as the desire to remain in one's comfort zone and avoid change, the tendency to seek scapegoats and assign blame, and the defensive attitude developed in response to the legal environment.

The change agents were skillful and up to the task. The DoM's chairperson had decades of management experience and was politically and culturally savvy. He would provide the necessary organizational support of the PSC's work. The PSC co-chairpersons were respected medical educators. In addition, one of the co-chairpersons possessed extensive research experience and understood the value and necessity of evidence in the improvement of patient care processes.

These change agents knew that they would need resources to bring about patient care safety changes. Original cost estimates included the salaries of the PSC members and programming changes to the medical center's clinical and management information systems. Fortunately, the medical center was among the most wired in the nation and so the infrastructure to support e-mail, data storage, and so on, in the patient care (i.e., clinical) information systems already existed. Nevertheless, the PSC would need approximately $300,000 annually to develop and implement patient safety initiatives.

The very announcement of the formation of the PSC served to unfreeze the previously existing environment. The DoM chairperson communicated his support of the PSC's efforts with discussions with colleagues, as well as management and staff within and without the DoM, of the dangerous lapses in patient care safety along with his dissatisfaction with the current state of affairs. These communications served to strengthen the driving forces. Critics of the efforts viewed the PSC as duplicating the efforts of existing departments and committees (Figure 18–4). However, the critics of the PSC were soon convinced that it was performing a worthwhile activity when the committee undertook the project of creating protocols to avoid potassium overdosing that, when administered, may result in a patient's death.

The PSC's initial charge was to examine lapses and problems in the delivery of safe patient care and identify trends and clusters that merited action. The responsibility of the PSC was subsequently

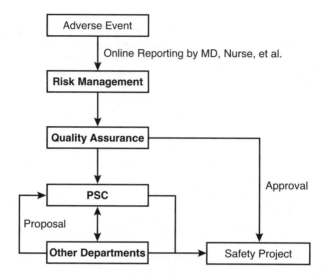

Figure 18–4 Adverse Event Work Flow

broadened to include the development of protocols for improving patient care. The participatory style of the PSC's leadership allowed all members and their respective departments to participate in the development and implementation of the agreed-upon new practices and procedures. The efforts of the PSC were communicated through educational events and status reports at its frequent meetings.

For example, the activities of the PSC involved providing objective data as to the current level of patient care before a project is undertaken and then providing periodic follow-up measurements. The original data and project results were presented by PSC committee members at medical conferences, patient safety seminars, quality fairs, and research forums. These communications reinforced the positive effects of the changes and served to reinforce acceptance as successful operating practices, thus promoting the refreezing of the operating environment with the new practices in place.

The PSC was intended as a means to the goal of safer patient care delivery. It provided an environment that welcomes problem reporting and patient safety initiatives. The PSC was the catalyst for developing and implementing projects to promote safer patient care. The number of projects and the quality of their results served as judge of the PSC's success. Projects successfully completed by the PSC include:

- Development and implementation of an on-line adverse-event reporting system.
- Development of a model for designing three-stage interventions to address patient safety problems (Figure 18–5).
- Reduction of the use of potassium and magnesium supplements.
- Development of an online narcotic conversion calculator and its deployment in clinical systems.
- Elimination of sliding-scale orders for insulin therapy.
- Reduction of use of serum amylase orders for diagnosis of pancreatitis.

Senior management support of a culture of learning and prevention and an organizational structure that promotes collaboration has provided an environment in which patient safety initiatives can flourish.

Identify and discuss Kotter's eight-step approach for successful organizational change in this case study.

SOURCE: Case developed by Richard Odwazny, Assistant Professor, and Robert McNutt, MD, FACP, Professor, Department of Health Systems Management, Rush University, Chicago, IL. Reprinted with permission.

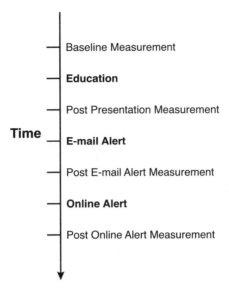

Time
- Baseline Measurement
- **Education**
- Post Presentation Measurement
- **E-mail Alert**
- Post E-mail Alert Measurement
- **Online Alert**
- Post Online Alert Measurement

Figure 18–5 Intervention Model

Exercise 18–1 Individual Readiness Assessment

INTRODUCTION

The Individual Readiness Assessment is an analysis of readiness for the change and potential sources of resistance and one component of the overall approach.

INDIVIDUAL READINESS ASSESSMENT

Resistance to change is natural and inevitable. A thorough analysis of the specific reasons why and how you will resist the change project is critical to increasing the probability of implementation success. Strategies and tactics can be developed to anticipate likely barriers and successfully manage the implementation project toward the accomplishment of important business objectives. Valuable information can be obtained by having this resistance assessment tool completed by Sponsors, Change Agents, and/or Targets and comparing the different results. In this manner, different Frames of Reference about the change can be surfaced and effectively managed.

INSTRUCTIONS

Each of the items on the following pages is to be rated on a scale from 1 to 5 with "1" meaning that you "strongly disagree" with the statement. A "5" indicates that you "strongly agree" with the statement. To the left of each item, place the number that represents your assessment of how you will react to your specific change. Your answers will be more accurate to the extent they reflect your perspective about the change.

(Continued)

Exercise 18–1 *(Continued)*

1	2	3	4	5
Strongly Disagree	Disagree	Neither Strongly Agree or Disagree	Agree	Strongly Agree

_____ 1. I am very clear about WHY the change is being implemented.

_____ 2. I believe that there is a strong need for the change.

_____ 3. I can easily see how this change can directly solve a problem for me.

_____ 4. I do NOT believe this change implies I have performed poorly in the past.

_____ 5. I see this change as having a LOW personal cost to myself.

_____ 6. This change has HIGH compatibility with the values and "unwritten rules" of the organization.

_____ 7. I see this change as having HIGH compatibility with my personal values.

_____ 8. I think there is a HIGH reward for successfully accomplishing this change.

_____ 9. I believe there will be no disruption of stable personal relationships after this change is implemented.

_____ 10. This change will have a positive impact on my job characteristics, such as status and/or salary.

_____ 11. Important habits and routine procedures are NOT disrupted by this change.

_____ 12. I feel the confidence necessary to accomplish this change.

_____ 13. I do NOT tend to focus on the old way of doing things.

_____ 14. I believe this change will have a positive impact on my power or the power of people important to me in the organization.

_____ 15. I see the change as reversible if it does not prove effective once it is implemented.

_____ 16. I do NOT believe this change will lead to less control over key aspects of my job.

_____ 17. I am very clear about what is specifically expected from me as a result of the change.

_____ 18. Generally this change will NOT cause a great deal of disruption in my work life.

_____ 19. I feel very involved in this change.

_____ 20. I believe that adequate organizational support and resources are provided to accomplish this change.

_____ 21. I think that adequate time is provided to accomplish this change.

_____ 22. I believe that the organization has been consistently successful in past implementations.

_____ 23. I am NOT experiencing a significant amount of work pressure and stress.

_____ 24. I believe that this change project will be implemented successfully.

_____ 25. Important Sponsors and Change Agents have a HIGH level of credibility with me.

INDIVIDUAL READINESS SCORE

1. Total your answers to all items.
   (Page 3 Total + Page 4 Total = Total Score)
2. Calculate your Average Item Score.
   (Total Score ÷ 25 = Average Item Score)

   _____ / 25 = _____

   Total Score   Average Item Score
3. Calculate your Individual Readiness Score.

   _____ × 20 = _____

   Average Item Score   Individual Readiness Score
4. Plot your Individual Readiness Score.
   Probability of Implementation Success

20	40	60	80	100
Very Low	Low	Moderate		High

Exercise 18–1 *(Continued)*

RESULTS

Your Individual Readiness Score represents the probability of implementation success for your current change project on the basis of your assessment of the level of Individual Readiness. Scores in the high range indicate a strong likelihood that you will be successful in this change as long as you continue to manage important sources of resistance. Scores in other ranges mean that you must develop strategies to eliminate or minimize significant sources of Target resistance to avoid the real costs of implementation failure and achieve strategic business objectives.

INDIVIDUAL READINESS PROFILE

	1 Very Low	2 Low	3 Moderate	4 High	5 Very High
1. Purpose	o	o	o	o	o
2. Need	o	o	o	o	o
3. Solve Problems	o	o	o	o	o
4. Imply Past Performance	o	o	o	o	o
5. Personal Cost	o	o	o	o	o
6. Organizational Compatibility	o	o	o	o	o
7. Personal Compatibility	o	o	o	o	o
8. Reward	o	o	o	o	o
9. Social Relations	o	o	o	o	o
10. Job Characteristics	o	o	o	o	o
11. Habits	o	o	o	o	o
12. Confidence	o	o	o	o	o
13. Old Ways	o	o	o	o	o
14. Shift Power	o	o	o	o	o
15. Reversibility	o	o	o	o	o
16. Loss of Control	o	o	o	o	o
17. Clear Expectations	o	o	o	o	o
18. Disruption	o	o	o	o	o
19. Involvement	o	o	o	o	o
20. Resources	o	o	o	o	o
21. Time	o	o	o	o	o
22. Past Implementations	o	o	o	o	o
23. Work Stress	o	o	o	o	o
24. Success	o	o	o	o	o
25. Credibility	o	o	o	o	o
Probability of Implementation Success	Very Low	Low	Moderate	High	Very High

---

SOURCE: © Implementation Management Associates, Golden, Colorado, 2001. Reprinted with permission.

Case Study 18–2 Healthy Lives: A Cost-Effective, User-Friendly Way to Improve Health and Productivity in Targeted Chronically Ill Workers

ABSTRACT: St. Mary's Health System, headquartered in Evansville, Indiana, is part of the Ascension Health National System. The system is composed of multiple entities, including a 450-bed medical center with more than 3,000 employees. The average age of employees is 44, the work force is predominately female, and the average tenure is 11 years.

St. Mary's Medical Center has a wellness center called Health Matters, which has performed health screening on employees and spouses since 1993. The system also has a preferred provider network, SelectHealth, which has more than 1,800 providers in a three-state area. The network has been accredited in Health Network and Health Utilization Management since 1999 by the Utilization Review Accreditation Commission (URAC).

St. Mary's Health System was experiencing annual, double-digit increases of more than 18–20 percent in medical claims costs for its health plan. Through analysis of this expenditure, modifiable healthstyle-related conditions such as diabetes, hypertension, obesity, and hyperlipidemia were targeted as an opportunity for improvement. This presentation shows how St. Mary's successfully triaged and educated about 75 percent of its employees and offered health promotion and disease prevention/management programs to 5 percent of its benefit-eligible population, who committed to modifying lifestyles to optimize health and minimize costs for individuals with hypertension, obesity, diabetes, and hyperlipidemia. These conditions were selected because: (1) Efforts can be concentrated on selected, measurable conditions, (2) these conditions occur frequently in high dollar medical cases, and (3) individuals can minimize the effects of chronic illness on productivity and quality of life by making a commitment to learn and better care for themselves.

Results after 18 months show significant improvements in financial, productivity, and clinical indices, which have been measured over the course of the program.

Historical Perspective/Cultural Assessment

Prior to the inception of Healthy Lives, St. Mary's had a wellness screening program from 1993 to 2001 named HealthStyle Plus! This program included basic laboratory tests and physical assessments. Participating employees and spouses received counseling on their results.

To incentivize good health, the hospital used the clinical results to categorize participants as low, mid, or high risk for purposes of health insurance premiums paid for benefits. Employees participating in HealthStyle Plus! received "credits" to offset insurance premiums in accord with their risk level. For example, if you smoked, were obese (body mass index of 30 or more), or had high lipids or high blood pressure, you would be classified as high risk and get the minimal reward. If married, the spouse had to participate, or the employee would automatically be placed in the high-risk category.

This old system had several problems. One, it rewarded individuals with good health and discouraged those with poor health from participating. Two, the program made the medical center vulnerable by incenting results rather than participation, once the Health Insurance Portability and Accountability Act (HIPAA) was passed in 1996. Three, employees worried about how poor health would affect their career. Four, the wellness program and the externally managed health plan worked in silos, limiting the possibilities of optimizing the health and medical resources utilized by the St. Mary's population. Five, healthy employees, rather than the individuals driving health plan costs and productivity, were targeted by HealthStyles Plus!

Communicating the Message for the Paradigm Change

The Plan

1. Data mine the wellness screening, medical claims, pharmacy claims, and productivity statistics to find the 20 percent driving health costs (Pareto Principle applies).
2. Identify the chronic health conditions that are modifiable by lifestyle changes and target those individuals who are ready to change.
3. Hold individuals accountable, not for health status but for behaviors within their control that influence health, performance, and medical costs.
4. Convince senior management and then the employees that this is a sound approach that will reward them with lower health plan costs and better productivity in their peers.

5. Utilize a systematic approach in triaging the health plan population, intervening and providing resources, measuring outcomes, and rewarding commitment to personal health.
6. Utilize the quality improvement process to identify systematic issues in benefit design, claims management, use of insurance, medical treatment, and educational or communication needs and prioritize and implement changes to address issues.
7. Provide feedback to the employer, physicians, and employees.
8. Market the program to other employers.

The Message

1. Employees who are chronically ill don't do their share of work, causing more overtime, poor morale, lower customer satisfaction, disability, turnover, and lost dollars through absenteeism and presenteeism. That is why health costs are only about 25 percent of what the chronically ill cost us.
2. Health is more than the absence of disease. It is about being the best that you can be. Healthy people have energy, endurance, strength, confidence, optimism, and a sense of well-being. Everyone deserves to feel this good.
3. Chronically ill people have problems because of bad genes or bad luck. The bad luck is in the form of inherited conditions, preventable illness, and complications, as well as lack of self care, emotional problems, or accidents.
4. Chronic illness is insidious and silent. Many people don't know they have a health problem, don't take needed medications, and don't take care of the problem because they think they feel fine, they are in denial, or they believe they cannot afford treatment and medication. Only when they start getting healthy do they realize how bad they once felt and the risk that they were taking.
5. Chronically ill people are often stressed, uninformed, and caught up in a vicious cycle, where they never budget time or money to care for themselves. They require a personalized approach to understanding their health needs, obstacles, and resources and help in creating and implementing their own health plan.
6. Good health is its own reward. Let's put our money to use where we will get the most benefit; that is, in helping the chronically ill health plan members learn about their health and take responsibility for improving it.
7. Make the reward within reach of all benefit eligible employees and spouses on the health plan who commit to taking personal responsibility for their health.
8. Keep results confidential. Release only aggregate results to management or to other publics. Include a confidentiality statement that binds the wellness and health plan to these standards.

The Culture

The system was recently redesigned to integrate the purchase of another hospital in the city and to compete with large national health plans in attracting employers to the SelectHealth network in the Tri-state area of Southern Indiana, Southeastern Illinois, and Western Kentucky. The hospital merger with all its issues of integration was a great factor. At the same time, insurance premiums were increased dramatically in 2003 and health plan management was contracted to SelectHealth to improve system's experience and reduce medical costs.

The incidence of obesity, hypertension, hyperlipidemia, and diabetes were increasing annually in the employees who were screened. In summary, medical costs were soaring and the system was in major flux, making the timing ripe for introducing a change that could correct the problem. (Major historical works on change process indicate that change is most readily accepted when a system is in flux. See *The Mob*, *Lewin's Change Model*, and most biographies on how dictators and politicians rose to fame and power.)

Assessment of Forces

In most situations, there are conflicting forces that drive and restrain the change process. A major problem for this program was to develop, market, and implement an integrated wellness/health promotion and disease management program within three calendar months. In this situation they were as follows in Table 18–2.

Table 18–2 Driving and Restraining Forces to Healthy Lives

Factor	Driving Forces	Restraining Forces
Model	1. Develop a simple model, targeting lifestyle illnesses that will reduce health costs for everyone. 2. Make the participant accountable. 3. Reward commitment to personal health. 4. Leadership wants change that will improve health and productivity.	1. Communicate a paradigm flip to employees. 2. Well people want to be rewarded. 3. Employees wonder why people with poor lifestyles get rewarded. 4. What if program can't be measured? 5. What if program doesn't work? 6. What if no one voluntarily participates?
Resources	1. Chronically ill will be able to afford medical care. 2. Money already budgeted. 3. Wellness and managed care staffs are experienced in program development, screening, and disease management. 4. Staff committed to work with available resources.	1. Fear that employees will say, "I counted on the money to reduce my health insurance premiums." 2. "Program isn't fair." 3. Must work with accounting to reallocate funds. 4. Need to create new program and integrate staffs from two different departments to develop and implement plan in three months. 5. Actual budget for new program unknown.
Infrastructure	1. Program leaders are well organized. 2. Employees accustomed to annual health screenings. 3. System needs to measure absenteeism and presenteeism that was complicated by the introduction of a Paid Time Off (PTO) system.	1. Need to develop database. 2. Establish baseline. 3. Create participant report cards. 4. Set up new program and reporting mechanism. 5. Need to find a reliable and valid tool for measuring absenteeism and presenteeism.
Leadership	1. System is in flux from merger. 2. System needs to stop the annual 18 to 20 percent increases in medical claims costs. 3. Leadership wants to make positive changes now. 4. This program could reduce health plan costs. 5. Some cheerleaders have been identified in different work areas.	1. Need to educate and get top-down support. 2. Must educate/convince leaders to participate and be resources for their employees. 3. Need employees to volunteer. 4. Need to report de-identified success stories. 5. What if physicians don't support the program or refuse to change practices?

Table 18–2 *(Continued)*

Factor	Driving Forces	Restraining Forces
Physicians	1. Physicians will do what is best for the patient if included in the plan and educated. 2. Medical Director and Physician Advisory Group for health plan are supportive. 3. Physicians will have more resources to achieve their goals with patients. 4. Medical Director is well respected by the medical staff and has strong communication with them.	1. Physicians need education to be part of the team. 2. Safety and follow-up issues with current, serious health issues. 3. Physicians must give permission for employees to participate in disease management program.
Project Design/ Outcomes Measurement	1. Commercial health risk analysis tool identified that minimizes scoring time and gives participants real time results. 2. Willing, salaried staff that have good relationship. 3. Staff is knowledgeable and experienced. 4. Consultant hired to expedite project.	1. No time or money for new information systems. 2. Three months to identify key measures, set up system to track improvements. 3. Need to accurately select baseline measurements and benchmarks. 4. Actual staff needs unknown.
Savings Potential	1. Improved health will translate into higher productivity, reduced absenteeism and presenteeism. 2. Medical costs will be reduced. 3. Healthy Lives participants will have improved health.	1. Database needs to be developed to capture clinical data. 2. Systematic method needed to track relevant medical costs through claims data. 3. Most health plans complain about inability to track actual costs. 4. What if baseline cannot be measured properly prior to intervention?
Communication	1. Consultant MD is experienced in writing a complex program in simple terms. 2. Consultant has charisma and experience. 3. Leaders in medical management and wellness have credibility with employees.	1. Logistics of reaching physicians, leaders, and employees and convincing them to participate in three months. 2. Challenge of using multimedia. 3. Need to send a message that encourages participation. 4. Challenge of reaching all parties. 5. Way to keep track of responses.

(Continued)

Table 18–2 *(Continued)*

Factor	Driving Forces	Restraining Forces
	4. Program staff is entrepreneurial; able to handle change.	
Personal Response	1. Participants will learn and be pleased with the experience. 2. Participants have time with health professional tailored to their needs. 3. Participants will be able to see actual results from their efforts.	1. There will be no volunteers. 2. Employees will not trust the program. 3. The proposed program might not work. 4. The new program might be disorganized. 5. All factors may not have been considered in development.
Health System Future	1. This program is innovative, and will distinguish our system for its excellence and leadership in addressing lifestyle problems that have become a national health crisis. 2. System needs to model wellness and disease management program before it is sold to other employers. 3. Employers want to see results and get relief from high medical costs. 4. Successful health systems attract commercial business.	1. System needs to be implemented successfully. 2. Results may not be positive; program may not work. 3. Difficult to measure "soft results"; i.e., how does a lower blood pressure save money that falls to the bottom line this year? 4. Employers want to see bottom line savings. 5. Employers want to understand what they are receiving for their investment and how the health plan is improving the lives of their employees; few systems know how to show results in dollars.

Implementation Plan

The leaders at the system level recognized the need for innovative changes in how employee health issues are identified and managed. They also wanted to stop the annual 18 to 20 percent increases in paid medical claims costs. The system hired a consultant that worked with the Healthy Lives team to develop the program. The sequence for major objectives was as follows:

1. Develop program and PowerPoint explaining program, including rationale.
2. August—Show senior management, accept input and make changes.
3. August—Present program to Leadership Team of all managers at monthly meeting.
4. September—Revise employee handbook to include Healthy Lives Program.
5. September—Develop forms and program methodology. Present design to senior management, including goals.
6. October—Present jointly with human resources at Open Enrollment Meetings so that employees learn about the changes in health screening, the new disease management program, and the incentives. Have a sign-up booth at open enrollment meetings to answer questions and enroll volunteers into disease management programs. Provide participants with handouts. Enroll participants in November wellness screening sessions.
7. November—Perform health screening and coach all disease management participants. Explain what participants must do for their particular health condition.
8. December—Present baseline statistics to system management team.
9. January—Incentivize those who participated in screening, coaching, and education.
10. February—First quarterly report submitted by disease management participants.
11. February—Reward participants who completed online education programs.

12. March—Send incentives to first quarter participants. Present first quarter results to management team in relation to goals for hypertension and diabetes.
13. May—Analyze second quarter reports.
14. June—Send second quarter incentives. Present two quarters of results to senior management team.
15. August—Receive third quarter reports.
16. September—Reward third quarter participants. Report results to senior management.
17. October—Announce 2004 program of hypertension, diabetes, lipids, and obesity and enroll participants.
18. November—Year-end screening for 2003 participants and 2004 screening for year two programs. Turn in fourth quarter disease management reports.
19. December—Receive fourth quarter incentive.
20. January—Start the cycle again. Report full year results.
21. July—Report financial results of plan for 2003, and productivity and progress for current participants.

Healthy Lives Program—Making the Changes

Healthy Lives is a corporatewide health promotion and disease prevention program that emphasizes hands-on assessment, education, personalized commitment, goal setting, and coaching for all employees and their spouses. The initial health assessment process allows population screening and early identification and intervention opportunities. Additionally, individuals with diabetes, obesity, hypertension, and hyperlipidemia are invited to participate in an intensive, personalized program to live a healthy lifestyle. The program is an on-site health initiative that blends health promotion with disease and case management to achieve remarkable results for participants.

This "case study" presentation reviews the steps and interventions that resolved problems.

The ActivHealth health assessment tool and online educational Personal Health Development programs developed by Duke University were licensed for use in Health Lives. Results of health screening were available in an access database from which queries could be generated by the vendor and by St. Mary's. Claims and pharmacy data were available to the health plan. An access database was developed to store clinical information, according to the critical measurements identified. The Work Limitations Questionnaire (WLQ) from Tufts New England Medical Center was the tool selected to monitor absenteeism and presenteeism.

Feedback Management and human resources have had feedback in the form of aggregate data compared to national benchmarks. The Year Two 2004 program includes hands-on quarterly coaching, where participants are being evaluated and coached on current progress in relation to pre-set goals. More exercise and nutrition classes have been added at Health Matters, and pharmacists have attended exercise classes to educate participants on disease-specific medications. Fitness and nutritional analysis has been added to 2004, at the request of participants.

This program has been very successful in improving the clinical and financial performance of Healthy Lives participants. The program was presented at the Ninth Annual Disease Management Congress in Boston in September, 2004 and has been successfully sold to other area employers.

Healthy Lives Results

Diabetes Program Results: Clinical results from year one were impressive. For example, at the end of the first year, 69 percent of diabetics achieved glycolated hemoglobin (HbA1c) levels of less than 7.0, compared to 43 percent at the beginning of the year. Statistically significant improvements in blood pressure, weight reduction, and compliance with national guidelines for monitoring the urine, eyes, and feet were also noted.

Hypertensive Results: At the beginning of the project, 57 percent of the hypertensive participants had blood pressure readings of less than 140/90. (Results are available in more detail and in graphics displays.) Seventy-five percent or more of participants in the hypertensive program achieved blood pressures of less than 140/90 for 9 of 12 months. They also had significantly improved results in other clinical measures.

In year two, beginning in November 2003, we started measuring participants using the WLQ, a Tufts–New England Medical Center productivity tool, to better assess the total costs of having a chronic health condition (see Table 18–3).

Table 18–3 Managing the Change Process

Process	Issues	Resolution
Outlining the Program and developing forms, processes, and baseline measures (August)	1. Process took more hours than anticipated. 2. Everyone had different ideas. 3. Search of literature showed congruence on major lifestyle health conditions; paucity of actual measures. 4. Medical claims database massive and time-consuming to analyze. 5. Outcome measures needed to be simple, focused.	1. Consultant served as facilitator in driving work. Both the director of health promotion, the medical manager, and the medical director had experience in change process. The team worked well together, split tasks, and spent extensive overtime to meet deadlines. 2. Use physician consultant and medical director to get support of senior management.
Selecting the Health Conditions	1. Conditions needed to be modifiable by lifestyle changes and quantifiable.	1. The MD consultant and medical director helped with the literature review. The Physician Advisory Council reviewed information and advised Healthy Lives staff.
Open Enrollment Presentation and Employee Handbook Changes	1. Educate senior management, leadership team, and human resources prior to open enrollment. 2. Response to programs was overwhelming and much greater than anticipated. 3. This totally new approach was hard to understand.	1. Accommodate those who meet criteria, assuming that some will not follow through with program requirements. Healthy Lives leaders had to prioritize time and arrange additional meetings to meet with participants to explain how the program works.
Health Screening	1. Participants were at all socioeconomic levels; some were barely literate, and others were educated but in denial. 2. It took longer to take the computerized assessment than planned.	1. Healthy Lives staff had to make adjustments as needed.

Table 18–3 *(Continued)*

Process	Issues	Resolution
	3. Many had limited computer skills.	
Structure	1. Some participants stated they could not progress without structure. 2. Many wanted to change, but did not know how. 3. Physician's releases needed.	1. Need for structure and hands-on help led to special exercise class for diabetics and hypertensives that followed American College of Sports Medicine guidelines. 2. Staff had to assist participants in getting releases and had to budget time/be available in classes as resources. 3. Additional needs for structure will have to be addressed in year two program.
Reporting	1. Database needed to be built for clinical information. 2. Data entry for health plan medical management needed to be streamlined, accurate, and complete. 3. Medical and pharmacy claims needed to be mined to determine health plan costs.	1. The medical director and medical manager wrote a letter explaining the program to physicians and presented the program initially and when results were available at a medical staff luncheon. Case managers worked with physicians to resolve individual participant problems.
Incentives	1. Changes in the budget caused the accountants to have problems in paying incentives. 2. Incentives were taxed.	1. The team was expanded to include other health plan professionals with experience in database design, projects, and claims analysis.
Physicians	1. Patients had to be educated about their health and screening results, so that they could discuss them with their physicians. 2. Written materials and formal education were needed.	1. This took member education and multiple meetings with finance. Rules had to be set to encourage compliance with rules, while not discouraging the newly motivated.

(Continued)

Table 18–3 *(Continued)*

Process	Issues	Resolution
Telling the Story	1. The program was multifaceted and complex. 2. Pressure to get results that can be marketed to other employers. 3. Measurement needs to be relevant and simple.	1. Access database allowed multiple sorts to identify outliers needing special attention. It also enabled rapid analysis of results. 2. Financial results were delayed for seven months to incorporate data on 2003 claims.
Measuring Productivity	1. The PTO system does not track the reasons for days off. 2. The system does not track presenteeism.	1. The health promotions director and the medical manager attended the 2003 Annual Institute of Productivity Management conference and were able to identify a tool, connect with the author, and secure permission to use this reliable and valid tool.

In year two, second-year participants have consistently higher results than the new program participants. For example, results in the hypertension program were as follows:

- Hypertensive patients in Healthy Lives cost the plan one-half as much as nonparticipants.
- Diabetics in Healthy Lives cost the health plan one-third less than nonparticipants.

Summary and Application of Healthy Lives Programs to Other Work Settings

The Healthy Lives Program has been very successful. This case study has focused on introducing a major change into a large health system. Results were successfully measured, but a presentation of these outcomes is beyond the scope of this case study.

General principles learned from this project are as follows:

A. Disease management is a continuation of the employer's commitment to workplace wellness promotion.
B. Disease prevention/management involves the following steps:
   1. Analyze the claims experience to identify the chronic health conditions that are most prevalent in the work population.
   2. Determine which conditions can be most effectively modified by lifestyle changes or modifications in work patterns.
   3. Further narrow the list by identifying the cost/benefit of implementing each program.
   4. Design a high-touch program that is result-oriented, simple, and based on self-responsibility and continuous learning in collaboration with the physician's plan of care for participants.
   5. Invite participants, and think of creative, tangible programs and incentives to keep them interested.
   6. Emphasize education and coaching, supported by helpful ideas and resources to make essential life changes.

7. Capture the spirit of the culture and strive to recruit company leaders to set the example.
8. Infuse a measure of fun and provide special one-to-one attention for individuals who are not progressing.
9. Measure the outcomes quarterly, using these results as a springboard for fine-tuning the approach to individual participants.
10. Add a productivity measure so that the full impact of illness can be calculated on absenteeism and presenteeism.
11. Evaluate self-concept and changes in health status, along with financial, clinical, and productivity measures to assess impact.

Principal Project Managers

Kishor R. Bhatt, MD, Medical Director, St. Mary's Managed Care Services

Dr. Bhatt completed medical school in India at M.P. Shah Medical College, where he also did a rotating internship. He then went to Metropolitan Medical Center in Minneapolis for a second rotating internship. From there he moved to the Bronx, where he became chief resident in pediatrics at Misericordia-Fordham in New York. After working in private practice in the Bronx, he moved to Southern Indiana, where he was Director of the Pediatric Clinic and later Chairman of Pediatrics at St. Mary's Medical Center. He also served as Chief of Staff at St. Mary's Warrick Hospital. Dr. Bhatt is board certified in pediatrics, serves as chief of pediatrics at St. Mary's Medical Center, has expertise in quality and utilization management, is currently in private practice, and works as the medical director for SelectHealth Network. He also has several systemwide appointments, where he serves as an advocate for healthcare quality, a peer educator in managed care, and a member of the hospital patient care evaluation committee and the managed care executive team.

Barbara E. Rutkowski, EdD, MN, Medical Manager, St. Mary's Managed Care Services

Ms. Rutkowski graduated with her Bachelor's and Master's degrees in nursing from the University of Florida and received her doctoral degree in Higher Education and Administration from Indiana University. She has authored four books (two were named American Journal of Nursing Books of the Year) and multiple professional articles and book chapters, and has published two national employment and labor law newsletters with her attorney husband for the past 19 years. Over the past 10 years, she has created and currently manages credentialing, quality, site visits, utilization, clinical risk, and case/disease management programs for St. Mary's Managed Care Services. The network spans the Illinois, Kentucky, and Indiana tri-state and has full URAC Health Network and Utilization Management Accreditation. Dr. Rutkowski has been active in community affairs and has spoken at conferences conducted by the Centers for Disease Control and Prevention and Centers for Medicare and Medicaid Services. She has recently served on a Joint Commission on Accreditation of Healthcare Organizations advisory group in managed care and is on the advisory board for the *Journal of Nursing Risk Management*. During her career, she has also presented hundreds of management workshops across the country.

Cynthia Williams, RN, BSN, Director of Health Promotion, St. Mary's Medical Center

Ms. Williams graduated from the University of Evansville with a Bachelor's degree in nursing. For the past 20 years she has been in health promotion. In 1992, she was promoted to Director of Health Promotion for St. Mary's Medical Center. In addition to overseeing the wellness program for employees, she has developed and implemented numerous creative wellness programs in business and industry throughout the tri-state area. Ms. Williams regularly does formal presentations at seminars, at company retreats, and at other businesses. Together with Ms. Rutkowski, she has created and beta-tested the Healthy Lives program.

Identify and discuss the 12 steps for implementing and monitoring a change management program.

SOURCE: Barbara E. Rutkowski, EdD, MN. Reprinted with permission.

REFERENCES

Borkowski, N., & Allen, W. (2002. Using organizational behavior theories to manage clinical practice guideline implementation. *The Journal of American Academy of Business, Cambridge, 1*(2), 365–370.

Carroll, L. (1865). *Alice's adventures in wonderland.* New York: Penguin Putnam.

Institute of Medicine. (1999). To err is human: Building a safer health system. Available at: http:www.iom.edu/report.asp?id=5575.

Kotter, J. P. (1995). Leading change: Why transformation efforts fail. *Harvard Business Review, 73*(2), 59–67.

Kotter, J. P. (1996). *Leading change.* Boston, MA: Harvard Business School Press.

Lewin, K. (1947). Frontiers in group dynamics. *Human Relations, 1*(1), 5–41.

Lippitt, G. L. (1973). *Visualizing change: Model building and the change process.* La Jolla, CA: University Associates.

Roethlisberger, F. J. (1941). *Management and morale.* Cambridge, MA: Harvard University Press.

Senge, P. M. (1990). *The fifth discipline.* New York: Doubleday.

Wheelen, T. L., & Hunger, J. D. (1998). *Strategic management and business policy* (6th ed.). Upper Saddle River, NJ: Addison Wesley.

OTHER SUGGESTED READING

Burke, W. W. (1987). *Organization development: A normative view.* Upper Saddle River, NJ: Addison-Wesley.

Bardwick, J. M. (1991). *Danger in the comfort zone.* New York: AMACOM.

Lewin, K. (1951). Field theory in social science. New York: Harper & Row.

Mone, M. A., McKinley, W., & Barker, V. L. (1998). Organizational decline and innovation: A contingency framework. *Academy of Management Review, 23,* 115–132.

Riggio, R. E. (2003). *Industrial/organizational psychology* (4th ed.). Upper Saddle River, NJ: Prentice Hall.

Sheehy, G. (1991). *New passages: Mapping your life across time.* New York: Random House.

Tomasko, R. M. (1987). *Downsizing.* New York: AMACOM.

Zand, D. E. (1995). Force field analysis. In N. Nicholson (Ed.), *Blackwell encyclopedic dictionary of organizational behavior.* Oxford: Blackwell.

Macrolevel—"The Organization"

Organization Theory and Design

Part VII includes four related topics. In Chapter 19, the history of organization theory is discussed, as is the importance of developing a learning organization. Chapter 20 describes the choices an organization makes that define how it relates to the external environment. The chapter examines the numerous issues associated with organizational strategy and how it relates to an entity's structure. Chapter 21 describes the contextual factors that a manager must consider relating to how the organization is structured to ensure that it can successfully interact with the environment. Chapter 22 discusses the internal characteristics of the organization that make up the structural dimension. The various elements within the structural dimension determine how the various parts of an organization will be organized for coordinating and controlling the entity's activities. What we learn from these four chapters is that organizational structures are a consequence of the simultaneous impact of multiple factors.

CHAPTER 19

Overview and History of Organizational Theory

Nancy Borkowski, DBA, CPA, FACHE

LEARNING OUTCOMES

After completing this chapter, the student should understand:

- ☛ The definition of organization theory.
- ☛ The definition of an organization.
- ☛ The components of an organization's formal structure.
- ☛ The factors that determine the stability and uncertainty of an organization's environment.
- ☛ The importance of the classic management theorists regarding the development of organization theory.
- ☛ The difference between closed and open systems.
- ☛ What is meant by the term "learning organization."

OVERVIEW

> Our society has become a society of organizations. Most social tasks are being done in and by organizations, and most public goals are achieved through them (Drucker, 1998).

Organization theory (OT) is commonly referred to as the study of the behavior and nature of organizations in their environments. Although OT emerged from the disciplines of sociology, economics, political science, and psychology, similar to organizational behavior (OB), its focus is the organization as a whole. In other words, OT relates to the macro-level versus the micro-level focus of OB—the study of individual and/or group behaviors in the workplace.

An organization may be defined as a collection of people working together (i.e., social entity) under a defined structure to achieve predetermined outcomes through coordinated activities (i.e., processes). Organization theory addresses the many issues associated with an organization's design and structure. Organization design may be viewed as the formal arrangement of departments, divisions, functions, and people interacting and linked together within an entity. As such, the concept of organization design is the process of creating the structure and developing the relationships to accomplish an organization's goals (Kast & Rosenzweig, 1985). Structure is the result of the design process, which is reflected by the clustering of these various departments, divisions, and so forth, to coordinate and control activities (and people) to achieve the organization's goals. Kast and Rosenzweig (1985, p. 234) defines an organization's formal structure as:

1. The pattern of formal relationships and duties—the organization chart plus job descriptions.
2. The way in which the various activities or tasks are assigned to different departments and/or people in the organization (differentiation).
3. The way in which these separate activities or tasks are coordinated (integration).
4. The power, status, and hierarchical relationships within the organization (authority system).
5. The planned and formalized policies, procedures, and controls that guide the activities and relationships of people in the organization (administrative system).

The formal structure of a company is reflected by its organization chart, which reveals the complexity of the organization. The complexity of an organization's structure is related to many factors. For example, the more differentiated and diverse the activities of the organization are, the more integration is required, resulting in a more complex structure. Factors affecting an organization's structure would be its size, technology, and strategies, all of which will be discussed in the following chapters.

One factor that greatly affects an organization's structure is its environment. As described in Chapter 18, organizations function within different environments. For example, the external/social environment indirectly affects all organizations. This includes sociocultural, political/legal, economic, and technological forces. The industry/task environment is more specific and includes those forces that an organization must continuously interact with and that directly affect the company's ability to achieve its predetermined outcomes (i.e., goals). These forces include suppliers, customers, and competitors. The number of forces an organization needs to deal with on a regular basis, how diverse these forces are, and how rapidly these forces are changing affect the stability or uncertainty of the organization's environment. The stability and certainty of the organization's environment have an impact on its structure. Burns and Stalker (1961) related that:

> Different types of organizational structure are suitable for particular environmental conditions. An organization with well-defined tasks and a rigidly hierarchical system of decision-making [*mechanistic* structure] is argued to be appropriate for stable environmental conditions. Where the environment is changing, an *organic* form of organizational structure is deemed more appropriate, in which tasks are flexibly defined and participants cooperate on the basis of expertise and not hierarchical positions.

Later in this chapter and in the following chapters, we will discuss how various factors affect an organization's structure, but first we will provide a brief overview of the history of OT so managers can develop a better understanding of why certain organizations select specific structures to achieve their goals.

HISTORY OF ORGANIZATION THEORY

The historical roots of OT can be found in the concepts developed during the Industrial Revolution in the late nineteenth and early twentieth centuries. It was during this period that Max Weber (1864–1920), a German sociologist considered to be the founding father of OT, developed a framework of administrative characteristics that allowed large organizations to play a positive role in the larger society by being "rational" and efficient.

Weber (1947) viewed an organization as a closed system (i.e., autonomous and isolated from environment forces) with rules and procedures enforced by an individual with rational/legal authority. Weber believed that manager/subordinate relationships should be impersonal with no reference to personal preferences, thereby ensuring that the manager did not permit emotional attachments or personalities to interfere with rational organizational decisions (Longest, Rakich, & Darr, 2000).

The six key administrative characteristics of Weber's rational and efficient organization, which is referred to as a bureaucratic organizational structure, are:

1. *Hierarchy of Authority:* To ensure clear communication of supervision and subordination positions (i.e., designations).

2. *Hiring (and promoting) of Technically Qualified Workers:* To ensure that hiring and promotions are based on merit rather than favoritism and that those hired view their positions as full-time, primary careers.

3. *Consistent System of Rules:* To ensure consistent and effective pursuit of organizational goals.

4. *Extensive Use of Written Documents:* To ensure that decisions are made and communicated through written rules and records.

5. *Functional Specialization and Division of Duties:* To ensure efficient operations, with each worker carrying out specific tasks and duties based on his or her skill and training.

6. *Separate Position from Worker:* To ensure that individual workers did not have "rights" to any aspect of his or her position, thereby eliminating the ability to pass the position on to friends or family once their contract ends.

Weber's rational bureaucracy model dominated social science thinking about organizations until World War II. It was at this time that others began to criticize Weber's ideas because his model ignored much of what really happens in organizations—conflicts, work-arounds, and informal leadership. The major issue, according to Selznick (1948 and 1957), was that "bureaucracies" were not and should not act like machines because they consisted of human beings and people will not imitate machines. In general, bureaucratic organizations are viewed as inefficient because of their functional design and slow decision-making capabilities. This generalization is erroneous. As previously noted by Burns and Stalker (1961), bureaucratic-type structures are suited for organizations in stable environments with routine tasks. However, according to Burns and Stalker, bureaucratic-type structures are not suited for organizations operating in industries with unstable environments and nonroutine tasks, for example, companies operating in the healthcare industry!

Another individual who had a major impact on OT was Henri Fayol (1841–1925), a French industrialist. Fayol (1949) developed a "set of rules" for managers to follow to be successful. His set of rules consisted of three parts: (1) activities of management, (2) principles of management, and (3) elements of management.

On the basis of his management/administrative experiences, Fayol argued that all activities within organizations could be divided into six main groups:

1. Technical (production, manufacturing, adaptation);
2. Commercial (buying, selling, exchange);
3. Financial (search for and optimum use of capital);
4. Security (protection of property and persons);
5. Accounting (stocktaking, balance sheet, statistics, costs);
6. Managerial (planning, organization, command, coordination, control).

According to Fayol, the six groups of activities are interdependent and it is the role of management to ensure that all six activities work smoothly to achieve the organization's goals.

The second part of Fayol's "set of rules" is the 14 principles of management. Although Fayol described these principles as flexible and adaptable, rather than rigid and absolute, he did stress that adherence to the principles by managers will contribute to a more effective organization (Miner, 2002). Fayol's principles of management are listed in Table 19–1, with division of work (specialization), unity of command, and scalar chain being the most important.

The third part of Fayol's "set of rules" is elements of management, which is composed of five activities. Fayol saw a manager's responsibilities as:

1. Planning
2. Organizing
3. Commanding
4. Coordinating
5. Controlling

As described in Table 19–2, these activities are more task- versus people-oriented (see Chapter 9, Behavioral Theories of Leadership). Although developed almost a century ago, Fayol's elements of management provide a useful framework for understanding the nature of managerial work and continues to be widely used in management training (Miner, 2002).

The third classic management theorist we will discuss is Frederick Taylor (1856–1915). As described in Chapter 1, Taylor (1911) developed the well-known framework of scientific management. On the basis of his work experiences, Taylor was primarily concerned with management of production workers to achieve maximum efficiency. Taylor's four basic principles of management were:

1. Develop a science for the work of each person. This involves determining how the work can best be performed by experimenting with it, conducting time-and-motion studies, and often applying mathematical formulas.

Table 19–1 Fayol's 14 Principles of Management

Principle	Description
Division of work	Division of labor or specialization limits the activities or tasks that attention must be given to by the worker and therefore allows for increased quality and quantity of output for the same amount of overall effort.
Authority and responsibility	Managers should exercise authority, both as it derives from the office held and as it derives from the intelligence, experience, and other personal qualities of the manager. In addition, responsibility must be commensurate with authority.
Discipline	Discipline is a condition for effective operation of a business. It consists of obedience, application, energy, behavior, and respect, all given on the basis of some formal or informal employment contract between the individual and the firm. To function as it should, discipline requires good managers, clear and equitable agreements, and the judicious application of sanctions such as warnings, fines, suspensions, and other, similar disciplinary actions.
Unity of command	An individual should receive orders with regard to a particular action from one supervisor only. Dual command is to be avoided.
Unity of direction	Unity of direction applies to coordination of effort and is a principle of organizations. A group of activities having the same objective should be placed under a single manager with a single plan.
Subordination of individual interests to general interest	For effective functioning, the interests of the organization as a whole must take precedence over those of individuals or groups. Subordination of interests is one basis for reconciling conflicting interests. In some instances, interests of a different order appear to have equal claims. Such conflicts must be reconciled rather than being permitted to continue. Possible means to this end are the firmness and good example of managers, fair agreements, and constant supervision.
Remuneration of personnel	Payments should be fair and equitable, should reward well-directed effort, and should not exceed reasonable limits.
Centralization	The amount of centralization, as opposed to decentralization, should be optimal for the particular concern. Contingency factors are firm size, personal character of the manager, manager's moral worth, reliability of subordinates, and conditions of business. The degree of centralization may vary considerably, depending on the relative potential effectiveness of the manager or subordinate.
Scalar chain	The line of authority from top management to the lowest ranks represents the scalar chain. Communication should occur up and down the scalar chain of authority. However, if following the chain creates delays, cross-communications can be allowed if agreed to by all parties and superiors are kept informed (Fayol referred to this as gangplank/horizontal communication).

(Continued)

Table 19–1 Fayol's 14 Principles of Management *(Continued)*

Principle	Description
Order	To avoid loss of material, there should be a place for everything and everything in its place. In addition, the prescribed place should be one that facilitates the carrying out of necessary activities. The principle of order applies not only to material things, but also to people. Thus there should be an appointed place for each employee, and each employee should be in that place with the appointed place appropriate to the task to be performed. This principle means good organization and selection, and it implies the existence of an organization chart.
Equity	Employees should be treated with kindness and justice, which together equal equity. The object is to elicit devotion and loyalty in return. Ideally, a sense of equity will permeate the whole scalar chain.
Stability of tenure of personnel	Employees and managers alike need time to settle into their jobs before they can achieve maximum performance (Fayol viewed high employee turnover as inefficient). Therefore, management should provide for job security and personnel planning. Stability of tenure promotes loyalty to the organization, its purposes, and values.
Initiative	Initiative is thinking out a plan and executing it, as well as having the freedom to do these things. Initiative of this kind should be encouraged; it is particularly valuable to an organization in difficult times. The manager who facilitates the initiative of subordinates is far superior to the manager who does not, because initiative can serve as a source of both satisfaction and motivation.
Esprit de corps	Essentially, this is a principle of unity. Harmony should be fostered and conflict minimized. Unity of command is one means to this end. Creating dissension among one's subordinates thwarts coordination and teamwork (e.g., Fayol was opposed to the divide-and-conquer technique). Verbal communication should be used whenever possible because, being two-way, it permits rapid resolution of conflicts. Written communication often fosters conflict.

SOURCE: *Organizational behavior: foundations, theories and analysis* (pp. 65–67), by J. B. Miner, 2002. New York: Oxford University Press. Reprinted with permission.

Table 19–2 Fayol's Five Elements of Management

Element	Description
Planning	Planning involves foresight, that is, assessing the future and making provisions for it. It requires the development of a plan of action based on contributions from throughout the business.
Organizing	The human organization is established to carry out managerial functions and implement the principles of management. Organizing involves developing an organizational structure and allocating human resources to ensure the accomplishment of objectives. Evaluation, especially of managerial personnel, is also part of the organizing function. Among the factors to be considered are health and physical fitness, intelligence, moral qualities, general education, management knowledge, knowledge of the other functions (technical, commercial, etc.), and specialized ability characteristic of the concern. Only the last requirement varies from one business to another; thus, managerial capabilities are highly transferable.
Command	Command activates the organization structure. It involves knowing the personnel thoroughly and eliminating incompetents; being knowledgeable about employer-employee agreements; setting a good example; conducting periodic organization audits; setting up conferences among one's chief assistants to establish unity of direction; avoiding an excess of detail; and generally fostering unity, energy, initiative, and loyalty.
Coordination	The function of coordination is to harmonize the various activities of an organization into a single whole. Basically, it is a matter of establishing rightful proportions for the parts, ensuring that these proportions are maintained, and adapting means to ends. Under such conditions, the various departments work in harmony with one another, communicating as needed, rather than operating in isolation as ends in themselves. The component units know their role in total effort and what interdependencies exist with other units. Departmental scheduling is constantly fine-tuned to external circumstances, rather than carried out without reference to organizational goals, loyalties, and needs for initiative. The prime method of achieving coordination is a periodic conference of department heads. Where this is physically not possible, an alternative is to use the liaison officers attached to the staff to coordinate departments. In either case, the need to facilitate horizontal communication is clearly evident.
Control	Control is the process of checking the realities of operations against plans and taking steps to correct deviations. It assumes the existence of up-to-date plans and the use of sanctions to achieve compatibility with them in a timely manner. Fayol notes that, if they are not devised correctly and monitored effectively, control systems may create duality of management. To the extent inspection is inherent in the control system, it should be impartial and objective.

Source: *Organizational behavior: foundations, theories and analysis* (p. 68), by J. B. Miner, 2002. New York: Oxford University Press. Reprinted with permission.

2. Scientifically select the best individual for the job, train that person to be able to perform the job better, and pay higher wages than ever before to reward the increased productivity.

3. Cooperate with the workers to ensure that the work is, in fact, done in the prescribed manner; make knowledge of the job (principle 1) and the worker selected (principle 2) come together. This should include, but not limited to, providing for increased earnings for those who follow the prescribed methods most closely.

4. Divide the work so that activities such as planning, organizing, and controlling are the responsibility of management; the worker, in contrast, has the responsibility for doing. This division is predicated on the assumption that most workers do not have the capability to create the science of their work.

Taylor believed that organizational efficiency was achieved by creating jobs that economized time, human energy, and other productive resources. As such, Taylor placed a strong emphasis on the exception principle. By establishing output standards, managers would only need to give their attention to those workers whose established standards were not met (or exceeded). Although Taylor preferred that managers dealt with one worker at a time, he was aware that group influences might produce changes in output (Miner, 2002). (See discussion of group norms in Chapter 14.)

The classic theories were well suited for the Industrial Age to create large, efficient organizations, but the "people" and "environment" components were missing. Although the human relations/behavioral management movement started to emerge in the 1920s as a result of the Hawthorne Studies (see Chapter 1), the bureaucratic approaches remained the primary focus for OT until the late 1970s and early 1980s. It was at this time that new directions for OT appeared in the literature; these theories emphasized that organizations were open systems interacting with and dependent upon unstable environments. Over the past 25 years, much research has been disseminated regarding the need for organizations to be flexible and adaptable in order to acquire the necessary resources to meet the needs of their changing environments. This is referred to as open-systems theory.

Open-systems Theory

Katz and Kahn (1978) developed a framework for open-systems theory that encompasses four phases: (1) inputs into the organizations, (2) the transformation of those inputs within the system, (3) outputs, and (4) recycling (see Figure 19–1). As previously noted, an organization is a group of people working together under a defined structure for the purpose of achieving stated goals through coordinated activities. These activities require the use of human, material, and financial resources. An organizations must be able to obtain the necessary input resources (i.e., employees, materials/supplies, capital, etc.) from its environment and efficiently transform the resources to outputs (i.e., goals). It is these outputs that provides for another external

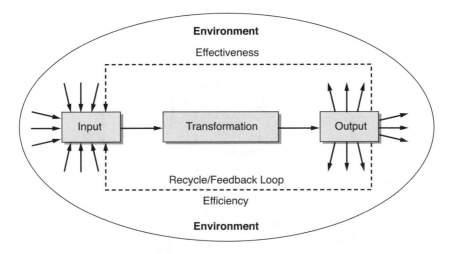

Figure 19–1

resource (i.e., dollars) so that the organization can again acquire the required input resources.

Organizations need to create more outputs than they consume. In addition, the organization must produce outputs that are needed and valued by purchasers (i.e., external environment). In other words, an organization needs to be both efficient and effective to survive. To achieve these results, an organization must be able to effectively interact with its environments (see Figure 19–2). An open-system organization is not passive. It needs to reach out and attempt to influence its environment, but at the same time the organization will be influenced by its environment. If the company's environment is stable, the organization can place more emphasis on efficiency (bureaucratic approach). When the environment is unstable, the company must emphasize both efficiency and effectiveness.

Today's healthcare environment is anything but stable. As reflected in Figure 19–2, a healthcare organization must interact with both the general and industry environments, in addition to numerous stakeholders with conflicting demands. For example, hospitals must accommodate demands for charity care while balancing criticism of cost shifting, for high-quality care while experiencing severe nurse shortages, and for providing jobs and decent wages with declining profit margins due to lower reimbursements from payors (Arndt, Bigelow, & Dorman, 1999).

On an annual basis, the American College of Healthcare Executives (ACHE) surveys hospital CEOs regarding the three most pressing issues affecting their hospitals to identify specific areas of concern. As reflected in Exhibit 19–1, financial issues remained the uppermost concern for hospital CEOs in 2007, with concerns related to quality and patient safety gaining prominence.

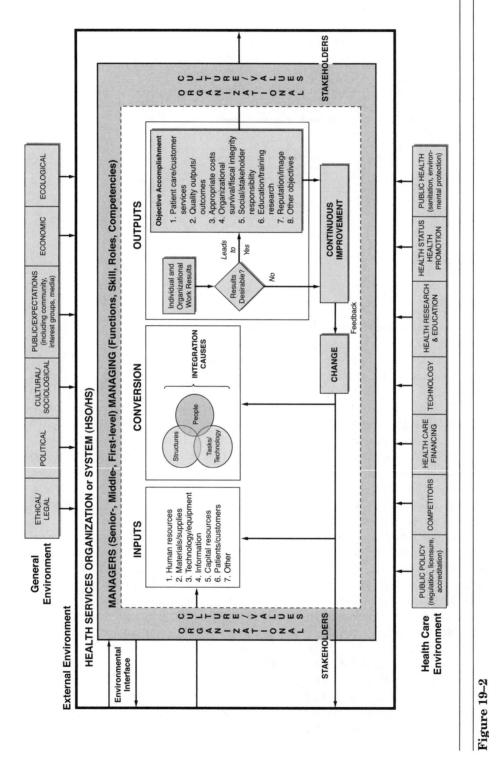

Figure 19–2

SOURCE: *Managing health services organizations and systems* (4th ed.) by B. B. Longest, J. S. Rakich, and K. Darr (2000). Baltimore, MD: Health Professions Press. Reprinted with permission.

Exhibit 19–1 Top Issues Confronting Hospitals

I. Top Issues Confronting Hospitals

Each of the issues in the following table is listed by the percentage of hospital CEO respondents who indicated it as one of the top three issues confronting their hospital.

Issue	2005 (%)	2006 (%)	2007 (%)
Financial challenges	67	72	70
Care for the uninsured	35	37	38
Physician/hospital relations	33	40	35
Quality	23	29	33
Personnel shortages	36	30	30
Patient safety	20	27	29
Governmental mandates	16	23	22
Patient satisfaction	18	16	17
Capacity	17	11	11

II. Specific Concerns Within the Top Issues

Within each of their three top issues, respondents identified specific concerns facing their hospital. Following are those concerns in order of importance for the top three issues identified in the survey.

Financial Challenges

Increasing costs for staff, supplies, etc.	74%
Medicaid	74%
Bad debt	73%
Medicare	71%
Inadequate funding for capital improvements	62%
Managed care payments	48%
Revenue cycle management	38%
Emergency Department	37%
Other commercial insurance	25%

Care for the Uninsured

Medicaid	82%
Underwriting costs	82%
Advocacy for funding	71%
Reaching out to all community members	28%
Response to other hospital closings	15%

Physician/Hospital Relations

Creating win-win collaborations	86%
Physician requests for payment for service to the hospital	83%
Competition with physician-owned facilities/equipment	77%
Medical staff structures/leadership	59%
Niche providers	53%

SOURCE: *Top Issues Confronting Hospitals*, 2007. Chicago, IL: American College of Healthcare Executives. Reprinted with permission.

According to Thomas C. Dolan, president and CEO of ACHE, "Creating, implementing and monitoring the systems to improve quality and patient safety have become a major focus of hospital CEOs. No longer treated as a delegated responsibility solely for clinicians, the entire hospital team—senior management, physician leaders and the board—are now actively working together to improve care." ACHE's annual survey results and Mr. Dolan's statement reflect the fact that healthcare organizations are complex and always changing because of their relationships with the many parts or constituents of the system. As such, healthcare managers must be flexible and willing to learn new things by consistently questioning the status quo. But this goal has been difficult to achieve in the past! As noted by Donald Berwick (2002), CEO of the Institute for Healthcare Improvement and one of the architects of the Institute of Medicine's *Crossing the Quality Chasm* report, "the quality chasm in health care reflects one crucial deficit: deeply embedded incapacities—a learning disability—at the heart of the health care industry. This disability is historical, cultural, and structural" (2001, p. 301).

Managers in today's unstable and complex healthcare environment need to understand that what worked in the past may not work in the future. As Albert Einstein said, "We can't solve problems by using the same kind of thinking we used when we created them!" Therefore, organizations need to "learn." In a learning organization, problem solving is key, as opposed to the traditional organization designed for efficient performance (see Figure 19–3). Learning organizations "promote communication and collaboration so that everyone is engaged in identifying and solving problems, enabling the organization to continuously experiment, improve and increase its capability" (Daft, 2007, p. 29).

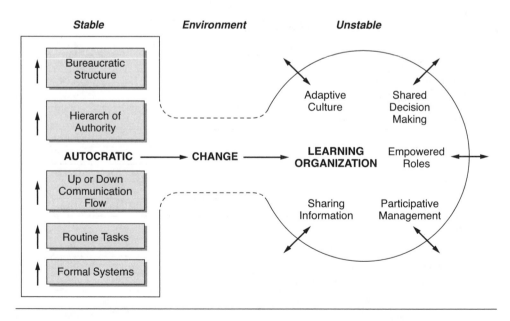

Figure 19–3

As noted previously, organizations are open systems that must interact with and be adaptable to the environment in order to survive. Over the past two decades, the rapid changes occurring in the healthcare industry have forced managers to reorient toward an open-system mindset and recognize that their organizations are part of a complex, interconnected whole (Daft, 2007). Open-systems theory assumes that all large organizations are made up of subsystems, each of which receives inputs from other subsystems and turns them into outputs for use by other subsystems of the organization (see Exhibit 19–2). The subsystems are interdependent and interrelated. The successful organizations must be able to achieve balance between their subsystems.

For example, the sales/marketing department of a national retail-based clinic company might grow very quickly as a result of patients' and insurers' need and want for efficient, cost-effective care for minor emergencies (versus going to hospitals' emergency departments). But if the human resources department of the organization is unable to keep pace with hiring qualified nurse practitioners to staff the miniclinics, the entire organization could break down. Thus, subsystems within an organization must maintain a state of balance as the organization adapts to environmental influences.

Exhibit 19–2 Subsystems of an Open-System

> Five subsystems were identified by Katz and Kahn (1978) as being important to the success of all organizations. Each of these subsystems may also be made up of subsystems.
>
> *Production subsystems* are the components that transform inputs into outputs. In most business organizations, all other subsystems are built around the production subsystem. In a hospital, for example, this subsystem would include the nursing, medical staff, pharmacy, and radiology departments.
>
> *Maintenance subsystems* maintain the social involvement of employees in an organization. Activities in this group include providing benefits and compensations that motivate workers, creating favorable work conditions, empowering employees, and fulfilling other employee needs.
>
> *Adaptive subsystems* serve to gather information about threats and opportunities in the environment and then respond with innovations that allow the organization to adapt to these conditions. For example, each section of a pharmaceutical company's research and development division would be part of an adaptive subsystem.
>
> *Supportive subsystems* perform acquisition and distribution functions within an organization. Acquisition activities include securing resources, such as employees and supplies from the external environment (i.e., human resources and purchasing departments). Supportive subsystems would also include those activities and efforts to transfer the product or service outside of the organization. For example, a hospital's supportive subsystems would include the medical records and patient billing departments.
>
> *Managerial subsystems* direct the activities of other subsystems in the organization. These managerial functions set goals and policies, allocate resources, resolve conflicts, and generally work to facilitate the efficiency of the organization.
>
> ---
>
> SOURCE: *The Social Psychology of Organizations*, by D. Katz and R. Kahn, 1978. New York: John Wiley & Sons. Reprinted with permission.

SUMMARY

This chapter provided an overview of organization theory and its historical roots based on the works of Max Weber, Henri Fayol, and Frederick Taylor. Since the Industrial Revolution, a wealth of information has emerged with the study of OT. We have abandoned Weber's original concept that organizations are closed-system and developed an understanding that organizations are part of a complex, interconnected whole. Organizations are open systems that must interact with and be adaptable to the environment in order to survive. The learning organization attempts to effectively interact with its environment by promoting communication and collaboration throughout the entity's subsystems. Communication and collaboration are achieved through the organization's design and structure. Organization design may be viewed as the formal arrangement of departments, divisions, functions, and people interacting and linked together within an entity, and structure is the result of the design process. The organization's structure is reflected by the clustering of these various departments, divisions, and so forth, to coordinate and control activities (and people) to achieve the organization's goals.

In the following chapters, we will explore the various elements within what is referred to as the structural and contextual dimensions. These two dimensions assist managers to better understand the components relating to the structure and design of organizations (and their subsystems) to achieve high performance.

We will begin our discussions with an overview of organizational strategy. It is only after an organization has developed its vision, mission, and objectives that it can be structured and designed to achieve these goals efficiently.

END-OF-CHAPTER DISCUSSION QUESTIONS

1. Define OT.
2. Define an organization.
3. Describe the components of an organization's formal structure.
4. Describe the factors that determine the stability and uncertainty of an organization's environment.
5. Explain the importance of the classic management theorists with regard to the development of OT.
6. Describe the difference between closed and open systems.
7. Describe what is meant by the term "learning organization."

END-OF-CHAPTER CASE EXERCISE

Visit the Web site of the Institute of Healthcare Improvements (IHI), a nonprofit organization dedicated to improving the quality of healthcare systems through education, research, and demonstration projects (www.ihi.org/ihi). Break into small groups, view the information found under Improvement Stories and Success Headlines, and discuss the achievements of selected health service organizations (HSOs) working to improve patient care.

- How are these HSOs demonstrating that they are "learning" organizations?
- How are they similar or dissimilar to your organization?

END-OF-CHAPTER CASE STUDY

Case Study 19–1   Merck: Is Merck's Medicine Working?

Richard Clark was flustered and unprepared when he was thrust into the CEO job at Merck & Co. on May 5, 2005. It was the darkest hour in the pharmaceutical giant's 114-year history. Merck was drowning in liability suits stemming from Vioxx, its arthritis drug whose total annual sales were $2.5 billion, which it had to pull from the market because of a link to heart attacks and strokes. Two other blockbusters worth a combined $7 billion in annual sales were facing patent expirations. And Merck's labs, which other companies once hailed as a bastion of scientific innovation, were crippled by a culture that buried good ideas under layers of bureaucracy. But in the morass, Clark saw opportunity. "A crisis is a terrible thing to waste," says the CEO.

The 35-year Merck veteran says he had "no clue" what his turnaround plan would be. What he did know: Getting back on track would take much more than a cosmetic restructuring or slash-and-burn layoffs. Clark had watched the company degenerate into a collection of fiefdoms more focused on advancing their own agendas than on getting the right drugs to patients. To revitalize drug development he would need to get Merck's 60,000 employees—scientists, regulatory staff, and salespeople—to work together.

Clark set out to blast open deeply blocked channels of communication. Over the years, Merck had fallen out of touch with customers. Clark wanted to get employees to stop thinking about their specific job functions and to instead focus on the diseases they were trying to conquer. So he began placing people in teams defined by therapeutic fields such as cancer and diabetes. He encouraged the teams to huddle with doctors who prescribe Merck's products, patients who take them, and even insurers that decide whether to pay for them. "It's a different way of doing business," says Clark, 61.

In essence, Clark turned Merck's drug development on its head. While he can't take credit for drugs that Merck discovered years ago, his disease-focused approach has pushed some products through Merck's pipeline at speeds that caught rivals by surprise. Januvia, a first-of-its-kind diabetes drug, hit the market in October, 2006, and HIV drug Isentress is on track to be approved by the Food & Drug Administration in October 2008.

It will be years before it becomes clear whether Clark's changes will produce a reliable stream of blockbuster drugs. Still, Wall Street has hope that there's a solid growth story at Merck, despite the Vioxx debacle. The company's stock has jumped 17% since January, outpacing the American Stock Exchange Pharmaceutical Index, which is up 4%. Analysts expect Merck's top line to grow 4%, to $23.5 billion this year, an achievement considering that sales growth had flatlined even before Vioxx imploded.

Different Dynamic

Virtually no one expected this from Clark. The low-key executive was promoted to CEO from a very unglamorous post at Merck: head of manufacturing. While Clark was well-known inside the company as a stickler for efficiency, outsiders feared he lacked the vision to restore Merck to its scientific glory days. "At the time we said: 'Who is he?'," recalls Morgan Stanley (MS) analyst Jami Rubin. The yawns grew wider when Clark announced plans to cut costs [$4 billion by 2009], a typical opening gambit by CEOs without grand plans. Then good news started flowing from Merck's labs, and Wall Street began to see that maybe something different was unfolding. "What's impressive is the speed with which he has galvanized an organization that was so depressed," Rubin says.

Uncertainty over the outcome of the Vioxx litigation casts a shadow over Clark's early progress, however. The company's strategy of fighting each suit separately is working so far: 10 out of 15 verdicts have gone its way. But Merck is still facing 27,250 Vioxx claims, and information expected to be released over coming weeks could bolster plaintiffs' claims against the company. Meanwhile, Vioxx has become a lightning rod in Congress, which has spent much of the summer debating tough new drug-safety legislation. Clark maintains Merck did nothing wrong in its handling of the product. Yet he acknowledges the sudden loss of the drug highlighted the company's need to find a more efficient way to fill its pipeline. "It really helped accelerate the change," he says.

Clark's struggle is emblematic of the difficult task facing all pharmaceutical CEOs. More than 70 big drugs will lose their patent protection by 2011, causing a collective loss of $100 billion in annual sales. The mapping of the human genome and advances that make it faster and easier to screen potential drug candidates should be lighting a fire under drug development, but they haven't so far. So pharmaceutical companies are grappling with new models. Pfizer Inc. is trying to become more inventive by looking outside and partnering with small biotechs. Johnson & Johnson—which has long maintained that the key to innovation is to preserve the independence of the companies it has acquired—has reconfigured its drug-development operations into three business units, so it can be more tightly focused. "We're all being challenged to rethink this," says Samuel O. Thier, a professor at Harvard Medical School and a Merck board member.

Despite the high-tech gloss on the pharmaceutical industry, most drug companies are still organized around an old industrial model. Typically a new product starts in research and is handed to manufacturing. Then sales comes up with a marketing plan. Finally, the drug gets passed down to regional managers around the world, who develop their own sales strategies. This hand-off model can lead to mistakes: Scientists might put years and millions of dollars into a drug, for example, only to find out that the audience is not as big as they imagined it to be. Worse, managers might not devote the necessary resources to the most promising ideas because they're blinded by the need to maximize their own units' profitability. Bringing disparate voices together from day one "is the way work should get done in companies," says Clark, drawing grids on a legal pad to make his point. "It's not up and down. You need people to work together."

Faster Path

One group of Merck employees was already experimenting with a disease-focused model before Clark became chief executive. They had come together to develop a diabetes drug that ultimately failed. But after hearing Clark talk about busting up the traditional approach to drug development, the team volunteered to pilot his new plan with Januvia, which was just about to go into pivotal clinical trials. They knew they had a potential blockbuster on their hands, because the drug offers a completely new way to attack diabetes. But rival Novartis was way ahead of Merck in testing a similar drug called Galvus.

In the past, Merck's science types might have spent years testing Januvia in combination with every other diabetes therapy patients might be taking so that the FDA would allow the drug to be pitched to the broadest possible audience. With advice from marketing colleagues, who were in tune with what diabetes patients and doctors were demanding, the diabetes group devised a faster path to victory: they decided that initially they would only test Januvia with the two most widely used diabetes drugs and as a solo therapy. "We didn't do studies that were nice to have," says Jay Galeota, general manager of the diabetes and obesity franchise. "We did studies that really represented where the product was most likely to be used."

Gathering input from customers such as doctors earlier in the process paid off in other ways. As Januvia moved along, reports emerged that Novartis' Galvus was causing some monkeys in the trials to suffer skin lesions. Conversations with doctors convinced Merck's diabetes team to design an extra monkey study to prove to the FDA that its drug was safe. The result: The agency approved Januvia without requiring a warning about the side effect. What's more, because there were manufacturing and marketing folks on the diabetes team who were constantly trading information about the approval time line and customer demand, Merck had Januvia on pharmacy shelves four days after the FDA gave it the green light. At the old Merck, it would have taken as long as a month to launch the product. Morgan's Rubin reckons Januvia and a related product will bring in $762 million in sales this year. Meanwhile, Galvus is still awaiting FDA approval.

Key Customer

Getting better products out faster is crucial, but paying attention to your biggest customer base—the insurance companies—is also important. Clark should know. He served as chief operating officer and then CEO of Merck's pharmacy benefit subsidiary, Medco, from 1997 to 2002, before it was spun out as an independent company. The experience drove home to him the immense power that insurance companies wield when they decide whether a new drug is worth paying for or whether it's not much different from older, cheaper alternatives.

Merck has always talked to insurers just before drugs hit the market, but Clark believes the discussion needs to start much earlier, when a new therapy is just an inkling in a scientist's brain. That way, Merck can be sure it is designing trials that directly answer payers' questions about safety and efficacy, especially in relation to what the comparative expense of a drug might be. "The value proposition has to be from the payer's perspective," Clark says. "If you don't listen to your customers you're going to wake up someday and not have them."

Mixing scientists with insurance executives is a little extreme. With the cost of drugs growing at double digits every year, payers come to the table with a built-in bias against new products, if not a little hostility. Yet Merck research and development chief Peter S. Kim has embraced the idea. Last September, for example, 200 Merck scientists went on a retreat. Along for the ride: a patient who suffers from rheumatoid arthritis and a top executive from insurer Aetna Inc.

The patient described her travails with steroids, which treat her disease effectively but also touch off side effects such as bloating. Merck is working on nonsteroid treatments with minimal side effects. Aetna suggested Merck look for clues to predict which patients respond best to which therapies. Tailoring the drug to the right audience would not only result in better outcomes for patients but also save insurers money in the long run. "As we figure out how to reinvent ourselves, understanding different perspectives is going to be a critical piece of the puzzle," says Kim, who joined Merck in 2001 from the Massachusetts Institute of Technology.

Kill Fee

If fraternizing with insurance executives sounds bizarre, consider this: Merck is rewarding scientists for failure. One of the hardest decisions any scientist has to make is when to abandon an experimental drug that's not working. An inability to admit failure leads to inefficiencies. A scientist may spend months and tens of thousands of dollars studying a compound, hoping for a result he or she knows probably won't come, rather than pitching in on a project with a better chance of turning into a viable drug. So Kim is promising stock options to scientists who bail out on losing projects. It's not the loss per se that's being rewarded but the decision to accept failure and move on. "You can't change the truth. You can only delay how long it takes to find it out," Kim says. "If you're a good scientist, you want to spend your time and the company's money on something that's going to lead to success."

Management consultants say rewarding misses as well as hits is the right idea, and one that the entire industry will need to adopt. "The earlier you determine when something should be killed, the better," says Charlie Beaver, vice-president at consultant Booz Allen Hamilton Inc. Still, he warns, changing a corporate culture from one that thrives on success to one that also accepts failure "is a very large hurdle to overcome."

While Clark is encouraged by the results of his changes so far, he's still haunted by the culture of complacency that left companies like his stuck in an innovation rut. "If you ever feel comfortable that your model is the right model, you end up where the industry is today," he says. "It's always going to be continuous improvement. We will never declare victory."

Discuss how Richard Clark, CEO of Merck & Co., is attempting to change the company into a learning organization. What were the driver(s) of this change? What were the environmental forces?

SOURCE: "Is Merck's medicine working?" by A. Weintraub, July 30, 2007. *BusinessWeek*, pp. 67–68, 70. Reprinted with permission.

REFERENCES

Arndt, M., Bigelow, B., & Dorman, H. G. (1999). In their own words: How hospitals present corporate restructuring in their annual reports. *Journal of Healthcare Management, 44*(2), 117–132.

Berwick, D. (2002). Quality chasm factors. *Health Affairs,* 21(5)1, 301–302.

Burns, T., & Stalker, G. M. (1961). *The management of innovation.* London: Tavistock.

Daft, R. L. (2007). *Organization theory and design* (9th ed.). Mason, OH: Thomson Southwestern.

Drucker, P. (1998). *Peter Drucker on the profession of management.* Boston, MA: Harvard Business School Press.

Fayol, H. (1949). *General and industrial management.* London: Pitman.

Institute of Medicine (2001). *Crossing the quality chasm: A new health system for the 21st century.* Available at: www.nap.edu/books/0309072808/html/.

Kast, F. E., & Rosenzweig, J. E. (1985). *Organization and management: A systems and contingency approach.* New York: McGraw-Hill Book Company.

Katz, D., & Kahn, R. (1978). *The social psychology of organizations.* New York: John Wiley & Sons.

Longest, B. B., Rakich, J. S., & Darr, K. (2000). *Managing health services organizations and systems* (4th ed.). Baltimore, MD: Health Professions Press.

Miner, J. B. (2002). *Organizational behavior: Foundations, theories and analysis.* New York: Oxford University Press.

Selznick, P. (1948). Foundations of the theory of organizations. *American Sociological Review, 13*(1), 25–35.

Selznick, P. (1957). *Leadership in administration: A sociological interpretation.* Evanston, IL: Row, Peterson.

Taylor, F. W. (1911). *The principles of scientific management.* New York: Harper and Brothers.

Weber, M. (1947). *The theory of social and economic organizations* (A. M. Henerson & T. Parsons, Trans.). New York: Free Press.

OTHER SUGGESTED READINGS

Chuang, Y., Giinsberg, L., & Berta, W. B. (2007). Learning from preventable adverse events in health care organizations: Development of a multilevel model of learning and propositions. *Health Care Management Review, 32*(4), 330–340.

Cunningham Wood, J., & Wood, M. C. (2002). *Henri Fayol: Critical evaluation in business and management.* New York: Routledge.

Fells, M. J. (2000). Fayol stands the test of time. *Journal of Management History, 6*(8), 345–360.

Lawler, E. E., & Worley, C. (2006). *Built to change: How to achieve sustained organizational effectiveness.* Willowbrook, IL: Jossey-Bass/John Wiley & Sons.

March, J. G., & Simon, H. A. (1958). *Organizations.* New York: John Wiley & Sons.

Society for Healthcare Strategy and Market Development of the American Hospital Association (2005). *Futurescan: Healthcare trends and implications 2005–2010.* Chicago, IL: Health Administrative Press.

CHAPTER 20

Strategy and Structure

Raymond S. Kulzick, DBA, CPA, CFE, FCPA

LEARNING OUTCOMES

After completing this chapter, the student should understand:

- ☛ The definition of organizational strategy.
- ☛ The role of the different levels of management in the strategic process.
- ☛ The three levels of strategy.
- ☛ The overall process of strategic planning, and the content and purposes of each step in the process.
- ☛ The relationship of structure and culture to the strategic planning process.
- ☛ The Miles and Snow organizational types and their environment–strategy–structure/process relationships.

OVERVIEW

Organizational strategy deals with the choices the organization makes that define how it relates, as a whole, to the external environment. Since the environment is in a constant state of change, strategy is an ongoing and continual process. However, effective strategy is not reactive to change after it occurs, but proactive in anticipating the need for change, planning appropriate change, and implementing that change consistently. Similar to structure, strategic choices are long term in nature and difficult to adjust effectively in the short term.

An understanding of strategy is critical to an organization achieving superior results in the long term. Selection and effective implementation of appropriate strategies are of even greater importance for healthcare organizations, as they operate in an industry that is subject to greater levels of stress, change, external threats, and pressures than organizations in more stable industries.

STRATEGY

Organizational strategy is both a process and a mind-set or way of viewing the environment. From a process standpoint, strategy is an integrated approach, including assessing the organization and its environment, developing and selecting long-term organizational direction, and implementing those strategies that will lead to accomplishing the organization's vision and objectives. The strategic process, however, also requires an executive mind-set that the organization can and will choose its own direction and be successful in achieving its own vision. The ideal strategic environment combines an appropriate executive mind-set with an effective strategic process.

By definition, strategy provides the means to accomplish the vision, mission, and objectives for the total organization. This focus on the organization as a whole, rather than individual units or parts of the organization, is a defining element of strategy. The other defining element of strategy is an external focus—a view that the organization does not stand alone, but is a part of and dependent on a wider outside environment. Understanding and planning appropriate responses to changes in this mostly uncontrollable environment is a key part of the strategic planning process.

In describing the process later in this chapter, strategy may seem to be just a series of sequential steps. In some organizations, it may be nothing more than that. But, to be effective, strategy needs to be an ongoing process; a continual cycle formulated and implemented at all levels within the organization. Strategy that is ingrained and integrated into day-to-day management is successful strategy. Strategy that is a set of books, no matter how well written, is a failed strategy.

An organization's structure and culture are among the most important long-term factors in the organization's accomplishment of its vision and mission. An appropriate match between the overall organization's direction, its chosen competitive strategies, and its structure and culture greatly increases its chances of long-term success.

Governance

Strategy is an essential part of the organizational governance process. Healthcare organizations may be for-profit, not-for-profit, or governmental entities. In all cases, an effective governance process is the key to ensuring that the aims of those providing long-term capital resources to the entity (respectively, stockholders, charitable organizations, and legislative bodies) are actually accomplished. An oversight body (such as a board) is established for the organization with primary responsibility to the stockholders or other providers of long-term capital.

In exercising their responsibility for oversight, they must consider both the long-term and short-term directions of the organization. The strategic planning process provides three key documents to the Board, through which they exercise control over the direction of the enterprise. These are the strategic plan, the medium-term plan (sometimes called a five-year plan), and the budget. By reviewing and approving these documents, the Board indicates its agreement with management's proposals for the future direction of the organization.

Management

Although executive management and the Board are ultimately responsible for determining strategy and accountable for its accomplishment, that does not mean that strategy should be a "one-person show." Development and implementation of effective strategy need the input and cooperation of all levels of management. The communication and coordination components of strategy are just as important as the content developed during the process. For this reason, operating managers, not staff personnel, should develop all plans and strategies.

During the assessment stage, management should seek wide participation to perform a thorough assessment. It is equally important that management actively seek input in the external and competitive assessments as during the internal analysis. The best strategic ideas, environmental perceptions, and competitive insights often come from middle- and lower-level managers who have closer contact with the organization's customers, vendors, and other external stakeholders.

Although input and feedback may be present at all stages, it is during the strategy development phase that the responsibility for the earlier stages (values, vision, and mission) is with executive management. This gradually expands to include more divisional management during the objectives and strategies stages. During the implementation phase, participation expands further from the divisional and higher functional levels in the medium-term plan to all levels of management by the annual objectives and budget stages. Finally, strategic evaluation is the responsibility of executive management.

THREE LEVELS OF STRATEGY

There are three interrelated levels of strategy, according to Hofer and Schendel (1978). The strategy-setting process addresses these sequentially. An understanding of the various levels of strategy can be helpful in understanding the strategic process and an individual manager's role within that process.

Level 1: Corporate Strategy: Corporate-level strategy answers the questions of what businesses the organization is in and what is the emphasis between those different businesses. As an example, a large healthcare enterprise may compete in both hospitals and walk-in clinics within Florida. The corporate office decides on these businesses and their scope, and then decides how much of the organization's limited resources to allocate to each.

Level 2: Business Strategy: Once the corporate strategy has defined the business and level of resource availability, business strategy is developed to define how the organization will compete within the defined business, given the resources the organization has been allocated. In our example, if the walk-in clinic division of the healthcare company has been assigned high growth objectives and relatively modest resource allocations, management may develop a business strategy of partnering with other businesses (such as a grocery or drugstore chain) rather than adopting a stand-alone facility strategy.

Level 3: Functional Strategy: After determining the corporate and business strategies, attention is directed toward creating effective and consistent functional strategies. Almost all implementation of strategy is accomplished at the functional level, as most organizations use a functional structure at some level (sometimes at the highest level and sometimes at lower, decentralized, levels). For those organizations having no functional structure at all, the lower units (such as teams or networks) still must have functioning strategies to guide them in carrying out the overall organizational strategies.

Within individual functions (such as operations or finance), numerous choices occur as to which functional strategy to implement (or whether the existing functional strategy requires change). In our example, the accounting functional strategy choice may be whether the hospital chain will do billing and collections from individual hospitals or from the corporate location.

These functional strategy choices repeat themselves throughout the organization. Consistent functional strategies that fully support the organization's chosen business strategy, lead to the targeted level of efficiency and effectiveness, and build on the organization's strengths are key to the successful implementation of the organization's corporate and business strategies.

The Strategy Process: Assessment

The strategic planning process contains four parts: strategic assessment, developing strategy, implementing strategy, and evaluating strategy. These four parts are highly interrelated and include several steps (see Figure 20–1). Since the typical cycle for the process is annually, all steps should be documented in writing, for clarity and future evaluation, as well as for efficiency in repeating the process the following year.

Values

The process begins with an assessment of the owner's values. This is accomplished through the organizational governance process. In an owner-managed business, this is a direct process of the owner–managers clearly stating their personal values related to the organization. In a larger organization or a not-for-profit or legislative-controlled entity, there are several steps. First, the "owners" select a Board of Directors (or Board of Trustees or similar body) that represents their values. The Board, in turn, appoints a top management team that reflects the owners' values. Much has been written recently about the governance process and the responsibilities of the Board to represent the owners' interests.

Values are personal in nature, but reflected in the values of the organization. These can be such things as a commitment to service to the community or a desire to deliver high financial returns to owners. A clear statement of these values is an essential first step in the strategic planning process. Decisions and trade-offs that are made at all other steps of determining and implementing strategy require consistency with the stated values, or at least a lack of inconsistency.

Internal Environmental Analysis

Next, management undertakes a thorough analysis of the organization's current internal environment. A frequently used approach is to analyze the organization's strengths and weaknesses. This would identify those aspects of the organization that are better than the industry's average (strengths) and those that are below industry averages (weaknesses). Examples of internal areas addressed in the analysis would be the various functions (such as finance, operations, and marketing), as well as organizational and managerial factors that cut across functions. This would include organizational structure,

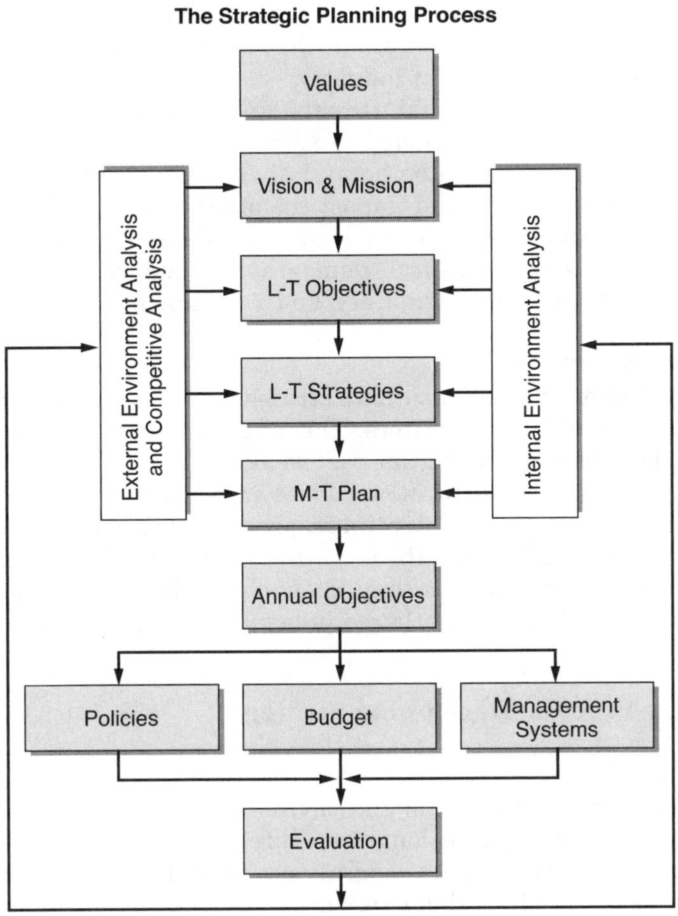

The Strategic Planning Process

Figure 20–1   The Strategic Planning Process

---

culture, historical context, stability of management, and nonfinancial control systems currently in place (such as Management by Objectives (MBO), Six Sigma, or Balanced Scorecard), as well as formal and informal planning systems. There are also other tools and approaches to perform this analysis.

As the figure shows, this analysis (as well as the external and competitive analyses) is completed over several steps in the strategy process. It begins with an analysis of the large, most significant factors and continues to a more detailed and thorough analysis as the strategic planning process moves from the highest level (Vision and Mission) to more specific and detailed analysis stages.

External Environmental Analysis

The external analysis is focused at two levels: the industry and the macroenvironment. Several tools exist to analyze the industry. For example, Michael Porter's Five Forces model (1980) looks at the structural forces within the industry. A trends analysis is also a common tool for industry analysis. In any case, it is important to understand the current structure of the industry and the major trends within that industry.

Reviewing the major external threats and opportunities is a common approach to macroanalysis, although a variety of other tools and techniques are also available. It may also be helpful at this stage to examine the major environmental trends that could impact the organization, either favorably or unfavorably. This would include analyzing trends and developments in the areas of economic; social, cultural, demographic, and geographic; labor and employment; political, legal, regulatory, and governmental; and technology.

Competitive Analysis

Before deciding on the organization's strategic direction, it is also important to understand the major competitors. This analysis would compare each competitor's market position, strengths, and weaknesses, as well as their current strategies and objectives. Also, it would be important to develop an understanding of each competitor's potential response to strategies the organization might be considering. As a goal, the organization should seek to know as much about each major competitor as they know about themselves. All competitor intelligence should always be gathered in legal and ethical ways.

The Strategy Process: Developing Strategy

Vision and Mission

After a thorough assessment of the environment, management proceeds to deciding the most appropriate long-term direction for the organization. The vision reflects the organization's aspirations; what it wants to become. This could be similar to "hospitals that care for the total person" or "providing convenient, value-priced, walk-in health care." The vision sets the tone and overarching direction for the rest of the strategy development phase, as well as providing the organization with an easily understood and unifying common purpose.

The mission has four purposes: defining the organization, providing direction (making the vision more specific), serving as a basis for resource allocation, and differentiating this organization from others competing in the same industry. It accomplishes these purposes by defining four aspects of the organization: the products and services, customers, markets, and philosophy (consistent with the vision).

Of these aspects, the most critical to effective strategy is a clear definition of the organization's markets: where and with whom they compete, both directly and indirectly, and a defined understanding of who the customers are. Customers can include both direct customers (for example, those that pay for the products and services, such as third-party payers) and indirect customers (for example, the patients themselves and patient referrers).

Long-term Objectives

Objectives reflect the desired end state. These are usually stated in three- to five-year terms. They can be of many types, but often reflect long-term objectives in the areas of growth, financial return, or customer perceptions (such as quality of care). An example of an objective for a hospital could be to "increase outpatient revenues from 10 percent of total revenues to 20 percent five years from now." Strategic long-term objectives reflect organization-wide objectives and not those of individual units or functions.

Long-term Strategies

Long-term strategies reflect how the objectives will be accomplished. They are corporate- or business-level strategies. For example, a strategy to carry out the outpatient revenue objective could be "to establish three new community clinics that would provide outpatient services within the current market area." Typical organizations should have no more than three to five long-term strategies.

Effective long-term strategies and objectives need to be critically evaluated on a number of criteria before acceptance. These criteria include: fit with the defined values, vision, and mission; consistency with external trends; feasibility of financial and managerial resources; organizational competencies to implement the strategies successfully; and potential impact on the competitive environment, including likely competitor counterstrategies.

The Strategy Process: Implementing Strategy

The key to a successful implementation of strategy is its integration with the daily operations of the organization. If strategy remains conceptual ideas, it has little chance of ever becoming fact. However, a well thought-out and thorough process of reflecting strategy in the daily decisions of middle and lower management substantially increases the likelihood of strategic ideas becoming strategic fact.

Medium-term Plan

Management looks mainly to annual plans and budgets as a guide in their daily decision process, so a "bridge" is necessary. The medium-term plan breaks down the three- to five-year long-term strategies and objectives into shorter, more actionable stages.

As well as breaking down long-term strategies and objectives into one-year time periods, major functional actions are mapped and sequenced and financial implications are considered. Most large strategic programs require a series of major actions within the various functional areas of the organization. The medium-term plan places these in their proper sequence. In our community clinics expansion example, locations would need to be determined before equipment is purchased or employees are hired and trained.

The final element of the medium-term plan includes a financial forecast for the five-year period, including the costs and expenses of the planned strategic actions. Of particular importance would be clear cash flow forecasts showing how the new strategies would be financed and repaid.

Annual Objectives

All functional and financial objectives from the medium-term plan are listed. This is the beginning point for expanding on these objectives. A hierarchy of objectives is then created from the top down, eventually establishing annual objectives for each budget unit within the organization. These objectives, if collectively carried out, would lead to accomplishing all strategic, financial, and functional objectives listed in the medium-term plan for the year.

Although this process must, of necessity, be top-down to assure strategic consistency throughout the organization, that does not mean there is no room for participation in this process. Once a department head has his or her objectives for the year, dividing these objectives among individual units and developing the specific methods of accomplishment should reflect a team effort within the department. Management by Objectives (MBO), as described by Peter Drucker (1974), can be a useful approach to accomplishing this.

Budget

Much has been written about the budget process, and there exists a wide variety of ways to execute budgeting. However, the only way to accomplish the strategic objectives is to build the budget around the annual unit objectives determined in the prior step. If, on the other hand, the budget is based on last year plus a percentage, it is decoupled from the strategic plan and the likelihood of strategic accomplishment is low (unless the strategy for this year is to copy last year).

In building a budget around the unit's annual objectives, staffing and spending levels necessary to accomplish the objectives are determined and then these amounts are budgeted. This would apply to both operating and capital budgets. If the strategy for the year requires substantial changes from "business as usual," this could mean that some units may lose 50 percent or more of their budgets, while other unit's budgets may double or triple. If management is not willing to reflect strategic priorities in the budgets, then resources are not being allocated on the basis of strategy, and without enough resources, key objectives will not be met.

Policies

In practice, the strategic process often neglects policies and procedures. This oversight can severely threaten strategic change. In making the daily decisions (that cumulatively either accomplish or fail to accomplish the organization's total strategy), middle- and lower-level managers rely on two primary guides: their budget (already discussed) and the organization's policies and procedures.

Policies accumulate over time, with older organizations having many more than younger organizations. These policies are often not well integrated and may even conflict with one another, since they are often issued in response to a negative event. For example, one day three patients' checks bounce, so a new policy banning the acceptance of checks is established. Since there is seldom any strategic input into policies, they can contain many land mines when attempting strategic change. Consequently, it is best practice to review all policies annually in terms of how they support the new strategic direction. If policies are found that hinder strategic accomplishment, they need to be either changed or abolished.

Management Systems

In addition to the budget and policies, some organizations may have other management systems in place. For instance, there may be a Six Sigma quality-improvement initiative, or MBO. If other systems exist within the organization, it is critical that they be integrated with the strategic planning system, so that they reinforce the strategic effort rather than dilute or even hinder strategic accomplishment. Of particular note is the Balanced Scorecard (Kaplan & Norton, 1996). This approach can be very helpful in the operational implementation of strategy if it is well integrated with the overall strategic planning process.

The Strategy Process: Evaluating Strategy

After year-end, and as the first step in the new strategy cycle, management evaluates the effectiveness of the prior year's strategies, including accomplishment of the year's strategic objectives.

This begins with a review of the major strategic assumptions in the year's plan and a determination of whether those assumptions were, overall, accurate. If there was a major change to one of the critical strategic assumptions, a meaningful evaluation is not possible and management may decide to shorten this step or, possibly, skip it entirely. In our community clinic expansion example, suppose the company had planned to open a clinic in October, but the bank that was to finance the clinic build-out and equipment was caught up in the subprime crisis and canceled our credit line in January. Because of the cautious lending environment, it took until September to obtain a new credit line with another bank. This delay of the clinic opening until the following year, due to a major problem beyond our control, does not reflect on the strategy's validity and may well cause management to delay the evaluation until the following year. It is important to caution, however, that this is not a place for management excuses, and such major events should be extremely rare.

If, as is most often the case, the assumptions did not change in any significant manner, then management must evaluate the strategic effectiveness. This evaluation can be of either a quantitative or qualitative nature (or a combination of both). Quantitative methods would look at the specific, measurable objectives that were to occur during the year and compare the plan to what actually happened. If in our clinic example, an objective was to increase outpatient revenue from 10 to 12 percent during the first year (on the way to the 20 percent long-term goal); management would objectively determine whether the 12 percent goal was met. On the qualitative side, if a goal was to improve depth of middle management (to handle the expansion) through intensive development efforts, management would subjectively assess whether that goal had been met.

If the annual strategy objectives were met overall and no major changes in the environment were forecast, usually the conclusion moving forward into the next year's cycle would be to continue with the current strategies and objectives. However, if the strategic analysis pointed to a shortfall, management would need to find the cause of the shortfall. There are two possibilities:

poor or excessively ambitious strategies, or poor implementation of the strategies. The bias at the executive level is to blame execution, while the bias at the operational levels is to blame the strategy. For an effective evaluation, biases need to be set aside and the analysis needs to be factual. Incorrect identification of the root causes of any shortfall inevitably leads to, at best, delay in fixing the problems and, at worst, severe financial consequences for the organization.

After completion of the strategic evaluation, the process begins anew in the next year's planning cycle with a review of the prior assessments and revisions, as needed.

STRUCTURE AND STRATEGY

Structure plays a dual role in the strategic planning process. It is an important consideration in the internal evaluation phase and a critical element in implementation. During internal evaluation, structure's effect on the organization's strategic focus, level of efficiency, integration of functions, and capacity to implement change is assessed. The structure chosen may also create (or eliminate) strategic competencies within functions. For example, centralized research and development departments are more likely to focus on new product breakthroughs and other long-term research at a strategic level. Decentralized research and development units, on the other hand, are more likely to focus on shorter-term process and product improvements at an operational level.

Once the assessment and strategy development phases have been completed, and the process moves into implementation, the organization's current structure must be assessed in terms of its appropriateness to implement the chosen strategic objectives. A critical issue in a decentralized organization, for example, would be whether the decentralization is on the same basis as the strategy. In our example, if the strategic direction is to customize services and delivery models at different community clinics, then the structure should be decentralized on the basis of geographic locations. If, on the other hand, the strategic direction is to serve as efficient "feeders" to the hospitals, then the structure would be much more centralized with few duplicated functions. These different strategic directions could well result in different structural alignments for various units such as credit, billing and collections, and diagnostic services.

If structural changes are needed in the organization as a result of changes in strategic direction (or ineffective prior implementation efforts), this change needs to be built into the medium-term plan. A change of structure is a major organizational change, requiring careful and thorough planning.

CULTURE AND STRATEGY

Similar to structure, organizational culture is also considered at both the internal assessment and implementation stages of the strategic planning process. During the internal evaluation phase, the organization's overall culture should be evaluated, as the organization's existing culture can be a major strength or weakness. It may also be useful at this stage to evaluate subcultures within units that may become critical to potential strategies. In our example, if there is a culture of constant conflict between doctors and other professionals within the surgical units of the hospital, that conflict may not be an issue for our example clinic expansion strategy if the culture is cooperative in the hospital's outpatient units. However, these culture issues need to be known in advance, so that during the implementation, managers, as well as professionals, for the new community clinics are drawn from the hospital's outpatient units and not from surgical units. If a strategic change is being considered, a thorough cultural analysis during assessment can prove very helpful later in the process.

During the implementation phase, culture can be a primary strategic consideration. If the existing culture is supportive of the new strategy, the odds of success are much higher than if the culture is neutral to the change. A neutral culture will require more management and change support, and possibly some organizational development efforts, during implementation.

Finally, a culture that is in opposition to the planned strategic change usually presents a major roadblock. A significant cultural change at the strategic level within an existing organization may be unrealistic, leaving us with few other strategic implementation options—none of them particularly good. If the new strategy is deemed essential to the organization, then implementation will need to move ahead. The best choice in these circumstances usually is to try to tweak the approach to implementation of the strategy (without changing the long-term objectives) to make it more palatable to the culture. Other choices are to use a high level of outsourcing (to companies with more appropriate cultures) or to just use force and threats to impose the change (usually a disastrous choice). If culture is going to be a problem, it may be worthwhile for the organization to revisit the strategic choice to be really certain that this is the direction they want to go.

MATCHING STRATEGY AND STRUCTURE

On the basis of research in 84 organizations (including 19 hospitals), Miles and Snow (1978) proposed four organizational types, in terms of their general characteristics, strategy sets, and internal characteristics and behavior. They proposed that a close relationship existed between a successful organization's internal characteristics, chosen competitive environments, and effective strategies. Later research (Zahra & Pearce, 1990; Brown & Iverson, 2004) has supported the major concepts of these typologies, although some specific functional matches have had mixed research results.

The four organizational types identified by Miles and Snow are defenders, prospectors, analyzers, and reactors. Miles and Snow point out that these organizational types may need some adjustment in particular types of industries.

Defenders

These organizations have narrow product/market domains, have industry-specific experienced executives, and do not search outside their defined markets for new opportunities. Their strategies are to penetrate deeper into current markets, to maintain prominence within their chosen markets, and to grow cautiously and incrementally.

Their structures are functional and stable with centralized controls and vertical information flows. They promote from within, focus on continual efficiency improvements, have formal job definitions, and use intensive (deep, detailed) planning systems. The politically dominant functions are finance and operations. Lincare Holdings is an example of an efficiency-focused organization with a narrow product/market domain. Sixty-seven percent of revenues are Medicare reimbursed, and their product line is restricted to provision of oxygen and respiratory therapy services to patients in the home.

Defenders, with a primarily internal focus, perform best in the stable environments that they seek and maintain. Major strategic risks for defenders are the continued viability of their narrow domains and their relative inflexibility to change if needed.

Prospectors

These organizations are continually searching for market opportunities and experimenting with potential responses to emerging environmental trends. Miles and Snow view this type of organization as the creator of change and uncertainty within markets. Their strategies look to a carefully monitored, broad product/market domain, which undergoes frequent change. Their growth is uneven and in spurts from new products and new markets.

Structures often change and tend to be product based. Information flows are to decentralized decision makers with results-oriented controls. There is low formalization in job descriptions and confrontation of conflicts, and the organization views its technology as people rather than machines. Efficiency is sacrificed for flexibility, with broad-based planning systems. The politically dominant functions are marketing and research and development. United-Health Group is an example of an organization with a frequently changing product/market domain, including consulting and processing services, plan administration, full range of risk-based health insurance plans, and pharmacy benefit management, as well as dental and disability solutions. Frequent structural changes occur that are reported as changes in their product and market domains.

Prospectors with a primarily external focus perform best in the unstable and changing environments that they seek out. The major strategic risk for prospectors is their inefficiency, and higher cost structure should their product domains become more stable and cost sensitive.

Analyzers

Analyzers operate in both stable and changing environments. In the stable environment, these organizations adopt efficient formal structures and processes, while in the unstable areas, they monitor competitors for successful ideas, adopting those that are most promising. Their strategies are successful imitation and being avid followers of change, using extensive market surveillance. Growth is usually through market penetration, but may also occur from product or market development.

The structure is normally matrix, with a functional organization in the stable areas, and a product organization in the unstable areas. Planning is both intensive and broad, with complex control systems that can make trade-offs between efficiency and effectiveness. Because of its dual nature and need for different structures and processes in the two areas, it is difficult in practice to maintain an analyzer organization. The politically dominant functions are marketing, applied research, and operations. A general hospital may pursue this strategy as it seeks to maintain efficiency (and low costs) in ongoing operations, but must also react to changes and instability in the technical, competitive, and reimbursement environments.

Analyzers, with their dual focus, perform best in mixed environments. The major strategic risks for analyzers are their need to straddle the middle and preserve power balances, which prevent them from aggressively pursuing either an efficiency or effectiveness strategy if the environment should shift strongly to one side or the other.

Reactors

These organizations have top managers who perceive change in their environments, but are unable to respond effectively. With an inconsistent strategy/structure relationship, they seldom adjust until forced to do so from external pressures. According to Miles and Snow (1978), this final organizational type is unable to succeed because of one of three strategic issues: (1) management cannot create a viable strategy; (2) management develops a strategy, but structure and processes are not appropriately linked; or (3) management continues with a strategy no longer suitable to the changed external environment.

Pfizer's inability to adapt to a changed regulatory and technological environment is an example of a reactor organization. Pfizer is now attempting to deal with longer (and tougher) new drug approval regulatory environment, patents expiring on major blockbuster drugs, generics obtaining an increasing market share, inefficient and high cost fragmented structures, and an organizational culture resistant to change. Other examples include many community hospitals that have been unable to adapt to a shift toward outpatient-based care models, more rigorous reimbursement policies, or demographic changes in their service areas.

The Miles and Snow (1978) typology demonstrates the close relationship and critical need to link strategy to both the external environment and internal structure and processes. Although there are other successful models in the healthcare sector beyond the four Miles and Snow present, the idea that the external environment, the strategy, and an organization's internal structure and processes must be carefully coordinated remains a central tenet of a winning strategy.

SUMMARY

Strategy plays a critical role in organizational success. Through a small number of major decisions, effective strategy guides the organization through changing environments, conflicting stakeholder demands, and uncertain economic and regulatory times. The strategic planning process provides an integrated approach to environmental assessment, strategy development, implementation, and evaluation. This top-to-bottom integrated strategic process can significantly improve the chances of an organization realizing its long-term vision.

The ideal situation is an organization that understands and selects a suitable competitive environment, develops strategies that match the chosen external environment, and designs organizational structures and processes best suited to implement those strategies.

END-OF-CHAPTER QUESTIONS

1. Discuss how the healthcare external environment differs from that faced by the average American company. Explain this in terms of both the industry and macro-levels.

2. Explain the differences in how personal values are reflected in an organization's values between an entrepreneurial firm and a large governmental agency. Do you think these differences change the typical values that each type of organization has?

3. Discuss at least three different types of healthcare organizations and how their differences could affect the strategic planning process that they use.

4. Using as an example a healthcare organization you are familiar with (or have researched), explain the competitive domain they have chosen, their strategies to compete, and their structure and processes. Are there mismatches? If so, what changes would you recommend?

END-OF-CHAPTER CASE STUDY

Case Study 20–1 Strategy, Stability, and Strength

Bronson's Journey to Excellence

Excellence has always been a focus of Bronson Methodist Hospital, a not-for-profit tertiary hospital based in Kalamazoo, Michigan. But it was not until 1999 that the organization adopted the Baldrige criteria and put into place a systematic approach to organizational excellence.

In the mid-1990s, as Bronson designed and prepared to move into a new, all-private-room facility, Bronson's leadership seized the opportunity to raise the bar on the quality of their internal processes so they could match the quality of the hospital's new state-of-the-art patient-care environment. The building project became a catalyst for moving the organization's culture from "good" to "great."

When the Baldrige criteria for healthcare became available in 1999, Bronson was poised and ready to begin using the model—a systems perspective for understanding performance management provided by the Baldrige National Quality Program (www.quality.nist.gov). We were attracted to this model because the Baldrige criteria are not prescriptive; they do not tell an organization what to do. Instead, the criteria challenge an organization to review and understand how it is doing things. This was precisely the formula for self-evaluation that Bronson was looking for to become a "great" hospital and sustain long-term success. Since implementing the Baldrige criteria, Bronson has achieved strong performance improvement and results in every key area measured, including low Medicare patient mortality, high overall patient, employee and physician satisfaction, and national recognition for workplace excellence. We have seen significant improvement in use of prophylaxis, registered nurse turnover rate, and the integration and use of technology; Bronson also has pioneered efforts to reduce waste and pollution. As a result of these and many other accomplishments, Bronson Methodist Hospital was named one of six recipients—from across American industries—of the Malcolm Baldrige National Quality Award in November 2005.

A critical component of the organization's success can be attributed to Bronson's Leadership System. In the past, we had been unable to clearly articulate exactly how we led the organization. Working with the Baldrige criteria compelled us to specifically delineate and document how the organization "fits" together in terms of strategy, performance standards, action, results, and accountability. As a result of this work, we created the Strategic Management Model to provide Bronson with a systematic approach that aligns all of our planning, including strategic, workforce, financial, capital, and information technology. Because strategy is the foundation for success, we have found that the consistent use of this tool has contributed greatly to our organization's evolution.

Focus: Bronson's strategy revolves around our Plan for Excellence, which captures the vision, mission, values, and service expectations of all staff and leaders (see Sidebar 2). It includes our strategies, the "3 Cs": clinical excellence, customer and service excellence, and corporate effectiveness. We use the plan extensively during employee, physician, volunteer, and other stakeholder interactions to effectively communicate the hospital's vision and actively engage them in achieving it.

In the early years of using the Baldrige criteria to focus our planning, we realized that the hospital's mission and vision also needed to be refined and focused. Our mission at the time was: *We are committed to improving the health of those we serve by providing services that are of value, that are comprehensive, and that are accessible through an integrated network of cooperating providers.*

As we talked with stakeholders, we realized that this mission seemed too "corporate" in its language and was difficult to understand. Furthermore, it only vaguely addressed community health and partnerships with other organizations, which was difficult to measure. We decided our mission should be succinct, direct, and measurable and address the needs of anyone seeking our services whether they are members of the community or not. Thus, our mission today is simply to: *Provide excellent healthcare services.*

This mission is easy to communicate, deploy, and measure. In a similar vein, we rewrote our vision, which was: *Bronson and its partners will be the system of choice in our region.*

The old vision focused on being the best in our area. But to truly raise the bar on organizational performance, it was critical that we benchmark ourselves against the best in the nation. As a result, our current vision is: *Bronson will be a national leader in healthcare quality.*

This vision has driven the organization and helped fuel performance improvement processes. The simplification of the mission and vision now keeps the entire organization focused and moving in a clear direction.

Re-evaluation: An important component of our Strategic Management Model is our Strategic Input Document (SID), which informs the planning process. The SID is a formal compilation of our assumptions about the environment and how those assumptions will affect Bronson during the year. We look at developments in the community; changes occurring in competing organizations; governmental issues on the local, state, and national levels; and the needs and wants of our stakeholders. While we always had considered these issues during our annual planning process, we had never formally documented them so that we could refer to them easily, prioritized our challenges, and most importantly, continuously re-evaluated them throughout the year. The SID is a simple yet critical process improvement. It helps us to react quickly to environmental changes yet stay on task with our plan.

Accountability: Before we adopted the Baldrige criteria and developed the Strategic Management Model, Bronson did not use scorecards to set targets and track our progress formally. As we implemented the Strategic Management Model, we designed detailed tactics based on metrics to achieve goals aligned with the 3 Cs. For example, the clinical excellence goal of reducing Medicare mortality—which is reported to our Board in an overall scorecard— cascades down to specific measurable activities on leader- and staff-level scorecards. We think of these detailed tactics as strings that are attached from Bronson's overall goals to every person in the organization. Thus the entire workforce, our employees and physician partners, know exactly how their efforts contribute to the organization's success. Not only do scorecards reinforce the responsibility that staff have in achieving the hospital's overall goals, but also—because of the metrics, which include a "meet," "exceed," and "far exceed" scoring criteria—staff know exactly where they stand at any given time. We monitor the impact of our efforts to improve accountability through our scorecards and employee and physician opinion surveys in which we ask them whether they understand our strategic direction and their role in reaching organizational goals.

Heightening the sense of accountability among staff also was made easier when we modified the vision and made a conscious decision to bring Bronson's strategic plan to light at all levels of the organization. Today, even our specific tactics are widely publicized throughout the hospital. Such disclosure has made a huge difference with the leadership team, employees, medical staff, and volunteers, who now feel connected to the vision.

Ownership: In the past, Bronson's strategic planning was primarily orchestrated by the vice president of Planning. In an effort to improve our results, we created Strategic Oversight Teams for each of the 3 Cs led by members of the executive team. The teams establish short- and long-term plans for their "C," develop the accompanying scorecards, and monitor results. With this approach to planning, we have better deployed ownership of the plan at the executive level and with leaders and key physicians who now feel as though they own the plan.

Integration: When we first began using the Baldrige criteria, we treated it as a separate process and convened a separate committee. This changed when we realized the true value of the Baldrige model is in integrating it into what you do everyday to run your organization.

Once we did this, we understood how it was going to make us a better business. By aligning the six categories of the Baldrige criteria, we learned the importance of examining the interrelationships among all facets of the organization. For example, through the process, we realized that we were approving capital purchases separately from our strategic planning cycle. Now, our capital and technology planning are wrapped into one process. Bronson holds a day-long retreat focused on reviewing and prioritizing clinical technology as part of developing the next year's strategic plan and budget. Prior to using the Baldrige criteria, many of our processes were people dependent.

Table 20–1

VISION		
Bronson will be a national leader in healthcare quality		

Clinical Excellence		
Achieve excellent patient outcomes		

Customer and Service Excellence	Corporate Effectiveness	
Enhance service excellence, staff competency, and leadership	Achieve efficiency, growth, financial, and community benefit targets	

Philosophy of Nursing Excellence	Values	Commitment to Patient Care Excellence
Respect Compassion Expertise Impact Pride	We believe in, and our actions will reflect: Care and respect for all people Teamwork Stewardship of resources Commitment to our community The pursuit of excellence	Healing with our knowledge Caring with our hearts Working together for Bronson patients and families

MISSION		
Provide excellent healthcare services		

Fortunately, we employed excellent people who did a great job of carrying out the work assigned to them; however, we realized that this was risky both in the short and long term. If those people left the organization, how would the processes be sustained? Tools like the Plan for Excellence, the SID, the Strategic Oversight Teams, and scorecards are now hardwired into the way we work; they are documented and repeatable. This helps ensure organizational stability and the high-quality service and excellent outcomes that we have achieved will be sustained in the future, regardless of any personnel changes.

Using the Baldrige criteria has dramatically changed how we serve our patients. Community preference for Bronson as the area's "best hospital" also is at a record high. Independent study data show there is a 32-point gap between Bronson and its closest competitor. This preference has translated into market growth as well: Inpatient volume at Bronson grew 34 percent between 2000 and 2005.

Since being named a Baldrige recipient last November, Bronson has received numerous phone calls and e-mails from organizations across the United States asking how to win the award. We tell them that there is no formula for winning; it is all about the journey to excellence and what each organization learns about itself along the way.

Using the Baldrige criteria has dramatically changed how we run our business, and we are very proud to now be considered a role model organization that others can learn from. But, for us, Baldrige is a journey without end. The tools it provides allow for continuous improvement that can strengthen and sustain any organization for years to come.

Strategy, stability and strength: Bronson's journey to excellence, by F. J. Sardone and S. Reinoehl, 2006. *Healthcare Executive, 21*(3), 16–20. Reprinted with permission.

Bronson Case Questions

1. Using the strategic planning model as a guide, discuss how Bronson currently carries out each step in the model.
2. Explain how Bronson links the various steps together. Are the steps in the same sequence as the model?
3. Discuss several changes you would recommend to Bronson to improve their strategic planning process.
4. Do you think Bronson is trying to become one of the three successful Miles organizational types? If so, which one. If not, why not?

REFERENCES

Brown, W. A., & Iverson, J. O. (2004). Exploring strategy and Board structure in nonprofit organizations. *Nonprofit and Voluntary Sector Quarterly, 33*(3), 344–400.

Drucker, P. F. (1974). *Management: Tasks, responsibilities, practices.* New York: Harper & Row.

Hofer, C. W., & Schendel, D. (1978). *Strategy formulation: Analytical concepts.* St. Paul, MN: West Publishing.

Kaplan, R. S., & Norton, D. P. (1996). Linking the balanced scorecard to strategy. *California Management Review, 39*(1), 53–79.

Miles, R. E., & Snow, C. C. (1978). *Organizational strategy, structure, and process.* New York: McGraw-Hill Book Company.

Porter, M. E. (1980). *Competitive strategy: Techniques for analyzing industries and competitors.* New York: Free Press.

Zahra. S. A., & Pearce, J. A., II, (1990). Research evidence on the Miles-Snow typology. *Journal of Management, 16*(4), 751–768.

OTHER SUGGESTED READINGS

Begun, J. W., & Kaissi, A. A. (2005). An exploratory study of healthcare strategic planning in two metropolitan areas. *Journal of Healthcare Management, 50*(4), 264–275.

Chan, S. (2002). The importance of strategy for the evolving field of radiology. *Radiology, 224,* 639–648.

Covaleski, M. A., & Dirsmith, M. W. (1981). MBO and goal directedness in a hospital context. *The Academy of Management Review, 6*(3), 409–418.

Crotts, J. C., Dickson, D. R., & Ford, R. C. (2005). Aligning organizational processes with mission: The case of service excellence. *Academy of Management, 19*(3), 54–68.

Ford, R. C., Sivo, S. A., Fottler, M. D., Dickson, D., Bradley, K., & Johnson, L. (2006). Aligning internal organizational factors with a service excellence mission: An exploratory investigation in health care. *Health Care Management Review, 31*(4), 259–269.

Kershaw, R., & Kershaw, S. (2001). Developing a balanced scorecard to implement strategy at St. Elsewhere Hospital. *Management Accounting Quarterly,* 28–35.

Rivers, P. A., Fottler, M. D., & Parker, M. (2005). Environmental assessment of the Indian Health Service. *Health Care Management Review, 30*(4), 293–303.

Steiner, G. A., & Miner, J. B. (1982). *Management policy and strategy* (2nd ed.). New York: Macmillan.

Williams, J., Smythe, W., Hadjistavropoulos, T., Malloy, D. C., & Martin, R. (2005). A study of thematic content in hospital mission statements: A question of values. *Health Care Management Review, 30*(4), 304–314.

CHAPTER 21

Organization Structures: Contextual Dimension

Nancy Borkowski, DBA, CPA, FACHE

LEARNING OUTCOMES

After completing this chapter, the student should understand:

- How each element of the contextual dimension relates to an organization's structure.
- The differences between mechanistic and organic systems.
- The advantages and disadvantages of the four basic organization structures.
- The importance of the various horizontal linkage mechanisms.
- What is meant by population ecology.
- What is meant by institutional theory and the three mechanisms associated with institutional isomorphism.
- The various strategies organizations use to develop and sustain interorganizational relationships.

OVERVIEW

As we learned in Chapter 10, effective leadership is contingent on the individual taking into account the internal and external constraints of the given situation. The same concept holds true for designing an organization's structure. For managers to effectively structure their organizations for high performance, they must take into consideration various internal and external constraints. Some constraints may be the organization's culture, the size of the organization, how the organization adapts to its environment, and differences among resources, operating activities, and strategies (see Chapter 20). Daft (2007) refers to these constraints as the contextual dimension of organizational design (see Table 21–1).

The contextual factors are important and interrelate to explain what goes on inside organizations. For example, when describing the size of the organization, what is the measurement used? Does the organization use number of employees, physical capacity (i.e., number of hospital beds), organizational inputs or outputs (i.e., 50,000 emergency room visits), or the organization's annual revenues or net assets? Although Kimberly (1976) suggests that these various measurements of size may be highly intercorrelated in some instances, managers must be clear as to the measurement used. Most of the research relating size to organizational structure has been based on the number of people employed by the organization. Blau (1968) found that increasing organizational size (number of employees) was related to increasing differentiation (number of levels, departments, etc., within an organization).

Table 21–1 Organizational Contextual Dimensions

Dimension	Description
Size	Size is reflected in the number of people in the organization. It can be measured for the organization as a whole or for specific components, such as a hospital within a health system or a division within a hospital. Because organizations are social systems, size is typically measured by the number of employees. Other measures, such as total patient revenue, total inpatient discharges, total outpatient visits, number of beds, or total assets, also reflect magnitude, but they do not indicate the size of the "people" part of the system.
Technology	Technology refers to the tools, machinery, and equipment (physical manifestation), as well as the accumulated knowledge (techniques and actions), used to transform inputs into outputs. It concerns how the organization actually produces the services and/or products it provides for patients and other customers and includes such things as advance information systems. An assembly line, a college classroom, and an overnight package delivery system are technologies, although they differ from one another.
Environment	The environment includes all elements outside the boundary of the organization. Key elements include the industry, government, patients, payers, suppliers, policymakers, and the financial community. The environmental elements that affect an organization the most are often other organizations. (See discussion regarding environment in Chapters 18 and 20.)
Goals and strategies	Goals and strategies define the purpose and competitive techniques that set the organization apart from other organizations. As fully described in Chapter 20, goals are the organization's intent and strategies are the plans of action that describe resource allocation and activities for dealing with the environment to accomplish the organization's goals. Goals and strategies define the scope of operations and the relationship with employees, patients, payers, and competitors.
Culture	An organization's culture is the underlying set of key values, beliefs, understandings, and norms shared by employees. These underlying values may pertain to ethical behavior, commitment to employees, efficiency, or patient service, and they provide the means that holds organizational members together. An organization's culture is unwritten but can be observed in its stories, slogans, ceremonies, dress, and design layout (see discussion regarding culture in Chapter 20).

SOURCE: *Organization theory and design* (9th ed., p. 20), by R. L. Daft, (2007). Mason, OH: Thomson South-Western. Adapted with permission.

Increasing differentiation is related to increased need for control and coordination. The widely cited Aston studies (Pugh et al., 1963; Pugh, Hickson, Hinings, Turner, & Lupton, 1968) found that increasing size is related to increasing structuring of organizational activities and decreasing concentrations of authority.

Technology is another important factor relating to an organization's structure. The contextual factor of technology has three components: (1) machine technology (i.e., facilities and equipment), (2) application of knowledge for effective performance of certain tasks and activities, and (3) organizational technology—the techniques used in the transformation of inputs into outputs (Kast & Rosenzweig, 1985). There are three questions that need to be answered when assessing an organization's technical system:

1. Are the organization's tasks and/or problem-solving needs standardized?
2. Is the organization's technical system simple or dynamic?
3. Is the organization's technical system staple or complex?

To answer the first question, Perrow (1967) provides us with the following guidelines: (A) if problem solving is standardized with few exceptions, it can be described as routine technology, (B) if problem solving is difficult with many exceptions, the technology is described as nonroutine. To assist in answering questions two and three, Kast and Rosenzweig (1985) relate that when considering organizational technologies, managers need to determine (1) the degree of complexity of the technology and (2) whether the technology is stable or dynamic. Organizational technologies can range from simple and staple (i.e., person-tool) to dynamic and complex (i.e., continuous process or advance technology). For example, a nurse practitioner diagnosing a patient for strep throat by obtaining a culture is simple and staple, whereas a team of surgeons performing a multiple organ transplant operation would be considered dynamic and complex technology. As more fully described in Chapter 22, Woodward (1965) and her associates found a correlation between technology and organizations' structures. The researchers stated that there was a close relationship between the type of technology, the average span of control, the number of levels of management, and the organization's success. The other contextual factors of environment, goals and strategies, and culture were discussed in Chapter 20 relating to their impact on an organization's structure.

Contextual dimension describes the organizational setting that influences and shapes the structure and design of the entity (Daft, 2007). In other words, given the situation, the organizational structure of a firm must "fit" with its environment and between its subsystems to achieve the company's goals. Since no two organizations are identical (different goals, cultures, size, etc.) managers need to appreciate that there is no one best way to structure an organization (Lawrence & Lorsch, 1967). For example, an organization making a standard product or offering a standardized service using the same processes and procedures will tend to use routine technologies and a bureaucratic structure to achieve maximum efficiency (i.e.,

Shouldice "Hernia" Hospital in Canada), whereas an organization with nonroutine activities dealing with unpredictable environments will use flexible technologies and a nonbureaucratic structure. Burns and Stalker (1961, 1994) termed these bureaucratic and nonbureaucratic structures mechanistic and organic systems, respectively.

MECHANISTIC AND ORGANIC SYSTEMS

Burns and Stalker (1961, 1994) developed the theory of mechanistic and organic systems when their research found that technology and market forces exerted pressures on organizations that made particular organizational forms desirable. The researchers found that mechanistic systems are suitable to stable conditions and characterized by repetitive tasks, clear hierarchy of control, vertical communication, and standardized technologies (see Table 21–2). Organic systems have the opposite characteristics and are therefore appropriate to changing conditions that introduce new problems and requirements for action (i.e., innovation). The organic system requiring a dynamic, changing structure is not feasible for all organizations. As such, Burns and Stalker noted that there are stages on the continuum between the two polar points (mechanistic and organic) and organizations may operate within both systems simultaneously (see Table 21–3). For example, a pharmaceutical company's research and development division may operate as an organic system, whereas the manufacturing division as a mechanistic system.

It is with an understanding of mechanistic and organic systems that we can explore an organization's structure, taking into consideration its complexity (i.e., size, goals, environment). As noted by Burton, DeSanctis, and Obel (2006, p. 57), "a poor choice of structure leads to opportunity losses which can be a threat to the organization's short-term efficiency and effectiveness as well as its long-term viability."

In Chapter 19, an organization's structure was defined as the clustering of its various departments, division, and so forth to coordinate and control activities (and people) to achieve the company's goals. Structure involves two issues: (1) how to organize the firm into smaller subunits and (2) how to coordinate the subunits so the firm's goals will be achieved (Mintzberg, 1979). How an entity has structured itself can be determined by viewing the company's organization chart. The organizational chart depicts the degree or level of vertical differentiation of the company (i.e., the depth of the hierarchy—top to bottom), vertical operational responsibilities (i.e., communication and coordination activities connecting the top and bottom of an organization), and sometimes, but not always, the horizontal linkages (i.e., communication and coordination activities across organizational departments). In this chapter, four basic structure configurations will be presented. We will discuss how these structures emerged and how and why they change over time. In Chapter 22, we examine the design of the organization's subunits on the basis of various parameters, such as task specialization, work standardization, and degree of formalization across the hierarchy.

Table 21–2 Characteristics of Mechanistic and Organic Systems

Mechanistic System (appropriate to stable conditions)	Organic System (appropriate to changing conditions)
The specialized differentiation tasks into which the problems and tasks facing the concern as a whole are broken down	The contributive nature of special knowledge and experience to the common tasks of the concern
The abstract nature of each individual task, which is pursued with techniques and purposes distinct from those of the concern as a whole	The realistic nature of the individual task, which is seen as set by the total situation of the concern
The reconciliation, for each level in the hierarchy, of these distinct performances by the immediate superiors	The adjustment and continual redefinition of individual tasks through interaction with others
The precise definition of rights, obligations, and technical methods attached to each functional role	The shedding of responsibility as a limited field of rights, obligations, and methods. Thus, problems cannot be avoided as someone else's responsibility
The translation of rights, obligations, and methods into the responsibilities of a functional position	The spread of commitment to the concern beyond any technical definition
The hierarchic structure of control, authority, and communication	A network structure of control, authority, and communication. Sanctions derive from presumed community of interest with the rest of the organization
A reinforcement of the hierarchic structure by the location of knowledge of actualities exclusively at the top of hierarchy	Knowledge about the technical or commercial nature of the task may be located anywhere. This location becomes the ad hoc center of authority and communication
A tendency for interaction between members of the concern to be vertical	A lateral direction of communication through the organization, resembling consultation rather than command
A tendency for operations and working behavior to be governed by the instructions and decisions issued by superiors	A content of communication that consists of information and advice rather than instructions and decisions
Insistence on loyalty to the concern and obedience to superiors as a condition of membership	Commitment to the concern's tasks and to the technological ethos of material progress and expansion is more highly valued than loyalty and obedience
A greater importance and prestige attaching to local than to cosmopolitan knowledge, experience, and skill	Importance and prestige attach to affiliations and expertise valid in the industrial and technical and commercial milieu external to the firm

SOURCE: *The management of innovation* (Rev. Ed., pp. 120–122), From T. Burns and G. M. Stalker, 1994. London: Oxford University Press. Reprinted with permission.

Table 21–3 Positions on the Mechanistic and Organic Continuum[a]

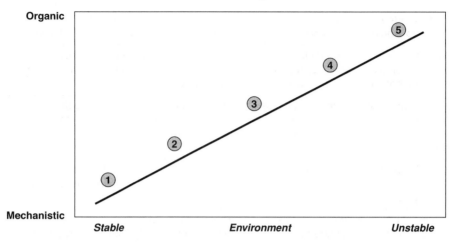

Mechanistic ◄───► Organic

Position 1	Position 2	Position 3	Position 4	Position 5
Well-defined hierarchy, bureaucracy structure with high degree of formational, horizontal differentiation (i.e., task/job definitions) and positional terms of reference, downward communications with little participation in decision making.	Bureaucracy structure but with some flexibility to meet operational contingencies.	Bureaucracy structure but use of horizontal linkages (i.e., cross depart-mental meetings, teams and task forces) to facilitate communication and coordination of operational activities.	Matrix type organization relying on teamwork to accomplish goals.	Learning organization (flexible structure) using project teams to ensure goal attainment; low complexity and formalization, uses all types of communications (upward, down-ward, lateral) to coordinate activities with high degree of participation in decision making based on expertise rather than position.

[a]Burns and Stalker noted that there are stages on the continuum between the two extremes points (mechanistic and organic) and that organizations may operate within both systems simultaneously.

ORGANIZATION STRUCTURES

A multiplicity of models exists regarding organizational configurations. Most of these models use variations of one or more of four basic organization structures. The four basic organization structures are simple, functional, divisional, and matrix (Miles & Snow, 1978). As noted, these four basic structures can be combined in different patterns and/or forms within an organization. Intraorganization variations can be found across organizational work units, departments, and divisions, as well as up and down in the hierarchy. For example, if an organization is designed with a divisional structure, within the division's subunits may be a functional, matrix, another divisional, or hybrid form of these basic structures (Burton et al., 2006).

Simple Structure

The simple organizational structure is very common, because in many industries, including health care, most organizations are small and therefore do not need a complex structure. Simple structures have the following characteristics: (1) centralized decision making, (2) low specialization (i.e., division of labor), and (3) high degree of informality (i.e., limited written rules, policies, and procedures). Although this simple structure may provide for job enlargement since employees are not bound by formality or division of labor, it also may lead to inefficiencies and conflicts if employees do not understand their roles and responsibilities. An example of a simple structure is a sole practitioner's (e.g., physician's) office. The physician is "senior management" who is responsible for making the practice's clinical and administrative decisions. Although there is a clear distinction between the roles of clinical and nonclinical professionals working in the office, administrative personnel usually multitask between front desk duties, obtaining needed referrals, coding, billing, and so on. Within small physicians' offices, policies and procedures are usually communicated verbally with little if any documentation except when required by local, state, or federal regulations.

Functional Structure

As the physician's practice grows, it may evolve into a functional structure with employees working in departments based on their roles and responsibilities (see Figure 21–1). This structure enhances the functioning of each subunit. For example, if all billing and coding employees work in the same department, they will increase their expertise by sharing knowledge and supporting one another. This structure allows the physician's practice to achieve efficiency because of the economies of scale. However, this structure makes communication and coordination between different departments more difficult, and it limits flexibility because of the centralization.

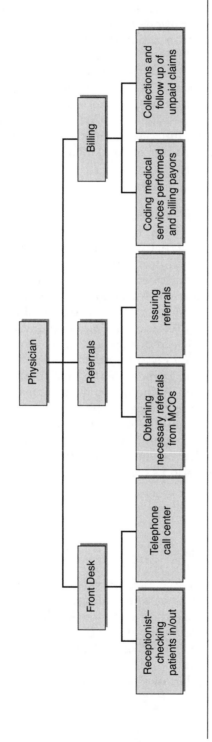

Figure 21-1

Divisional Structure

A divisional structure divides the organization's operations into product/service or customer segments or geographical locations. For example, a managed care organization may be divisionally structured by its customer segments—Medicare, Medicaid, and commercial members. Each division is responsible for product/service lines, customer bases, or geographic locations with its own supporting functional units, such as finance, marketing, and human resources. A divisional structure is decentralized, which allows for flexibility and quick responses to environmental changes. However, this structure results in duplication of resources because each division has the same administrative operations. In addition, it does not support the exchange of knowledge between people working in the same profession (i.e., human resources, marketing, finance) because employees are working in different divisions.

An example of a divisionally structured organization is HCA, Inc., a for-profit company that owns and operates approximately 179 hospitals and approximately 104 freestanding surgery centers in 21 states, England, and Switzerland. HCA is grouped into broad geographical and/or service-related segments: Western Group, Central Group, Eastern Group, Outpatient Services Group, and the Financial Services Group. The geographical groupings are further divided into divisions (see Figure 21–2). For example, the Eastern Group includes approximately 52 HCA hospitals in Florida, southern Georgia, North Carolina, and South Carolina. The Florida operations includes the North Florida division (10 hospitals), the East Florida Division (12 hospitals), and the West Florida Division (15 hospitals). By creating a divisional structure, HCA is able to balance economies of scale as being the largest for-profit hospital company in the world (e.g., information technology, billing, and group purchasing are "corporate" services to the divisions) and each division's ability to focus on patients and customers at the local level. Flattening the corporate hierarchy

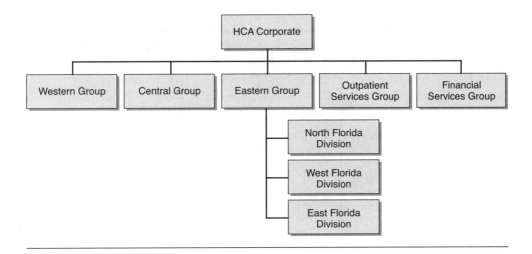

Figure 21–2

makes sense for HCA, as the company implements its strategy to integrate its hospitals and ancillary facilities in each of the local markets in which it operates (Galloro, 2005).

Matrix Structure

The matrix structure combines the functional and divisional structures. The matrix organization was developed for the purpose of improving management's control over a product or project within a multifunctional firm (Scott & Davis, 2006). The matrix structure is reflected on an organizational chart with the various products/projects (each with a nonfunctional orientation) on the horizontal axis, and the functional contributors to those products/projects on the vertical axis. Because of the "cross representation" (i.e., product/service and function), an employee will be accountable to both a product/project manager as well as a functional manager. For example, a hospital may organize itself under clinical service lines while still maintaining permanent functional units (see Figure 21–3). The cardiovascular services line is assigned a clinical service line (CSL) manager who is responsible for directing the operations of all medical and surgical cardiac care, including the hospital's cardiac catheterization laboratory. As such, some nurse employees would have two managers: a functional manager (director of nursing) and a CSL manager.

This type of structure is not easy to implement because of the dual authority. However, the matrix structure eliminates the duplication of skills and

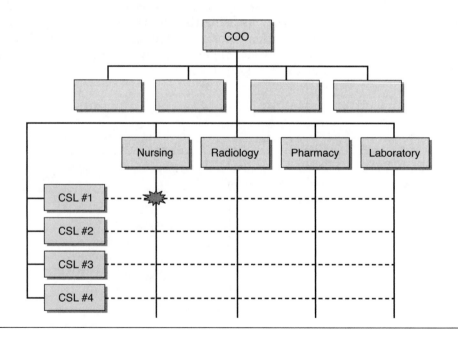

Figure 21–3

responsibilities by identifying functions or common components that are shared by multiple divisions, services, or products within an organization. Matrix organizations provide clear accountability within a specific business function and allow more efficient allocation of specialized skills. By taking advantage of the shared services and skills, and not having to develop and manage those skills, the service/product line manager can better focus on his or her goals (see Case Study 21–1, "SSM St. Joseph Hospital").

Case Study 21–1 SSM St. Joseph Hospital

In 1996, the financial situation at SSM St. Joseph Hospital of Kirkwood, Missouri, was in crisis mode. But SSM Health Care had no intention of closing the facility. The organization planned to use St. Joseph's resources and strong history in the community to turn the situation around. Radical structural changes made the hospital stronger and more efficient. At the heart of this turnaround was a move away from centralized nursing. St. Joseph organized a decentralized structure around clinical service lines with one core objective—to provide the best patient care possible.

Senior management realized that the hospital could not be all things to all people. They were steadily losing market share in pursuit of full service. The hospital needed to change, if it was going to survive. Senior management knew that to survive in its very competitive market, they had to define who "we were and determine our niche." In 1996, St. Joseph started the process by taking stock of its situation:

- It was a small community hospital in southwest St. Louis County, Missouri.
- It was one of six hospitals in SSM Health Care, the third largest major not-for-profit hospital system in the city.
- In St. Louis, 74 percent of its 39 hospitals are part of a network system, compared with the national average of 44 percent.
- St. Joseph's main competitors—both of which are within a 5-mile radius—are part of the two largest hospital systems in the area.
- The hospital had 281 licensed beds, an average daily census of 100 patients, and 750 full-time employees.
- According to the St. Louis–area Business Health Coalition, 9,904 hospital beds are available in the metropolitan area, including the outlying Illinois suburbs. The coalition estimates that 3,708 beds are excess capacity when hospitals are considered full or at 80 percent occupancy.

On the basis of its situation, St. Joseph chose to move away from its traditional nursing structure and implement the CSL model. The hospital organized itself around four CSLs: surgical, cardiovascular, women and children, and senior services. For each of these CSLs, a clinical director was assigned who had a nursing background. The CSL directors, who reported to the chief operational officer, were responsible for:

- overseeing his or her CSL
- developing a business plan that included strategies on promoting growth
- improving operational efficiencies
- planning ways to improve customer satisfaction and clinical outcomes

In addition, the hospital formed a nursing leadership team (NU) that included all clinical directors with nursing unit/departments from emergency department services, nursing service operations, and home health care. The team's challenge was to guide everyone through this cultural transition while performing at the same high level. The CSL structure helped limit territorial issues and foster positive growth for the hospital by enabling departments to work together.

For example, because of rapid patient turnover, patient rooms needed to be emptied and cleaned quickly for new admissions. The housekeeping department couldn't meet the new demand. As soon as the problem surfaced, the CSL director met with the housekeeping director and other staff members and developed a housekeeper float role to solve it.

In comparing a functional structured organization with St. Joseph's new matrix organizational structure, one senior manager commented that the patient turnover problem's quick response and change would have been challenging in a centralized organization with clear departmental lines. Territorial issues would have taken center stage in more traditional structures, which would obstruct problem solving. However, "when people come together around patient care, they don't have to deal with maintaining departments. Their priority becomes determining what the patient needs and then providing care to the patient. When we focus on patient care, employees agree that the solution to every issue and the reason behind every dollar spent center on adding value and enhancing patient or physician satisfaction. And that agreement empowers employees to achieve the organization's success."

Epilogue: Less than 10 years after implementing its matrix structure, SSM St. Joseph received the 2005 Missouri Quality Award, became the first winner of the Missouri PRO Quality Award, and a 2007 recipient of the Premier Award for Quality in the area of acute myocardial infarction (AMI) or heart attack.

SOURCE: "Clinical service lines bring patients into focus," by G. Green, 2000. *Nursing Management, 31*(3), pp. 40–43. Reprinted with permission.

The value of the matrix structure is its flexibility in responding to environmental pressures (Miner, 2002). Because the matrix structure increases interdependencies, increased communication and collaboration are required. New patterns of behavior must be learned if managers and employees are to function effectively in a matrix structure. As Miner (2002) suggests, this can be facilitated through a team-building process aimed at identifying expectations, objectives, leadership, roles and responsibilities, decision modes, communication, and conflict-resolution modes (see Chapter 16—Teams and Team Building). In addition to team building, employee development will be needed to provide knowledge and skills relevant to the matrix structure. Because of the complexity of the matrix structure, Miner (2002, p. 496) states that three conditions must be present for an organization to consider this form:

1. Two or more critical sectors, such as functions, products, services, markets, or geographical area, must be highly salient for goal accomplishment at the same time.

2. The need to perform uncertain, complex, and interdependent tasks must exist, so that a sizable information-processing capacity is required.

3. There must be a need to realize economies of scale by using limited human resources effectively.

Because of the complexity of the matrix structure and the major role and power conflicts that can occur, some organizations use horizontal linkages to achieve coordination and communication across departmental units.

HORIZONTAL LINKAGES

Horizontal linkages are methods employed by an organization to overcome the barriers found in the functional structure, such as lack of coordination and poor information flow. Although horizontal linkage mechanisms are usually not reflected in the firm's organization chart, they are nevertheless part of the organization's structure (Daft, 2007). Organizations can use any one or many of the following structural alternatives to improve horizontal coordination and information flow (Daft, 2007, pp. 95–99):

- *Information Systems:* Computerized information systems can enable managers or frontline workers throughout the organization to routinely exchange information about problems, opportunities, activities, or decisions (see Case Study 21–2).

- *Liaison Role:* An individual is located in one department, but has the responsibility for communicating and achieving coordination with another department.

- *Task Forces:* A temporary committee composed of representatives from each department affected by a problem (see Chapter 16, "Teams and Team Building")

- *Full-time Integrator:* The integrator is responsible for coordinating several departments but does not report to nor is assigned to one of the functional units. An integrator needs excellent interpersonal skills, because in most cases he or she has little authority but all the responsibility! (See Case 21–3.)

- *Teams:* Teams are used when activities among departments require coordination over a long period of time (see Chapter 16, "Teams and Team Building").

Case Study 21–2   Using Computerized Information Systems as a Horizontal Linkage

The following example illustrates how organizations can use computerized information systems as a structural alternative to improve horizontal coordination and information flow across departments or divisions.

In a recent study of 251 providers and 359 information technology members of the Healthcare Informatics Research Panel (Trends in Healthcare Financial Systems, Vendome Group, 2007), accurate charge data were noted as the most significant reimbursement challenge. For example, in an organization that chooses a registration system that is not truly integrated with its patient accounting application, patient financial services employees may need to correct a lot of bad data before they can submit claims. As such, providers are adopting a multipart strategy to address this challenge, including improving the front desk collection process as well as coding and documentation, and aligning charge capture at the point of care.

Charity Hospital's outpatient department receives a referral from a physician's office through its advance-revenue-cycle information technology system. The physician's office refers a patient using an online "scrip" system that transmits the patient's information directly to the hospital: demographic and insurance information; diagnosis code and text description; test, therapy, or treatment ordered; and preferred scheduling options.

Both the scheduling and registration systems are loaded with the information received from the physician's office. If diagnosis and clinical information are sufficient, medical necessity screening is automatically invoked. If insurance and demographic information is sufficient, real-time benefits and eligibility checks are also automatically launched.

In case of a diagnosis or procedure mismatch, or missing or incomplete information, this information is "worklisted" for exception-based follow-up. When benefits confirmation is received, corresponding registration data fields are updated automatically.

Master patient index matching is also invoked. When a match is obtained, the patient's electronic health record is activated and linked to the current episode of care. If there is no match, a set of workflow rules guides the registrar through the steps necessary to prevent the creation of a duplicate master patient index entry.

The scheduler or registrar then confirms the requested schedule online and reserves the treatment or examination room. Next, a pop-up box or worklist entry alerts the registrar that the Health Insurance Portability and Accountability Act (HIPAA) eligibility transaction has been received. Using advance connectivity software, the registrar confirms the patient's deductible, co-payment, and health savings account balance. Using the out-of-pocket estimator, the registrar then calculates the patient's portion of the total charges and communicates that information to the patient via telephone or secure e-mail.

Simultaneously, the system checks the patient's address, medical credit score, and prior payment history. If a concern is identified, the account is worklisted for a financial counselor to contact the patient.

When the patient arrives on the scheduled date, the registration system presents a previously scanned image of the patient's identification and insurance cards to the registrar, who then only has to compare the patient's cards with the stored images, updating them as necessary.

The patient e-signs all the necessary forms and the registrar collects the previously estimated out-of-pocket payment from the patient's health savings account. The patient then proceeds to the treatment location.

SOURCE: "Beyond bolt-ons: breakthroughs in revenue cycle information systems," by D. Hammer and D. Franklin, 2008. *hfm*, pp. 52–60. Copyright 2008 by the Healthcare Financial Management Association. Reprinted with permission.

Case Study 21–3 Clinical Nurse Leaders—Lateral Integrators of Care

A new nursing role—the clinical nurse leader, the first new nursing role advanced nationally in more than three decades—currently is under development in more than 180 pilot healthcare delivery sites across the United States and Puerto Rico.

The clinical nurse leader (CNL) is a master's-prepared nurse who assumes accountability for healthcare outcomes for a specific group of clients within a unit or setting. As such, CNL's role is that of a lateral integrator for the patient care unit. As the lateral integrator of care, the CNL's expected or emphasized core competencies are the ability to (1) communicate and collaborate with other members of the interdisciplinary healthcare team, (2) contribute to the assessment and reduction of risk, (3) manage and coordinate care at the microsystems level, and (4) use quality improvement methods.

The CNL acts as the lateral integrator of care by working with physicians and all other disciplines providing patient care services, such as social workers, respiratory therapists, nursing assistants, dietitians, pharmacists, and rehabilitation therapists. In this role, the CNL facilitates, coordinates, and oversees the care provided by the entire healthcare team for a specific group of clients within a unit.

In a hospital inpatient setting, the CNL would typically report to a nursing unit manager and be responsible for patients in a predetermined number of beds. In that situation, any formal authority of the CNL would be delegated by the unit manager.

SOURCE: "Opportunities for improving patient care through lateral integration: the clinical nurse leader," by J. W. Begun, J. Tornabeni, and K. R. White, 2006. *Journal of Healthcare Management, 51*(1), pp. 19–25. Copyright 2006 by the American College of Healthcare Executives. Reprinted with permission.

As previously mentioned, there is no one best way to structure an organization; however, most firms use one or more (i.e., hybrid) of the basic structures to achieve their goals. This is evident within the healthcare industry, where most organizations share great similarities regarding their structures. Why is this so? The answer may be found within the population ecology and institutional theories.

POPULATION ECOLOGY

Population ecology is a theory about the "survival of the fittest" in populations of organizations (Carroll & Hannan, 2000). A population is defined as a set of organizations engaged in similar activities with similar forms (i.e., technology, structure, products/services, goals, and personnel). Hannan and Freeman (1977, 1989) related that long-term change in the diversity of organizational forms within a population occurs through the selection process rather than adaptation because most organizations have structural inertia (i.e., tendency to maintain its internal structure regardless of other factors or concerns) that hinders adaptation when the environment changes. Hannan and Freeman argue that there are many limitations on the ability of organizations to change. The limitations come from substantial investment in facilities, equipment, and specialized personnel, limited information, established viewpoints of decision makers, the organization's own successful history that justifies current procedures, and the difficulty of changing corporate culture (Daft, 2007, p. 183). Because of these barriers, true transformation tends to be a rare and unlikely event for organizations (Hannan & Freeman, 1989).

Those organizations that are unable to adapt, and therefore become incompatible with the environment, are eventually replaced through competition with organizations that do meet the environment's demands (see Figure 21–4).

Stinchcombe (1965) noted that if two populations of organizations occupy the same market niche while differing in some organizational characteristic, the population with the less fit environmental characteristic will be eliminated.

As a result of the selection and retention process, organizational forms within a population become consistent over time. Consistency of form relates to legitimacy of an organization. Legitimacy is described by Suchman (1995, p. 574) as

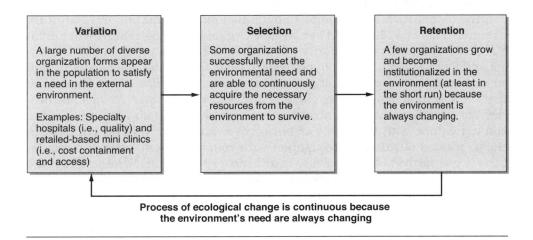

Process of ecological change is continuous because
the environment's need are always changing

Figure 21–4

"a generalized perception or assumption that the actions of an entity are desirable, proper or appropriate within some socially constructed system of norms, values, beliefs and definitions." The legitimacy of an organization is the focus of institutional theory. Although institutional theory differs from population ecology in the fact that institutional theory explores how organizations adapt to their environment and how population ecology theory examines the relationships of organizations to their environment from the selection perspective, both theories help to explain why healthcare organizations share structural-form similarities.

INSTITUTIONAL THEORY

DiMaggio and Powell (1983, p. 147) observed that "structural changes in organizations are less and less driven by competition and that bureaucratization and other forms of organizational change occur as the result of processes that make organizations more similar without necessarily making them more efficient." This process of "homogenization," referred to as institutional isomorphism, is described as the constraining process that forces one unit in a population to resemble other units that face the same set of environmental conditions. DiMaggio and Powell proposed that there are three mechanisms through which institutional isomorphism change occurs: coercive, mimetic, and normative.

Coercive isomorphism may result from pressure from other organizations on which a focal organization is dependent or it may be caused by the cultural expectations within the society where the organization functions. Perhaps more than any other type of business, it is external environmental forces that bring change to the healthcare industry. For example, the Leapfrog Group, a consortium of large employers, uses its collective purchasing power to require hospitals to implement certain standards relating to patient safety and quality-of-care issues; the largest purchasers of hospital services, federal and state governments, use their funding status to determine what medical services are provided to which patient groups in what settings (i.e., inpatient or outpatient); and regulators such as the Joint Commission on Accreditation of Healthcare Organizations and Medicare Peer Review Organizations determine what organizational and medical standards will be followed within the industry. DiMaggio and Powell (1983, p. 154) hypothesized that "the greater the dependence of an organization on another organization, the more similar it will become to that organization in structure, climate, and behavioral focus." As such, healthcare entities adapt their organizations to fit the needs of their funding agencies and regulators, with little time or resources available for innovation. Delbecq (1995) pointed out that preoccupation with reimbursement rules and regulations (e.g., reactiveness) may cause healthcare organizations to lose sight of the pervasiveness of the need for continuous change (e.g., proactiveness).

Mimetic isomorphism is a response to uncertainty. In situations in which a clear course of action is unavailable, organizations tend to model themselves after similar organizations in their field that they perceive to be more successful. Arndt and Bigelow (2000) state that in the case of hospitals, there is considerable uncertainty about technology (i.e., true impact on patients' health) and performance measures due to continuously changing laws and regulations that require providers not only to meet strict medical standards but also to provide proper care at all times to avoid liability actions. The more uncertain the relationship between means and ends, DiMaggio and Powell (1983, 154) hypothesized, "the greater the extent to which an organization will model itself after organizations it perceives to be successful. However, this modeling effect may cause a decrease in variation and diversity within the industry. As DiMaggio and Powell explain, "new entrants which could serve as sources of innovation and variation, will seek to overcome the liability of newness by imitating established practices within the field" (p. 156).

The third mechanism, normative isomorphism, is the result of professionalization, which includes two areas. First, members of professions receive similar training that socializes them into similar world views. Second, members of professions interact through professional and trade associations, which further diffuse ideas among them. The robustness of graduate health services administration programs is important for the development of organizational norms. Accreditation by the Commission on Accreditation Healthcare Management Education (CAHME) [formerly the Accrediting Commission on Education for Health Services Administration (ACEHSA)] assures that a program meets the standards developed by the profession and the health services industry. These standards are determined, in part, by CAHME's sponsoring organizations, which represent the healthcare industry's major professional trade associations and educational institutions. As such, the same standards influence the professional throughout his or her career (educational program followed by membership in professional associations). However, according to Hamel (1998) and Morrison (1999), this may lead to a lack of diversity in leadership and management. Hamel states "all too often . . . conversations become hard-wired over time, with the same people talking to the same people about the same issues year after year. After a while, individuals have little left to learn from each other" (p. 13).

Seizing opportunities involves change within an organization. Change can be problematic for mechanistic/bureaucratic/functional structured organizations because change requires new forms of coordination, information exchange, transfer of goods and services, and measurement (Stevenson & Jarrillo, 1986). But change is essential for survival. As Delbecq (1995, p. 1) points out,

> Healthcare organizations that will emerge as leaders within the industry will have incorporated not only radical changes to deal with new patterns of reimbursement, but also simultaneous changes in core medical services—changes that not only incorporate new technology, but also push down costs. They will also have to cope with radical changes in information and quality systems.

In 2001, the Institute of Medicine (IOM) made the following recommendations for revamping the nation's healthcare system to improve patient care:

- Healthcare providers, payers, policymakers, purchasers, and patients should commit to a national effort to raise healthcare quality to "unprecedented levels";

- Providers, patients, and payers should agree to a "redesign" of the processes by which care is delivered;
- The federal government should identify "priority conditions" that need to be addressed first and provide resources to "stimulate innovation" and "initiate the change process";
- Healthcare organizations should support fully the changes needed to improve care;
- Participants in the healthcare industry should foster an environment for change in healthcare delivery by creating an "infrastructure to support evidence-based practice," facilitating the use of information technology, and aligning "payment incentives" to encourage quality.

How can healthcare organizations drive this change process versus reacting to changes imposed by others? Hamel (1998) suggested that there are five areas an organization can develop to achieve strategy innovation, a term used to describe the capacity to reconstruct the existing industry model in ways that create new value for customers and produce new wealth for all stakeholders. The five areas identified are: (1) new voices, (2) new conversations, (3) new passions, (4) new perspectives, and (5) new experiments.

As noted by Hamel (1998), new voices provide previously underrepresented constituencies (e.g., young people, newcomers to the organization) a larger share of voice in the strategy creation process, making it a pluralistic process. Hamel explained that new conversations create dialogue across all organizational and industry boundaries. "Opportunities for new insights are created when one juxtaposes previously isolated knowledge in new ways" (Hamel, p. 13). New passions release individuals' deep sense of discovery to search for new wealth-creating strategies. Hamel suggested that individuals will eagerly embrace change when given the opportunity to participate in creating their organization's future. New perspectives allow individuals to reinvent their industry and their organization's capabilities by searching for new opportunities to fulfill environmental needs. Only by experimenting with new forms will organizations learn which ones satisfy the environment's needs.

One method used by organizations to adapt to their environment is by creating interorganizational relationships. Interorganizational relationships allow an entity to keep its core form but provide the organization with necessary resources and flexibility for adaptation.

INTERORGANIZATIONAL RELATIONSHIPS

Interorganizational relationships are resource transactions, flows, and linkages that occur among two or more organizations (Daft, 2007, p. 172). These relationships are strategies used by organizations to reduce their dependence on the environment and/or to share resources. Interorganizational relationships may be between or among organizations that provide similar services (i.e., horizontal integration) or between or among dissimilar but related organizations to provide a continuum of services (i.e., vertical integration). We will examine these relationships through resource dependency theory and the use of collaborative networks.

Resource Dependency Theory

Resource dependency theory states that all organizations exchange resources with the environment that are essential for their survival and that organizations will attempt to acquire these resources without creating dependencies (Pfeffer & Salancik, 1978). In other words, organizations seek to establish relationships with other organizations to obtain scarce resources by attempting to (1) minimize their own dependence on other organizations and/or (2) by increasing control over resources that maximize the dependence of other organizations on themselves (Ulrich & Barney, 1984). By achieving either or both of these outcomes, the organization increases its power with other organizations. The goal of resource dependency theory is for the organization to have sufficient power to influence the environment so that scarce resources are available to it (Pfeffer, 1981).

According to Pugh and Hickson (1996), the amount of dependence on a resource is based on two factors: (1) importance of the resource to the organization and (2) how much discretion or monopoly power those who control a resource have over its allocation and use. For example, hospitals need nurses for patient care and colleges and universities provide the education for Bachelor of Science in Nursing (BSN) degrees. As such, hospitals are dependent on higher education institutions for their current and future nursing workforce. Physicians control which hospital their patients will be admitted to for services. Hospitals need high occupancy rates to remain financially viable, so they are dependent on physicians to admit their patients to their facilities. Surgeons decide at which facility they will perform their surgical cases. Hospitals, as well as outpatient surgery centers, are dependent on surgeons for their essential resource, patients for surgery! On the basis of resource dependency, healthcare organizations will develop short-term and long-term strategies to address their dependency issues. For example, a hospital may use an outside agency to provide skilled nurses to cover its short-term shortages. This strategy would be cost prohibitive in the long run. As such, hospitals may offer scholarships to students pursuing their BSN degree in exchange for a work commitment after graduation. Some hospitals have provided funding for nursing faculty positions so more students could be admitted into the various nursing programs [i.e., Associate of Science in Nursing (ASN), BSN, Master of Science in Nursing (MSN)]. Others, such as Baptist Health South Florida (Baptist), have established, in partnership with a local college, an on-site nursing educational program. In 2001, Baptist capitalized on an opportunity to partner with a local college by helping the college manage the long waiting list for entrance of candidates into their nursing programs. The college faced the same challenges as many educational facilities across the nation—limited classroom space, too few faculty, and inadequate funding to meet these needs through their own campus resources. This initial partnership became the model for other future partnerships within the community for advanced nursing education (BSN and MSN) and demonstrated the presence of a strong outreach program between the community and Baptist. The on-site program provided classroom space on the hospital's campus, adjunct faculty that were Baptist nurse employees, and funding, thereby allowing an additional 90 students annually to enter the program. These students received full scholarships and stipends while they attended the nursing program on the Baptist Hospital campus, completed their clinical rotations at a Baptist facility, and received faculty support from incumbent employees. Once they completed their program, these nurses were given preferential employment opportunities. In less than three years, the number of newly graduated nurses hired per year by Baptist increased from approximately 80 nurses in 2000 to 136 nurses in 2003 (see www.baptisthealth.net).

As previously noted, the goal of resource dependency theory is for the organization to have sufficient power to influence the environment so that scarce resources are available for it. That is exactly what Baptist achieved! By having the on-site nursing program, it influenced its environment and now has a direct source of future nurse employees. In addition, by providing classroom space, adjunct faculty, and funding for other full-time faculty positions, the local college has increased its dependence on Baptist! Resource dependency can create win–win opportunities for all parties, as reflected with the Baptist and local college partnership. Collaboration is another interorganizational relationship that can create win–win opportunities.

Collaborative Networks

Collaborative networks are organizations that join together to become more competitive and to share scarce resources. For example, in 1994, a group of community health centers (CHCs) discovered that by linking together and creating a network they could receive the advantages and expertise of a large health system while remaining independent. This unique and powerful alliance, Health Choice Network (HCN), is a national model of a successful collaboration among 33 CHCs and one of several Health Resources and Services Administration (HRSA)–sponsored health center–controlled networks. HCN's mission is to provide high-quality service, support, and expertise to its member organizations and to act as a vehicle for strategic efforts that strengthen its community member partners. The shared functions integrated through the network are: finance; information technology, including electronic health records; clinical support, including disease management programs; and managed care contracting. In today's healthcare environment of cost containment, reduced reimbursement, and advancing technologies, collaborative networks are becoming more common as organizations attempt to remain competitive in their environments.

Co-opetition

A relatively new concept that has emerged in the healthcare industry is co-opetition, which refers to alliances formed between competitors. The term "co-opetition" is used to describe the relationship when organizations are competing against and cooperating with each other simultaneously. Although relatively new to healthcare, the practice of co-opetition has been quite common in other industries. For example, U.S. milk producers and distributors who compete with each other over various brands in milk and dairy products launched a joint advertising campaign "Got Milk?" Their goal was to reestablish milk as a primary source of nutrition and breakfast food in an effort to fight the pressure of substitution from other nondiary and breakfast foods. As such, these "co-opeting" alliances are not only used to extend or complement each organization's capabilities, but also to eliminate potential threats to the "partners" (Chalhoub, 2007).

According to Ernest and Young (2004), co-opetition is one of the more powerful trends driving change in the industry. This is illustrated by the following scenario:

> Hospital A and Hospital B are competitors in the area. Each has 50 percent of the inpatient cardiology market, and each has a group of dedicated cardiologists who compete against the others to provide outpatient cardiology imaging services.[1] To ease this competition, Hospital A and its cardiology group joint ventures with an outpatient center that has new cardiac CT/MRI equipment. This equipment streamlines the work of cardiologists by allowing on-the-spot reading of the imaging so that more tests can be ordered if needed. As such, the center provides convenience for patients and their families. This patient-centered approach shifts business from Hospital B and other service providers in the area. Although Hospital A and its cardiologists still compete on providing echocardiograms, they are generally ahead of others because of the inpatient and outpatient business they pull in from their co-opetition (LeTourneau, 2004, p. 82).

Co-opetition is multifaceted in terms of what it means to hospitals today (see Case Study 21–4). The key to effective co-opetition is mutual trust among the partners. If it is approached with open communication and awareness of a larger context, it can represent win–win opportunities for all involved parties.

Case Study 21–4 Partnerships: Rx for Hospitals

As hospitals search for ways to cut costs and improve efficiency, many are looking to combine efforts. Already this month, two pairs of Metro Detroit hospitals reached affiliation agreements.

After more than a year of negotiations, Pontiac hospitals St. Joseph Mercy Oakland and North Oakland Medical Centers (NOMC) announced a formal affiliation. Details have yet to be ironed out, but the two hospitals agreed to combine services and facilities, which will save money and add purchasing clout.

One day after that announcement, Botsford Hospital in Farmington Hills and Sinai Grace Hospital in Detroit announced they also had reached an agreement on physician training. The affiliation allows Detroit Medical Center–owned Sinai Grace and independent Botsford to share federal funds for postgraduate training positions.

"Part of our mission always has been medical education," Botsford President and CEO Paul LaCasse said. "(The affiliation) does fulfill that portion of our mission that talks about supporting osteopathic medical education and the education of young physicians in the state."

---

[1]In recent years, hospital physicians have been building their own freestanding outpatient surgery or diagnostic centers. Services offered at these centers compete with the hospitals' most lucrative businesses, and because most physician businesses only deal with people who have health insurance, they do not help relieve hospitals from uninsured/underinsured patient loads.

The announcements come at a time when established Metro Detroit hospitals are bracing for increased competition from new ones that are set to open soon. "It's this weird world of hospitals where you see both collaboration and competition," said Alwyn Cassil, a spokeswoman for Washington, DC–based Center for Studying Health System Change.

The effectiveness of an affiliation, she said, often depends on whether the individual hospital leaders can share a common vision. "(Success) depends on what the ground rules are, how certain the leadership is in going in this direction and how committed they are to making it work," she said. "Oftentimes, things come down to personalities and personal relationships."

The Botsford–Sinai Grace agreement began July 1 and will be reviewed each year. The two hospitals are working to develop specific details and programs, LaCasse said, to be implemented next July. But both sides are on the same page, he said.

"We will spend the next couple months determining which programs would be good to establish and grow in a collaborative fashion," LaCasse said. It's too soon to predict how the affiliation will play out, LaCasse said, but it could result in training more than 20 additional primary care physicians each year—a growing need in Southeast Michigan, because more physicians are choosing specialty paths. "We both had the same objective and that is to advance osteopathic medical education and fulfill a need in the community," LaCasse said. "There is a physician shortage that will only get worse. This affiliation allows us to train primary care specialists."

The Botsford-Sinai Grace affiliation came together quickly—after just two months of discussions, LaCasse said. But the Pontiac hospital discussions have been more complicated.

Novi-based Trinity Health, the nation's fourth-largest Catholic health-care system, owns St. Joseph Mercy Oakland, a consistently profitable hospital. NOMC, which has lost money since 1999, is independent.

Discussions between those two hospitals—which, at one point, also included POH Medical Center in Pontiac—were broader and perhaps more imperative than the Botsford–Sinai Grace talks. With new suburban hospitals set to open, many healthcare experts have said Pontiac's hospitals must work together to survive. That group includes St. Joseph President and CEO Jack Weiner.

"My belief is the best interest of the people of Pontiac would be for the three hospitals to come together," Weiner said in May. "As a healthcare executive who took an oath to serve the community, I would feel very bad if I can't accomplish what should happen for the community."

Although POH is absent from the affiliation, Weiner has achieved part of his goal.

NOMC will close its neonatal intensive care and pediatrics units and let St. Joseph handle child deliveries. NOMC will open a 40-bed acute care unit for patients whose needs fit neither a hospital nor nursing home.

It's a necessary step to assure NOMC's viability, President and CEO John Graham said.

"We believe it will be more beneficial to the community to collaborate rather than compete," he said. "We are excited to work with a large multistate health system to drive economics of scale, and to have access to clinical and administrative services and expertise in addition to educational resources."

St. Joseph is a 428-bed hospital, while NOMC has 366 beds. Botsford has 330 beds, and Sinai Grace 404.

Source: "Partnerships: Rx for hospitals," by J. Briggs, August 9, 2007. *Oakland Business Review*. Reprinted with permission.

SUMMARY

In this chapter, four basic structure configurations were presented as a conceptual framework that managers can use to understand how structures emerge, and how and why they change over time. In Chapter 22, we will narrow our focus to an organization's internal characteristics or design parameters. These characteristics, such as formalization, specialization, and centralization, interact with and are reflective of the contextual dimension of the organization.

It is when these various characteristics are clustered together that the organization's overall structure is formed.

END-OF-CHAPTER QUESTIONS

1. Describe how each element of the contextual dimension relates to an organization's structure.
2. Discuss the differences between mechanistic and organic systems.
3. Discuss the advantages and disadvantages of the four basic organization structures.
4. Describe the importance of the various horizontal linkage mechanisms, and discuss when each one would be used within an organization's structure.
5. Describe population ecology and how it differs from institutional theory.
6. Describe the three mechanisms associated with institutional isomorphism and how each one affects organizations' homogeneity.
7. Discuss the various strategies organizations use to develop and sustain interorganizational relationships.

END-OF-CHAPTER EXERCISE

Create an Organizational Chart

Jackson Health System (JHS) of the Miami–Dade County Public Health Trust is a complex, vertically and horizontally integrated academic and tertiary healthcare system.

In March 2004, JHS faced a dire situation. Net income losses increased almost tenfold between 2001 and 2004, with the system reporting losses of $7.4 million in FY02, $47.4 million in FY03, and $85.2 million in FY04. JHS's downward financial spiral was caused by a number of factors, one being its organizational flaws. JHS's operations and infrastructure were in disarray. Like many healthcare organizations, JHS had evolved into a complex structure with layered management across numerous corporate entities, businesses, and cost centers.

JHS knew it had to radically transform operations if it was to continue to fulfill its mission to deliver value to its customers through a combination of service excellence and financial strength. A massive operational and financial overhaul was needed, and the result was "reCreate Jackson."*

Visit Jackson Health System's Web site at http://www.jhsmiami.org/. Using information found on the Web site, (i.e., executive member team, annual

---

*For an overview of the "recreate Jackson" project, see M. O'Quinn and K. C. Mulqueen (July 2007). "Recreate Jackson," a turn around tale, *hfm*, pp. 82–87.

report, facilities, etc.) construct JHS's organizational chart through the vice president level.

In groups, compare each member's organizational chart. Discuss the similarities or dissimilarities of each member's organizational chart.

END-OF-CHAPTER CASE STUDIES

Case Study 21–5 Bayer AG of Germany

Bayer AG of Germany—the company best known in the United States for its Bayer aspirin products—is one of the largest and oldest chemical and healthcare products companies in the world. Because of massive sales gains and increased activity overseas in the early 1980s, Bayer announced a reorganization in 1984. Bayer had been successful with a conventional organizational structure that was departmentalized by function.

However, in response to new conditions the company wanted to create a structure that would allow it to achieve three primary goals: (1) shift management control from the then-West German parent company to its foreign divisions and subsidiaries; (2) restructure its business divisions to more clearly define their duties; and (3) flatten the organization, or empower lower-level managers to assume more responsibility, so that top executives would have more time to plan strategy.

Bayer selected a relatively diverse matrix management format to pursue its goals. It delineated all of its business activities into six groups under an umbrella company called Bayer World. Within each of the six groups were several subgroups made up of product categories such as dyestuffs, fibers, or chemicals. Likewise, each of its administrative and service functions were regrouped under Bayer World into one of several functions, such as human resources, marketing, plant administration, or finance. Furthermore, top managers who had formally headed functional groups were given authority over separate geographic regions, which, like the product groups, were supported by and entwined with the functional groups. The net effect of the reorganization was that the original nine functional departments were broken down into 19 multidisciplinary, interconnected business groups.

After only one year of operation, Bayer management lauded the new matrix structure as a resounding success. Not only did matrix management allow the company to move toward its primary goals, but it also had the added benefits of increasing its responsiveness to change and emerging opportunities, and of helping Bayer to streamline plant administration and service division activities.

Bayer AG of Germany's reorganization occurred in the early 1980s. Research the company and determine whether the organization's continues to operate under a matrix structure. If yes, what if any structural changes have occurred in the past 20 years? If no, what organizational structure does the company currently use and why?

SOURCE: Bayer AG, *Encyclopedia of Business* (2nd ed.)—*Man-Mix*. Retrieved May 27, 2008, from the *Advameg Inc.* Web site: http://www.referenceforbusiness.com/encyclopedia/Man-Mix/Matrix-Management-and-Structure.html

Case Study 21–6 Organizational Structure: A Driver of Performance

Would you build a house without laying a foundation? The result would be four walls lacking any grounding and with little stability. Similarly, it is impossible to build a high-performing organization without first constructing a strategy. Nonetheless, across all industries, less than 10 percent of strategic plans are executed and realized. How can this happen if the primary responsibility of management is to develop and execute strategies that will help the enterprise realize its vision and mission?

Hospitals that *do* successfully execute strategies share a key common element: an organizational structure that insists upon clear role focus, fosters accountability, and requires manageable spans of control. Moreover, high-performing hospitals and healthcare systems design their management structures to execute strategies. They consider organizational structure as they would any other resource (e.g., capital, workforce, physicians) and deploy it according to the strategic needs of the company. In short, hospital strategies should not just inform organizational structure, but should determine it.

One of the most performance-driven healthcare companies in America today utilizes this approach to organizational design. Several years ago, executives at this large healthcare system realized that their ambulatory strategies were not keeping pace with market demands. Accordingly, a single corporate position was created with responsibility for outpatient services at all of the system's hospitals. This new job, and the new structure, was born out of strategic need and focused accountability. The result was an enhanced focus on outpatient development, streamlined outpatient decision-making processes, and, ultimately, improved hospital ambulatory services performance.

Considerations in Restructuring Your Organization

Look at your current organizational structure. Assess your strategic initiatives and how you will execute your plans on the basis of the current decision-making structures and accountabilities. Such an assessment will encompass an analysis of management requirements and should include a review of the following focal points:

- Strategic plan.
- Organizational control structure.
- Management responsibilities.
- Physician leadership.

An example of an organization that has employed this form-follows-function approach is St. Joseph Hospital.

Strategic Plan

St. Joseph's strategic plan includes three major initiatives:

- Develop cancer, cardiac services, and neurosciences as distinctive, market-leading service lines.
- Expand the outpatient strategy to include new facilities in two markets within St. Joseph's primary service area.
- Significantly upgrade quality and patient safety throughout St. Joseph's facilities.

These initiatives are fairly typical for metropolitan tertiary hospitals; what distinguishes high-performing organizations, however, is successful execution—and the structure that enables it.

Control Structure

Control structures need to encompass patient care functions, patient care support functions, and administrative support functions. The way these functions are aligned varies dramatically between organizations and defines both culture and accountabilities within the hospital. At St. Joseph Hospital, leadership responded to a change in the hospital's strategic plans by also revising the control structure. The new, revised strategy shifted the hospital's major spheres of organizational responsibility, prompting a leadership structure that was reflective of the institution's goals:

- An outpatient executive dedicated to the growth of outpatient centers, with line accountability for staff in the outpatient areas.
- A service line dyad for each major program that links a clinical director with a physician leader. The dyad is accountable for service line development and profitability.
- A clinical quality structure headed by the Chief Medical Officer with direct oversight and reporting from clinical quality and patient safety personnel.

In the traditional environment, the control structure is organized in a purely functional way that does not respond to the business of healthcare: the provision of high-quality care within a service line. Patients do not seek nursing services, radiology, or physical therapy or the other traditional departments within a hospital. Instead, they want care to treat their heart condition, cancer, or other illness or injury. In the traditional departmental control structure, it is difficult to implement service line strategies that bridge multiple departments because there is not a direct line of accountability between the service line director and the department managers. The department managers are held accountable for the performance of their department, rather than the performance and growth of the service line, leading to competing priorities.

This structure creates a "silo" mentality that optimizes performance within narrowly focused units but in which a patient and physician perspective is disconnected, inconvenient, and confusing. These service lines (e.g., cancer, heart, and so forth) should represent the new control structure of your hospital, since they ultimately drive hospital performance. High-performing organizations look to service line or discrete clinical program areas to help define the control structure (organizational reporting and hierarchy structure) of their hospital.

In Figure 21–5, a traditional hospital organizational structure is compared to that same organization that adapted its structure to implement its key strategies:

Managerial roles within hospitals rarely change following development of a new strategy such as a shift to a service line focus. This stagnancy is counterproductive: As you implement key strategies around growth, clinical services, quality, and safety, the control structure of your organization must change to reflect your strategies. One of the biggest complaints that physicians, staff, and managers make about hospital leadership is the slow pace of decision making. This is probably a symptom of larger control structure issues. If your control structure does not reflect your strategy, you are probably suffering from an inefficient decision-making process involving too many sign-offs.

A leadership structure for an oncology service line is presented in Figure 21–6 as an example of a service line leadership group. This group makes the key decisions for the service line, and their reporting relationships are depicted in the multidisciplinary executive-level organizational chart.

Management Responsibilities

Management responsibilities include those functions that must be regularly executed; these responsibilities vary according to the control structure. There are administrative management (staff) functions required by all control centers and additional responsibilities related to the management of patient care (line management) functions. Building on our example of St. Joseph's, a management structure might include site administrators for each ambulatory site and functional managers within each service line (for example, cath lab manager reporting to the cardiac dyad, radiation therapy reporting to the cancer dyad, and so forth).

Management responsibilities should be determined on the basis of your strategy and plan for execution through the modified control structure.

Physician Leadership

Just as the administrative organizational structure must reflect strategic objectives, so must the physician leadership structure. In many academic organizations, there are formal physician leadership structures (e.g., department chairs, service or section chiefs) that include employed physicians rather than traditional elected members of the medical staff. If you are contemplating a service line initiative, you must adapt your physician leadership structure to accommodate different responsibilities and objectives.

Strong physician leaders from a range of clinical areas within the service line are critical to driving change and engendering support from the medical staff. If you are committed to effective, service line–based management, hiring a medical director for each major line may be a logical step to ensuring credibility with affected physicians and accelerating service line development. You should also consider a management or advisory role for nonemployed physicians.

Engineering a Structure Built for Success

Good leaders do not put their employees in a position where they are destined to fail. Success requires clear lines of authority and accountability, and those in authority need the right tools to meet performance expectations. Some organizations have created a "matrix" service line management structure, appointing a vice president of a clinical service without formal line authority or control

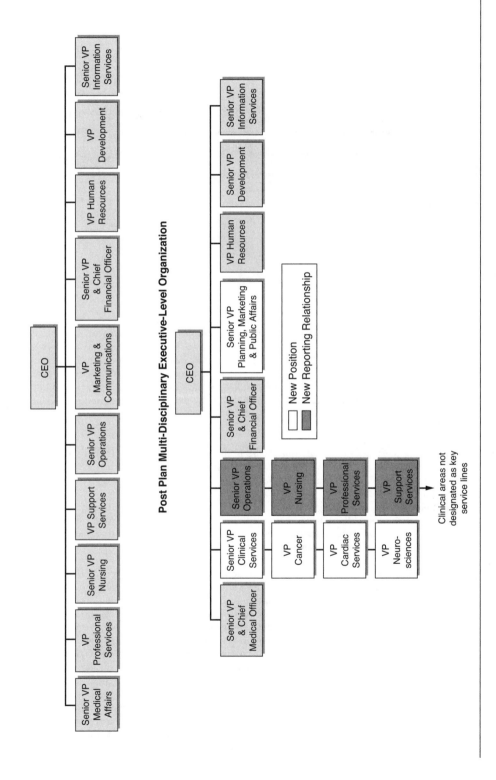

Post Plan Multi-Disciplinary Executive-Level Organization

Figure 21–5 Traditional Functional Executive-level Organization

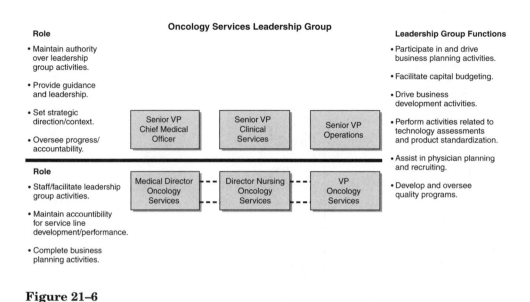

Figure 21–6

over the deployment of resources. Others have created mixed models, where the head of a service line may have direct control over functions that directly relate to the service (e.g., radiation oncology reports to cancer and the cath lab to cardiology) but indirect influence over shared services (such as radiology or inpatient care). This influence often comes in the form of operational councils or committees where multiple users of these services have an opportunity to explain their needs and priorities. While either structure can work, keep in mind that the leader is more likely to succeed if there is greater control—and thus, accountability—for the resources and the performance of those resources within that service line.

Lessons Learned

Strategic planning does not end when the report is finalized; it must also include a revised organizational structure. If you aren't willing to take the time to reconsider and assess your management structure as you explore your strategic direction, then don't waste your resources on strategy development.

Implementation of changes in organizational structure, reporting relationships, span of control, and role focus requires a thoughtful, measured, and sensitive approach. And you must be prepared for the effect of changing individuals' jobs and responsibilities. As your organizational structure changes, some of your managers will feel disenfranchised and perhaps move on to other opportunities.

This raises a tough question. Do you design the structure and jobs around your valued people, or design the structure and positions with a focus on performance and then assign the right people to those roles? The right answer is a combination of both. Performance-driven organizations employ talented and effective managers in roles that foster accountability and decision making to achieve the organization's strategic goals. They leverage the talent they currently have, but do not design important roles around the strengths, weaknesses, and/or desires of managers. You also need to recognize instances in which your current resources lack the appropriate seasoning or skill set to fill the positions and when it is necessary to make a strategic hire.

Having the right people in the right roles is a critical step, but you must cement changes in your organizational structure by tasking your management team with developing business and operating plans under the new rubric. For example, when migrating to a service line structure, require that the service line management team develop a business plan to hardwire the new strategy and structure and provide a canvas upon which the new team can paint the future. The process of drafting and revising a business plan will help the management group not only refine its focus, but also begin working as a team.

Discuss

1. How organizational structure impacts performance of new strategies;
2. Key considerations when redesigning your management structure;
3. Effective service line management and leadership structures;
4. How to "hardwire" new reporting relationships.

SOURCE: ECG Management Consultants, Inc. Copyright 2007 by ECG Management Consultants, Inc. Reprinted with permission.

REFERENCES

Arndt, M., & Bigelow, B. (2000). The transfer of business practices into hospitals: history and implications. In J. D. Blair, M. D. Fottler, & G. T. Savage (Eds.) *Advances in Health Care Management: Vol. 1*, pp. 339–368. New York: JAI/Elsevier Science.

Bayer AG of Germany (2007). Encyclopedia of Business (2nd ed.). Farmington, MI: Thomson Gale.

Begun, J. W., Tornabeni, J., & White, K. R. (2006). Opportunities for improving patient care through lateral integration: The clinical nurse leader. *Journal of Healthcare Management, 51*(1), 19–25.

Blau, P. M. (1968). The hierarchy of authority in organizations. *American Journal of Sociology, 73*, 453–467.

Briggs, J. (2007, August). Partnerships: Rx for hospitals. *Oakland Business Review*.

Burns, T., & Stalker, G. M. (1961). *The management of innovation: Strategy, structure, and managerial skill.* New York: Free Press.

Burns, T., & Stalker, G. M. (1994). *The management of innovation: Strategy, structure, and managerial skill.* London: Oxford University Press.

Burton, R. M., DeSanctis, G., & Obel, B. (2006). *Organizational design: a step-by-step approach.* New York: Cambridge University Press.

Chalhoub, M. S. (2007). A framework in strategy and competition using alliances: Application to the automotive industry. *International Journal of Organization Theory and Behavior, 10*(2), 151–183.

Carroll, G. R., & Hannan, M. T. (2000). *The demography of corporations and industries.* Princeton, NJ: Princeton University Press.

Daft, R .L. (2007). *Organization theory and design* (9th ed). Mason, OH: Thomson South-Western.

Delbecq, A. L. (1995). The hidden competitive weapon supporting innovation in health care. *Physician Executive, 21*, 18–23.

DiMaggio, P. J., & Powell, W. W. (1983). The iron cage revisited: Institutional isomorphism and collective rationality in organizational fields. *American Sociological Review, 48*, 147–160.

ECG Management Consultants, Inc. (2007). The strategic imperative of adapting the hospital's management structure. Available at: http://www.ecgmc.com/ insights_ideas/pdfs/IN_Adapting_Hospitals_Management_Structure.pdf.

Ernest & Young, LLP. (2004). Practical governance: Co-opetition—The new governance challenge. Available at: http://chairmanssociety.org/images/PG_ 2004.pdf.

Galloro, V. (2005, October). HCA tries to think small: company to reorganize hospitals into three groups. *Modern Healthcare*, p. 12.

Green, G. (2000). Clinical service lines bring patients into focus. *Nursing Management, 31*, 3, 40–43.

Hamel, G. (1998). Strategy innovation and the quest for value. *Sloan Management Review, 39*, 7–14.

Hannan, M. T., & Freeman, J. (1977). The population ecology of organizations. *The American Journal of Sociology, 82*(5), 929–964.

Hannan, M. T., & Freeman, J. (1989). *Organizational ecology* (pp. 3–27). Cambridge, MA: Harvard University Press.

Health Choice Network (2008). http://www.hcnetwork.org/.

Institute of Medicine (2001). *Crossing the quality chasm: A new health system for the 21st century*. Committee on Quality of Health Care in America, Institute of Medicine. Washington, DC: National Academy Press.

Kast, F. E., & Rosenzweig, J. E. (1985). *Organization and management: A systems and contingency approach*. New York: McGraw-Hill Book Company.

Kimberly, J. (1976). Organizational size and the structuralist perspective: A review, critique and proposal. *Administrative Science Quarterly, 21*, 571–597.

Lawrence, P., & Lorsch, J. (1967). *Organization and environment*. Homewood, IL: Irwin.

LeTourneau, B. (2004). Co-opetition: An alternative to competition. *Journal of Healthcare Management, 49*(2), 81–83.

Miles, R. E., & Snow, C. C. (1978). *Organizational strategy, structure, and process*. New York: McGraw-Hill Book Company.

Miner, J. B. (2002). *Organizational behavior: Foundations, theories and analysis*. New York: Oxford University Press.

Mintzberg, H. (1979). *The structuring of organizations*. Englewood Cliffs, NJ: Prentice Hall.

Morrison, I. (1999). Leadership and white space: The struggle for strategy innovation in healthcare. *Health Forum Journal, 42*, 18–25.

O'Quinn, M., & Mulqueen, K. C. (2007). "Recreate Jackson," a turn around tale. *hfm*, 82–87.

Perrow, C. (1967). A framework for the comparative analysis of organizations. *American Sociological Review, 32*, 194–208.

Pfeffer, J (1981). *Power in organizations*. Marshfield, MA: Pitman Publishers.

Pfeffer, J., & Salancik, G. (1978). *The external control of organizations: a resource dependence perspective*. New York: Harper & Row.

Pugh, D. S., Hickson, D. J., Hinings, C. R., Lupton, K. M., McDonald, K. M., Turner, C., et al. (1963). A conceptual scheme for organizational analysis. *Administrative Science Quarterly, 8*, 289–315.

Pugh, D. S., Hickson, D. J., Hinings, C. R., Turner, C., & Lupton, T. (1968). Dimensions of organizational structure. *Administrative Science Quarterly, 13*, 65–105.

Pugh, D. S., & Hickson, D. J. (1996). *Writers on organizations*. Thousand Oaks, CA: Sage Publisher.

Scott, W. R., & Davis, G.F. (2006). *Organizations and organizing: Rational, natural and open systems perspectives*. Upper Saddle River, NJ: Prentice Hall.

Stevenson, H. H., & Jarrillo, J. C. (1986). Preserving entrepreneurship as companies grow. *Journal of Business Strategy, 7,* 10–23.

Stinchcombe, A. L. (1965). Social structure and organizations. In J. G. March (Ed.), *Handbook Organizations* (pp. 142–193). Chicago, IL: Rand McNally.

Suchman, M. C. (1995). Managing legitimacy: strategic and institutional approaches. *Academy of Management Review, 20,* 571–610.

Ulrich, D., & Barney, J. B. (1984). Perspectives in organizations: Resource dependence, efficiency, and population. *Academy of Management Review, 9*(3), 471–481.

Woodward, J. (1965). *Industrial organization: Theory and practice.* London: Oxford University Press.

OTHER SUGGESTED READINGS

Boblitz, M. C., & Thompson, J. M. (2005). Assessing the feasibility of developing centers of excellence: six initial steps. *hfm,* 72–84.

Borkowski, N., & Gordon, J. (2006). Entrepreneurial organizations: The driving force for improving quality in the healthcare industry. *Journal of Health and Human Services Administration, 28*(40), 531–549.

Burns, L.R. (1989). Matrix management in hospitals: Testing theories of matrix structure and development. *Administrative Science Quarterly, 34*(3), 349–368.

Hall, R. H. (1996). *Organizations: structures, processes, and outcomes* (6th ed.). Englewood Cliffs, NJ: Prentice Hall.

Kaplan, R. S., & Norton, D. P. (2006). How to implement a new strategy without disrupting your organization. *Harvard Business Review 84,* 3.

Miller, D., & Friedson, P. H. (1980). Momentum and revolution in organizational adaptation. *Academy of Management Journal, 23*(4), 591–614.

Perrow, C. (1986). *Complex organizations: A critical essay* (3rd ed.). New York: Random House.

Ruef, M., & Scott, R. S. (1998). A multidimensional model of organizational legitimacy: Hospital survival in changing institutional environments. *Administrative Science Quarterly, 43*(4), 877–904.

Scott, R. W., Ruef, N., Mendel, P. J., & Caroma, C. A. (2000). *Institutional change and healthcare organizations: From professional dominance to managed care.* Chicago, IL: University of Chicago Press.

CHAPTER 22

Organization Design Parameters: Internal Characteristics

Nancy Borkowski, DBA, CPA, FACHE

LEARNING OUTCOMES

After completing this chapter, the student should understand:

- ☞ The five organizational parts of an organization as described by Mintzberg.
- ☞ How the five organizational parts relate to the simple, machine bureaucracy, professional bureaucracy, divisional, and adhocracy structural configurations.
- ☞ The importance of communication to the coordination and control of organizational activities.
- ☞ How each element of the structural dimension relates to organization design.

OVERVIEW

> The core issue [of the quality chasm in health care] is fragmentation, and the solution lies in forms of assembly and cooperation that the prevailing structures in health care cannot achieve. Disciplines divide from disciplines, organizations from organizations, events from events. Patients cross over these boundaries time and again, and their needs get lost in the disorder—DAVID BERWICK (2002).

Burton, DeSanctis, and Obel (2006) describe an organization's complexity as the property or characteristic of its structure based on the breakdown of subunits by two dimensions: vertical differentiation and horizontal differentiation. "It is the height and width of the organization's hierarchy. The vertical differentiation reflects the depth of the hierarchy—top to bottom—and the horizontal differentiation refers to the degree of task specialization across the hierarchy" (p. 69). In Chapter 21, we examined the organization and the factors that affect its overall structure (i.e., vertical differentiation). Now we will focus on the formal division of the organization into subunits (i.e., horizontal differentiation) based on various parameters. These parameters are shaped by the following questions (Mintzberg, 1979, p. 66):

1. How many tasks should a given position in the organization contain, and how specialized should each task be?
2. To what extent should the work content of each position be standardized?
3. What skills and knowledge should be required for each position?
4. On what basis should positions be grouped into units and units into larger units?
5. How large should each unit be, and how many individuals should report to a given manager?

6. To what extent should the output of each position or unit be standardized?
7. What mechanisms should be established to facilitate mutual adjustment among positions and units?
8. How much decision-making power should be delegated to the managers of line units down the chain of command?
9. How much decision-making power should pass from the line managers to the staff specialists and operators?

The preceding questions or parameters relate to the basic issues of structure design. Daft (2007) organizes these questions into the structural dimension of organizational design (see Table 22–1). These design parameters, or "internal characteristics," create the basis for an organization's structure.

The design parameters determine how the various parts of an organization will be organized to coordinate and control the entity's activities. In his seminal work on organizational structures, Mintzberg (1979), one of the leading scholars in organization theory, breaks down organizations into five basic but interrelated parts: (1) strategic apex, (2) middle line (i.e., middle management), (3) operating core, (4) technostructure, and (5) support staff (see Figure 22–1 and Exhibit 22–1).

Table 22–1 Structural Dimension of Organization Design

Dimension or Parameter	Description
Formalization	The amount of written documentation in the organization. Documentation includes procedures, job descriptions, regulations, and policy manuals.
Specialization	The degree to which organizational tasks are subdivided into separate jobs (also referred to as the division of labor). If specialization is high, each employee performs a narrow range of tasks. If specialization is low, each employee performs a wider range of tasks in their job (i.e., job enlargement).
Hierarchy of authority	This is also referred to as span of control and describes (1) who reports to whom and (2) the number of employees reporting to a supervisor. When spans of control are narrow, the hierarchy will be tall, and when spans of control are wide, the hierarchy will be shorter.
Centralization	The decision-making position or level in the hierarchy. If decision making is at the top of the hierarchy, the organization reflects centralized decision making; when decision making is delegated to lower hierarchy levels, it is referred to as decentralized decision making.
Professionalism	The level (or average number of years) of formal education and training of employees.

SOURCE: *Organization theory and design* (9th ed., pp. 17–18, 20), by R. L. Daft, 2007. Mason, OH: Thomson South-western. Adapted with permission.

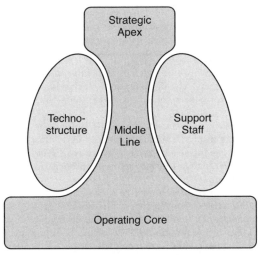

The Five Basic Parts of Organization

Figure 22–1 The Five Basic Parts of Organization
SOURCE: *The structure of organizations* (1979) by H. Mintzberg. Englewood Cliffs, NJ:
Prentice Hall. Reprinted with permission.

On the basis of varying configurations of the five basic parts of an organization, Mintzberg states that most (if not all) entities will fall into one of five structural designs (see Figure 22–2). Table 22–2 details the key dimensions of Mintzberg's five structural configurations and how each one relates to the five basic parts of organizations.

The five organizational parts allows managers to better understand the complexity of and the interrelationships between the subsystems within an organization. How the five organizational parts form is based on the company's environment, mission, size, and so on, as well as its requirements to coordinate and control its activities to accomplish its goals.

Proper use of communication forms and methods by managers is essential for the coordination and control of an organization's activities. Communication activity and frequency increase as activity and/or task variety increase. As discussed in Chapter 4, the form, method, and direction of communication changes depending on if the manager is dealing with routine activities and/or tasks (vertical communication) or nonroutine activities and/or tasks (horizontal communication). To better understand the importance of proper communication, let's examine the increasing need and direction for communication when interdependence between or among departments regarding an organization's workflow exists. Interdependence refers to the extent that organizational units depend on one another for resources or materials to accomplish their tasks. There are three types of interdependence: pooled (minimal), sequential (medium), and reciprocal (high) (Thompson, 1967). Pooled interdependence means that each organizational unit is relatively independent because work does not flow between or among units. With pooled interdependence, there is a low need for coordination, with most of it

---

Exhibit 22–1 Five Basic Parts of Organizations

The *strategic apex* is what we would refer to as "senior management." Senior managers are responsible for ensuring that the organization effectively serves its mission, serve the needs of the organization's various stakeholders, and manage the organization's relationships with its environment.

The *middle line or middle management* is the chain linking the strategic apex to the operating core. This chain runs from the senior managers just below the strategic apex to the first-line supervisors (e.g., the nurse supervisor), who have direct authority/supervision over the operating-core members. In general, this chain of authority is scalar; that is, it runs in a single line from top to bottom.

The *operating core* is the heart of every organization, the part that produces the essential outputs that keep it alive. The operating core of the organization encompasses those members who perform the basic work related directly to the production of services and products. The members perform four prime functions: (1) securing the inputs for production; (2) transforming the inputs into outputs; (3) distributing the outputs that result from the transformation process; and (4) providing direct support to the input, transformation, and output functions.

The *technostructure* includes the staff that serves the organization by affecting the work of others. These employees design the systems by which work processes and outputs are standardized in the organization. Technostructure employees are removed from the operating work flow—they may design it, plan it, change it, or train the people who do it, but they do not do it themselves. As such, technostructure employees spend a good deal of their time in informal communication.

An organization's *support staff* comprises those employees who perform support services to the organization outside of its operating workflow, such as public relations and legal counsel. Although an organization can outsource many of these functions, the existence of support staff reflects the organization's attempt to encompass more boundary activities in order to reduce uncertainty and to control its own affairs.

The structuring of organizations, by H. Mintzberg, 1979. Englewood Cliffs, NJ: Prentice Hall. Adapted with permission.

---

being accomplished by standardizing activities. Since there is a low need for coordination, communication between units is minimal with formalized rules and procedures. Sequential interdependence relates to a one-way flow of resources, where the output of one unit becomes the input of another unit (e.g., assembly line). With sequential interdependence, there is increased independence and sharing of resources; therefore, there is an increased need for coordination between organizational units. Because this is a one-way flow of resources, managers can use task forces as the coordinating horizontal linkage, with frequent communications relating to planning, schedules, and feedback. Reciprocal interdependence requires increased coordination and control because of the high level of independence and sharing of resources between organizational units. Reciprocal interdependence means that the output of unit one becomes the input for unit two, which transforms the input and sends it back to unit one as its input. Hospitals are an excellent example of reciprocal interdependence because they provide coordinated services to patients (Daft, 2007). Assume a patient is admitted to a hospital for a knee replacement operation. The patient will move

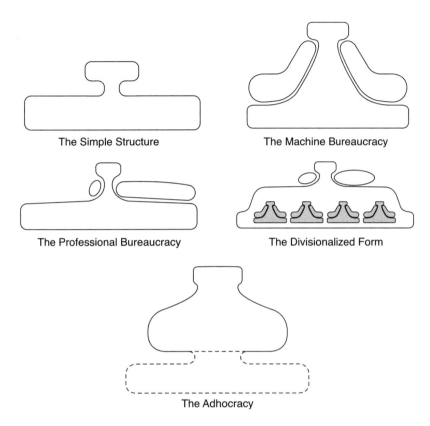

The Simple Structure

The Machine Bureaucracy

The Professional Bureaucracy

The Divisionalized Form

The Adhocracy

Figure 22–2
Source: *The structure of organizations* (1979) by H. Mintzberg. Englewood Cliffs, NJ:
Prentice Hall. Reprinted with permission.

back and forth from radiology, surgery, the ICU, medical/surgical floor, physical
therapy. To achieve this high level of coordination, a horizontal organizational
structure would be recommended, as well as the use of permanent teams to
assure open and frequent communication between and among organizational
units to deal with any problems or issues. However, managers be aware! The culture of health care can directly and strongly oppose this "shared" communication
even at the very local levels. "The people who run one floor of a hospital often
don't know or don't want to know how the people on another floor of the same
hospital handle a particular process, procedure, or problem" (Halvorson, 2007, p.
87). George Halvorson, chairman and CEO of Kaiser Foundation Health Plan
and Hospitals, uses the change of nurse shift information transfer process,* a
universal basic task as an example to illustrate his point:

---

*To read more about the nurse shift transfer process change at South Sacramento Medical Cen-
ter, a Kaiser Permanente hospital, go to the Institute of Healthcare Improvement's Web site at
www.ihi.org, and select "Shifting to a Higher Standard" under Medical-Surgical Care improvement stories.

Table 22-2 The Key Dimensions of Mintzberg's Five Structural Configurations

Structural Configuration	Prime Coordinating Mechanism	Key Part of Organization	Main Design Parameters	Contingency Factors	Example
Simple	Direct supervision (i.e., one individual takes responsibility for the work of others)	Strategic apex	Centralization, organic structure	Young, small, unsophisticated technical system, simple, dynamic environment, possible strong power needs of top manager	Sole practitioner's office or small outpatient health center
Machine Bureaucracy	Standardization of work processes (i.e., every work process follows a predefined path and a set of rules)	Technostructure	Behavior formalization, vertical and horizontal job specialization, usually functional grouping, large operating unit size, vertical centralization and limited horizontal decentralization, action planning	Old, large, regulating, non-automated technical system, simple, stable environment, external control	Health-related manufacturing company, such as a vitamin manufacturing company
Professional Bureaucracy	Standardization of skills (i.e., everyone has the same knowledge and qualifications)	Operating core	Training, horizontal job specialization, vertical and horizontal decentralization	Complex, stable environment, nonregulating, unsophisticated technical system	Hospital and academic medical centers

(Continued)

Table 22–2 The Key Dimensions of Mintzberg's Five Structural Configurations (*Continued*)

Structural Configuration	Prime Coordinating Mechanism	Key Part of Organization	Main Design Parameters	Contingency Factors	Example
Divisional Form	Standardization of outputs (i.e., measures for the outcome of product and/or services; however individuals have freedom to achieve the results in a variety of ways as long as the end result conforms to the results standard.)	Middle line	Market grouping, performance control system, limited vertical decentralization	Diversified markets (particularly products or services), old, large, power needs of middle managers	National or regional healthcare provider
Adhocracy	Mutual adjustment (i.e., individuals coordinate their own work)	Support staff	Liaison devices, organic structure, selective decentralization, horizontal job specialization, training, functional and market grouping concurrently	Complex, dynamic environment, young, sophisticated and often automated technical system	Healthcare organization using a matrix structure

SOURCE: *The structuring of organizations*, by H. Mintzberg, 1979. Englewood Cliffs, NJ: Prentice Hall. Adapted with permission.

Hospitals are open twenty-four hours a day so multiple shifts are needed for each work site and unit. At the end of each shift, the nurses from the prior shift take some time to brief the new set of nurses about each patient in the relevant work unit. That's a very good thing to do. It's essential for continuity of patient care. It's a job that has to be done three times a day—hopefully very well, because the quality of the information sharing affects the quality of care for each patient.

Unfortunately, that process is not always done either well or efficiently. It can take a lot of time. The communication process itself can too easily create factual errors. It's a typical type of care linkage deficiency—one that we may more readily expect from outpatient clinical care, but one that is somehow a bit more surprising when it happens in an institution as formal and highly organized as a hospital. In the real world, each floor in a hospital is likely to have its own separate information transfer process, "invented here, by us." People don't typically try to found who has the best process for transitioning that information. Process improvement as a desirable cultural value doesn't show up at all on a lot of health care radar screens.

For the nurse shift transfer process, simply implementing an easy-to-use, standardized, well thought out, carefully designed information checklist for the use with each patient can cut the transfer time from nurse to nurse from over half an hour per shift change to less than fifteen minutes while reducing communication errors about individual patients hugely. Patient care improves. Nurse efficiency improves. Care linkages improve. The nurses who are tired and worn out at the end of their shifts get to go home a bit earlier. And everyone wins!

Now that we have a greater understanding of the five interrelating parts of an organization and with the need for proper communication to coordinate and control an organization's activities, we will continue our discussion of each design parameter that makes up the structural dimension of organizational design.

ELEMENTS OF THE STRUCTURAL DIMENSION

The design parameters that make up the structural dimension of organizational design are: formalization, specialization, hierarchy of authority, centralization, and professionalism.

Formalization

Formalization is the degree to which the organization communicates how the work will be performed, who will do the work, and under what circumstances or constraints the work will be done. This is usually measured by the amount of written documentation in the organization. Documentation includes procedures, job descriptions, regulations, and policy manuals. Monitoring and feedback systems (i.e., budgets, production measurement systems, performance reviews) serve to reinforce the degree of formalization. However, as Burton et al. (2006) point out, there can be high formalization within an organization even though rules, policies and procedures, and so on are not "written down." Rules can be communicated through training procedures, modeling of behavior, or verbalized codes of working that people are expected to learn over time. In highly formal organizations, there are penalties for "breaking the rules!" (See Chapter 14 for a discussion regarding group norms.)

When an organization lacks a set of strongly written or unwritten accepted rules of conduct, formalization is considered to be low. When formalization is low, there is high variance in the methods and procedures used to govern the organization's work (Burton et al., 2006). In this situation, employees must use their own judgment in deciding how the work will be performed. This flexibility is appropriate when employees are dealing with situations where there are no "preprogrammed" answers. Organizations that have low formalization are usually those that deal constantly with new situations for which precedents do not exist, such as scientific research (Hall, 1996).

All organizations but the very small ones need some degree of formalization to avoid chaos. However, too much formalization may cause an organization to become bureaucratic, which may prohibit creativity and innovation. Most organizations operate in between relatively high formalization or relatively low formalization (Burton et al., 2006).

Specialization

Specialization refers to the degree to which organizational tasks are subdivided into separate jobs (i.e., division of labor). If specialization is high, each employee performs a narrow range of tasks. If specialization is low, each employee performs a wide range of tasks in his or her job.

Dividing work into specialized tasks and organizing them into distinct departments was one of the basic foundations of Weber's rational bureaucracy model (see Chapter 19). Weber's (1947) idea of functional specialization applied both to persons within an organization and to relations between larger units or divisions of the organization. Weber argued that such specialization is essential to a rational bureaucracy and that the specific boundaries separating one functional division from another must be fixed by explicit rules, regulations, and procedures (Miner, 2002). In addition, the principles of Taylor's (1911) scientific management included subdividing work into measurable and manageable units to achieve "maximum efficiency" of an entity's operations. This required managers to (1) divide the work into separate tasks, (2) develop a science for each person's work, (3) initiate controls to ensure the work is done in the prescribed manner, and (4) train the person to be able to perform his or her job better.

The growth and current status of medical specializations provides an excellent example of division of labor. Today there exist over 60 medical specialties and subspecialties that are formally recognized by training and certification. In his book *Divide and Conquer: A Comparative History of Medical Specialization*, George Weisz (2006) provides the historical content of the creation of specialists from generalists, giving attention to the cultural and institutional dimensions of this process. For example, Weisz relates that hospitals played an important role in influencing the legitimization and value of medical specialization by providing the venues for treating illnesses and pursuing clinical research and opportunities for clinical training. Support of specialization continues today with hospitals creating centers of excellence around selected service lines, such as cardiology, oncology, and orthopedics. In addition, there also exists a wide variety of specialized organizational forms that support medical specialization, such as specialty hospitals, free-standing renal disease units, retail-based urgent-care centers, neighborhood health centers, and home health agencies. As Scott, Ruef, Mendel, and Caronna (2000) pointed out, these specialized organizational forms are reflective of the practice of service "unbundling," whereby a cluster of services once performed in a generalized community-based hospital is disaggregated and re-formed as separate units. This unbundling reinforces the specialization of medical practice. In addition to medical specialties, nurses can and do specialize, although this is more closely related to locus of practice than to differences in training. For example, nurses can specialize (and receive certification) in the areas of child-care nursing, gerontological nursing, maternity nursing, medical–surgical nursing, nurse anesthesia, nurse midwifery, nurse practitioner studies, nursing administration, nursing education, oncology nursing, psychiatric nursing, public health nursing, and rehabilitation nursing.

Kast and Rosenzweig (1985) noted that the more specialization within an organization, the greater the requirement for sophisticated methods of coordination and integration of activities. This leads to increasing levels of organizational complexity, making the role of managers more difficult! The following vignettes in Exhibit 22–1 describe quality-of-care issues that may arise as a result of the lack of coordination and integration of specialized services of a hospital's subsystems. The vignettes illustrate the fragmentation of today's U.S. healthcare system as a result of specialization. Managers need to develop the proper coordination and control mechanisms to achieve the system "redesign" goals stated in the Institute of Medicine's 2001 report, *Crossing the Quality Chasm: A New Health System for the 21st Century* (see the present book's Opening Remarks).

Hierarchy of Authority

Hierarchy of authority refers to a manager's span of control. Span of control describes (1) who reports to whom and (2) the number of employees reporting to a supervisor. If an organization is structured so that on average each manager has few people reporting to him or her, the resulting shape will be tall and narrow (see Figure 22–3). If the average span of control for each manager is increased, the resulting shape is flatter and the number of levels in the hierarchy will be less (Miner, 1973).

As companies grow larger, they tend to increase the number of hierarchic levels, with a pronounced positive relationship between size (as measured by the number of employees) and levels (Hickson, Pugh, & Pheysey, 1969). An interesting side note is the effect of flat and tall structures on employees' job satisfaction. A comprehensive survey of over 1,500 managers in both tall and flat organizations revealed that for the group as a whole, those in flat structures were no more satisfied than those in tall structures (Porter & Lawler, 1964). However, in smaller companies (under 5,000 employees) there was a

Exhibit 22-2

Vignette One

Howard came into Hospital A's outpatient renal dialysis center for hemodialysis on Tuesday, Thursday, and Saturday afternoons. One day the renal dialysis nurse noticed during a routine foot check that Howard had an ulcer on his left foot that would require daily wound dressings for at least three weeks. The renal dialysis nurse called the hospital's home health division to schedule a home care nurse to change the dressing on Howard's nondialysis days. The home care nurse asked the renal dialysis nurse, "Where are you calling from again?" The renal dialysis nurse repeated that she was calling from the hospital's outpatient renal dialysis center. There was a pause, and then the home care nurse responded, "Well, that explains why Peter is never home on Tuesday and Thursday afternoons for us to check his blood sugar. I didn't know he was on dialysis! You know, we've been seeing him for six months at the request of the hospital's diabetes clinic—does the diabetes nurse manager know?"

Vignette Two

Mary was admitted for surgery to Hospital B on Monday after her weekly treatment at the hospital's community-based hemodialysis center. During her hospitalization she received dialysis in the hospital's inpatient hemodialysis unit. On Friday afternoon, after her treatment, the surgeon discharged her from the hospital. On Monday morning when Mary was late for her hemodialysis appointment, a nurse from the hospital's community hemodialysis unit called the hospital's inpatient unit. The unit secretary said, "Mary was discharged on Friday, didn't you know?" "No, we didn't, we're part of the hospital's outpatient division and therefore do not receive discharge notifications." The nurse called Mary's home but there was no reply. The nurse became concerned and called 911. The paramedics found Mary unconscious at home and immediately brought her to the hospital's emergency room. Shortly after readmission, Mary had a cardiac arrest and required resuscitation. Mary later told the hemodialysis nurse, "After I was discharged, I went home by taxi and managed to crawl up the stairs to my apartment—there's no elevator, you know, and dialysis always makes me feel tired, so I went straight to bed. When I woke up I was too weak to get to the phone in the living room to call for help." Mary remained in the hospital as an inpatient for three weeks and required intradialytic parenteral nutrition (IDPN) for three months.

SOURCE: "Access within a fragmented healthcare system: A nurse's perspective on Romanow," by E. F. Ravenscroft, 2005. *Nursing Leadership—Online Exclusive*. Copyright by Longwoods Publishing Company. Adapted with permission.

---

tendency for the flat structure to be associated with greater job satisfaction; in the larger companies this relationship was reversed, that is, job satisfaction was greater in the tall structure (Miner, 1973).

Early theorists believed that organizations should have narrow spans of control. For example, Fayol (1949) believed that when the work was nonroutine, the span of control for each manager should be fewer than 6 employees, and when the work was routine, he recommended a span of 20 or 30 employees for each manager. Over the years, considerable research has been done regarding spans in various organizations, and certain factors are consistently associated with the size of the spans of control. The most widely cited research in this area is Woodward's (1965) work with various manufacturing companies in the United Kingdom. Woodward found that there was a close relationship between the type of technology, the average span of control, the number of levels of

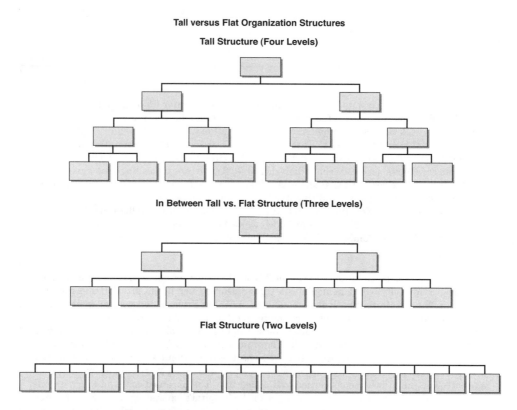

Figure 22–3 Tall versus Flat Organization Structures

management, and the organization's success (see Figure 22–4). The small-batch and unit-production firms (e.g., ship-building or aircraft-manufacturing firm) usually had three levels of management. When these organizations had three levels, they were more likely to be successful as compared to others that had more or fewer levels. In large-batch and mass-production firms, the typical and desirable number of levels rose to four. In the continuous-process firms (e.g., chemical or petroleum manufacturers), the average levels of management were six. Organizations in the continuous-process category with fewer or more levels in the hierarchy were usually less successful. As previously noted, Woodward's work was related to industrial companies' use of technology. However, service organizations' technologies also influence organizational structure as a result of interdependence, as discussed earlier in this chapter.

All things being equal, a wide span of control is more efficient because it requires fewer managers. However, it is important to recognize that, at some point, effectiveness will decline. Therefore, Miner (1973) provides us with certain generalizations regarding span of control:

- The optimal span for most situations is in the range of 5 to 10.
- Larger spans (e.g., 8 through 10) are most appropriate at higher levels in an organization where the greater resources for diverse decision making are needed.

	Span of Control					
	Up to 20	21 *to* 40	41 *to* 60	61 *to* 80	*Over* 80	*Total Employees*
Production System Unit and Small Batch						
All firms	7	12	4	0	1	24
Above-average success		5				5
Below-average success	2		3			5
Large Batch and Mass Production						
All firms	1	7	13	6	4	31
Above-average success			5			5
Below-average success	1	2		1	2	6
Continuous Process						
All firms	18	7				25
Above-average success	6					6
Below-average success	1	3				4

Figure 22–4

- The size of the core operations span is influenced by both the type of technology and the costs associated with smaller spans. Spans below 10 may not be economically feasible because of the number of managers required in spite of other potential advantages.
- In establishing a span of control for a specific situation, factors such as the desirability of group solidarity, the need for job satisfaction, the amount of control required, the nature of the work, the stability of the environment, and the extent of operational support for the manager (i.e., assistants) must be taken into account.

Centralization

Centralization is the degree to which decision making is concentrated with the senior management team at the top of the organization's hierarchy. Decentralization is the extent to which decision-making authority is moved down the organization structure and shared with many employees. Generally, when the organization's operating activities are of a relatively routine nature with a high degree of uniformity, there is likely to be considerable centralization of decision making. When the work is less routine and where many individuals with professional specialization and training are involved, decision making is delegated to lower levels and to the professionals (Hage & Aiken, 1969; Hall, 1962). For example, in organizations employing professionals, a decentralized form would be required for day-to-day operating decisions. As Miner (1973) noted, professionals, such as physicians, attorneys, accountants, and consultants, must make their own decisions regarding their patients and/or clients with reference to the particular circumstances existing at a point in time.

Attempts to centralize such decisions often result in a considerable loss of professional staff to the organization. Furthermore, the requisite knowledge and information is typically available at the level of the practicing professional.

A high degree of decentralization is appropriate (1) when an organization is operating in an unpredictable environment, which is constantly changing and characterized by high risk, or (2) when an organization becomes large and complex in terms of product/service lines and/or markets. In these situations, the organization needs to respond quickly to new cues in the environment whenever they arise. A very centralized decision structure could easily result in outdated responses or in no response at all! However, even under those conditions that make decentralization most desirable, the practice should not be carried to the point where senior management becomes relatively powerless (Miner, 1973). When this occurs, organizations become much less effective (Tannenbaum, 1968). Therefore, even when an organization may be considered decentralized, a number of decision-making activities should remain centralized at the top level. Some of these activities, in addition to strategic planning, would be setting company-wide policies, finance, accounting systems, some research, activities relating to mergers and/or acquisitions, approval of capital expenditures above certain dollar amounts, senior management selection and compensation, negotiating with unions for collective bargaining settlements, and public relations. For example, ProMedica Health System, the country's most integrated health system, operates as a decentralized system with the corporate office providing the organization's overall strategic direction. In Exhibit 22–3 are excerpts of an interview with Alan Brass, CEO and President of ProMedica Health System, published in Deloitte Health Care Review (2004), as he explains how a decentralized organization with consistency in implementing strategic goals has resulted in ProMedica being recognized in 2007 as the nation's best-performing healthcare system (see Evans, 2008).

To determine whether an organization's decision making is more centralized or decentralized, one needs to view who is making operational decisions. As reflected in the ProMedica example, if strategic decisions are made at the top level of the organization but operational decisions are made by the subunits, the organization would be considered decentralized (Burton et al., 2006). In addition, centralized organizations have more levels of management with narrow spans of control, whereas decentralized organizations have fewer levels of management with wide spans of control.

The current trend is toward broadening decentralization by delegating decision-making authority to those employees closest to the organization's patients, clients, or customers. Delegating gives employees more freedom of action to implement positive changes that directly impact their and the organization's performances. However, as Miner (2002) points out, managers need to proceed with caution when delegating decision-making authority. There have been several studies conducted to determine the effectiveness of delegating decision-making authority. Miner (1973) reported that in simulation studies it was found that although some employees will go well beyond the freedom delegated to them, others will not use the freedom that is given. Thus, delegating decision-making authority may be less important to the final outcome than the individual tendencies of employees to make their own decisions or defer to their managers. As dis-

Exhibit 22–3

ProMedica is composed of over 70 corporations and joint ventures, serving 27 counties throughout Ohio and Michigan. It is made up of 10 acute-care hospitals and more than 282 ambulatory-care centers and diagnostic centers. It employs over 15,000 individuals. More than 2.5 million patients are served by ProMedica annually and are cared for by more than 2,900 physicians (see: http://www.promedica.org/)

ProMedica serves its communities through five divisions—ProMedica Ambulatory and Acute Care; ProMedica Physician Group; ProMedica Health, Education and Research Corporation; ProMedica Continuing Care Services Corporation; and ProMedica Insurance Corporation. According to Alan Brass, ProMedica's CEO and President, "All the business units except continuing care are decentralized. The air and land transport network, durable medical supplies, visiting nurses, and other components of the continuing care can be managed more efficiently if they cut across the counties that ProMedica serves.

According to Brass, "ProMedica's corporate office does certain things and the operating units do other things. We want the boards of our different regional hospitals and our different regional businesses to be responsible and accountable. That can happen only if we believe in and follow a decentralized model." For example, the corporate office produces "an extremely strong five-year strategic plan, one that includes input from the community and is fully communicated, reviewed, and assessed constantly, so that the executive officers and their decentralized boards know the plan as well as the CEO." The local officers and boards then take responsibility and accountability in their own communities for the system's facilities and services, continuum of care, and standards of quality.

ProMedica's 70 corporations, 282 sites, 350-plus managers, and 15,000-plus employees operate under the strategic plan. "You have to know who you are and where you are. Unless an integrated delivery system (IDS) is consistent in applying its strategic plan throughout the organization, it cannot maintain and sustain itself in this day and age. In putting together an IDS the size of ProMedica, which is getting larger and larger, you really need to be very, very consistent in application," Brass asserts.

"The consistency of application starts at the CEO level, but it goes up and down. It goes up to the board, and it goes down to all of the executive officers, managers, and supervisors." Brass says that, "in March and April, we formulate strategies for the company and all of its business units. I'm the first one out of the gate saying to the 14 presidents, 'Here is what I have; here's what I want to see done next year; here's what I want to work toward; here's what I want to see you building into your plan.' They take those strategies and move them into their local business units and add the strategic thrusts that are appropriate for their areas . . . Whether in the case of board nominating processes, planning processes, or financial decision processes, we rely on the decentralized model very extensively." For example, in figuring out revenues, the regional presidents need to work with their financial officers and the parent company's chief financial officer to figure out what their reimbursements will be and whether there will be policy changes that will affect their bottom lines.

For Brass and for ProMedica, "it is very important in 'growing' a company to make sure that the culture of its various components fits together. It is crucial to be explicit and forthright in communicating what the parent company is looking for, what is important and what is not important." That philosophy relates to the principles of decentralization, consistency, teamwork, and concentration on quality and delivery that Brass says drive ProMedica.

cussed in Chapter 5 relating to job design, some employees are unwilling to take the risk of making decisions and being held accountable. They may claim that their freedom of action is restricted when, in fact, it is merely that they do not want to accept responsibility for their own decisions. As such, if delegation is to improve organizational effectiveness, employees must be recruited or developed who are willing to accept delegation and make decisions (Miner, 1973).

Professionalism

Professionalism refers to the level or average number of years of formal education and training of employees. The higher level of professionalism and the more professionals employed within an organization, the greater the need for a decentralized structure. There is a large body of literature on professional organizations and the sociology of the professions (Friedson, 1984; Larson, 1977; Parsons, 1968; Scott, 1982). Much of the sociological theory on professionals has pertained to the mechanisms of control over professionals, including socialization in the profession, a desire to serve others, control by professional peers within and outside of the employing firm, reputation in the community, bureaucratic controls from the hierarchical supervision within firms, and client control (Hodgson, 2002; Sharma, 1997; Tolbert & Stern, 1991).

Management of highly motivated and largely autonomous professionals is always challenging. As such, managers need to develop an understanding of the professional's culture (i.e., why they act the way they do) to reduce conflicts and resistance to change within the organization. For example, when an organization's interests, standards, or procedures conflict with the opinions of peers in the profession, professionals will usually side with their profession, because most professionals identify more closely with the profession than with the organization (Alvesson & Willmott, 2002; Bolton, 2004). This has been referred to as the "clash of cultures" between corporate culture and professional culture. The corporate culture reinforces the conflict between professionals and managers by formalizing roles, relationships, and procedures that are inimical to professionals' predispositions. For example, managers need to coordinate and control the diverse activities and individuals that contribute to organizational goals. However, professionals expect to maintain self-control over the application of their field of knowledge, establish their own agenda, and be controlled by no less than their peers (Clegg, 1981; Hodgson, 2002). This professional culture of self-control and autonomy are the results of professionals' prolonged training and socialization into their profession. This lengthy and rigorous process causes professionals to govern themselves by an internalized set of social–regulative rules and norms (Philip, Padsakoff, Williams, & Williams, 1986; Raelin, 1986). For example, physicians tend to emphasize preserving independent medical decision making to uphold their ethical obligations to provide the best care possible, regardless of cost, while healthcare managers are interested in standardizing healthcare delivery because of concerns over rising healthcare costs, medical errors, and wide variations in physicians' practice patterns. These attempts at standardization have resulted in confusion, frustration, and conflict and between physicians and managers because professionals will resist attempts to exert control over them or in any way limit their freedom to make important decisions independently (Friedson, 2001; Kleinke, 1997; O'Connor & Lanning, 1992; Raelin, 1986). As such, managers need to establish an environment that effectively reduces the tension between the needs of physicians (i.e., clinical autonomy and independence) and the needs of the organization (i.e., control of resources and variations in patients' outcomes) (Marcus, 1985: Meyer & Tucker, 1992).

SUMMARY

Mintzberg (1979, p. 2) states that

> Every organized human activity—from the making of pots to placing of a man on the moon—gives rise to two fundamental and opposing requirements: the division of labor into various tasks to be performed, and the coordination of these tasks to accomplish the activity. The structure of an organization can be defined simply as the sum total of the ways in which it divides its labor into distinct tasks and then achieves coordination among them.

It is a manager's responsibility to first determine the necessary activities to achieve the organization's goals objectives, followed by dividing the activities on a logical basis into departments that perform the specialized functions, and finally to implement the systems necessary to coordinate and control the activities and individuals who perform the tasks. This is a challenge considering all the variables that must be considered and evaluated—the environment, technology, strategies, processes, and so on. As noted by Hall (1996), organizational structures are a consequence of the simultaneous impact of multiple factors. Structure should reflect the organization's situation—age, size, type of technology needed for its services or products, the extent to which its environment is complex and dynamic. However, on the basis of decades of research, there are a few rules of thumb that managers can use. Larger organizations need more formalized structures—more rules, more planning, more detailed job descriptions—as do those in stable environments and those in mass production. Organizations in more complex environments need higher degrees of decentralization; those diversified in many markets need divisional instead of functional structures (Miller & Friesen, 1984). The higher the routineness of job functions, the more mechanistic the structure, and the greater the interdependence of activities or processes, the more organic the structure. How does this all come together? The ideal state occurs when the company's strategy, perfectly suited to the current external environment, is matched by the organization's design and structure, which allows for the optimal implementation of the entity's strategy. However, managers need to always consider one important factor: the organization's culture. There's an old saying in business that "culture trumps strategy very time." The most carefully thought-out design will not accomplish the company's goals unless it is supported by the organization's culture. This would include not only the formal rules and procedures that govern employees but also the practices and communication they actually follow, and the congruence of the values the organization espouses and actually practices (Monteiro, 2002).

END-OF-CHAPTER QUESTIONS

1. Describe the five organizational parts of an organization and their significance to organizational design.
2. Discuss the relationships of the five organizational parts of an organization to simple, machine bureaucracy, professional bureaucracy, divisional, and adhocracy structural configurations.
3. Discuss why the proper communication form and method is necessary to coordinate and control organizational activities.
4. Discuss the contingency factors associated with simple, machine bureaucracy, professional bureaucracy, divisional, and adhocracy structural configurations.
5. Describe each element of the structural dimension and how it relates to organization design.

END-OF-CHAPTER EXERCISE

As noted in the Opening Remarks to this book, there have been urgent calls for redesigning the U.S. healthcare system as a result of quality-of-care and patient safety issues that relate to how the healthcare system is structured and how organizations are designed (Institute of Medicine, 1999, 2001). An emerging consortium "Stepping Up to the Plate" (SUTTP) Alliance consisting of nine leading medical specialty societies, with the support of the American Board of Internal Medicine (ABIM) Foundation, the Agency for Healthcare Research and Quality (AHRQ), the Institute of Healthcare Improvement (IHI), the National Committee for Quality Assurance (NCQA), and others, are working to develop principles and initial standards to design a system of coordination between sites of care with the goal of reducing medical errors, gaps in care, and waste.

Using SUTTP's Issue Brief #6,* "White Space or Black Hole: What Can We Do To Improve Care Transitions?" as background information, in groups discuss how Hospital A and Hospital B from the two vignettes in Exhibit 22–2 could be redesigned to better coordinate and control the organization's activities to achieve improved quality of care.

---

*SUTTP's Issue Brief #6 can be downloaded from the ABIM Foundation's Web site at www.abimfoundation.org.

END-OF-CHAPTER CASE STUDY

Case Study 22–1 Mitigating Hazards Through Continuing Design: The Birth and Evolution of a Pediatric Intensive Care Unit

Introduction

A recent report (2000) published by the Institute of Medicine (IOM) found that medical errors kill as many as 100,000 people each year in American hospitals. The report argues that many medical errors stem from structural problems in healthcare organizations and the U.S. healthcare system, suggesting that increasing patient safety is (at least in part) an organizational design problem. To the surprise of interested healthcare managers and professionals, the literature on organizational safety and design offered little guidance on how to design a safe hospital and on designing organizations for hazardous environments more generally.

William Howard Taft Children's Hospital Pediatric Intensive Care Unity

Pediatric intensive care is a complex and unpredictable domain. The potential for treatment-induced complications abounds. Children often react differently than adults. Even minor procedures such as injections or intravenous line insertions can cause patients to become agitated and move in unpredictable ways.

To meet the challenges associated with treating children in critical condition, William Howard Taft Children's Hospital (WHTCH) established a new pediatric intensive care unit (PICU) in 1988. WHTCH is the tertiary children's hospital for a geographic area more than three times the size of Vermont. The population is 2.5 million, with 500,000 under the age of 15. In 1988 WHTCH brought in a pediatric intensivist as the director of the new PICU. A second intensivist joined the unit a year later, and these two physicians headed the unit until 2000, when they both left the hospital. During their tenure, the PICU grew from an initial size of 8 beds to 25 beds with an average daily census of 21 children, including an average of 9 on ventilators. By 1999, the PICU had more than 1,300 admissions per year, making it one of the largest PICUs in the United States in terms of both number of beds and admission rate.

The Evolution of Organizational Design in the Pediatric Intensive Care Unit

The Setting

Many medical organizations follow a model of treatment that delineates the attending physician as the primary decision maker, more or less solely responsible for the care of his patients and the management of their medical outcomes. Therefore, if one physician establishes a care plan but is unavailable when another physician sees the patient, the second physician may change the care plan without any interaction with the first. Because traditional physician roles in this model are highly individualistic, the teamwork aspect of care is often missing. In this model, physicians may be unaware that each one works differently and there is no incentive for doctors to forge agreed-upon plans. The physician answers to the patient, not to another physician, and medical doctors rarely accept advice from peers on how to practice medicine.

Furthermore, while a physician's relationship to other doctors is one of independence and individual responsibility, her relationship to nurses and other healthcare personnel is usually one of hierarchy and authority. This model dictates unidirectional planning and communication, with the physician as director in a vertical hierarchy. The physician remains the "final common pathway" for decision making regarding the patient's care. In the PICU director's experience, many physicians underscored their authority through belligerence and criticism, leading nurses and other support staff to live in fear of physicians. He had seen that the culture of fear encouraged nurses to think independently as little as possible and focus instead on avoiding physician notice. In this environment, nurses, therapists, and residents quickly learned that the path of least resistance was to follow physician instructions to the letter. The PICU director observed how interactions among physicians and staff unnecessarily complicated patient care.

The Birth of a Pediatric Intensive Care Unit

With these experiences in mind, the first pediatric intensivist came to WHTCH as PICU director in 1988. At this time, the PICU did not exist as a distinct unit within the broader 627-bed medical center. Prior to this, critically ill children were either treated in the adult ICU or transferred to other hospitals with pediatric facilities. With the intensivist's arrival, the adult ICU donated eight beds and the PICU began to function independently.

From the beginning, the new PICU director saw founding a new unit as an opportunity to diverge from the traditional design of critical-care units as he had seen it. He was a navy combat veteran from the Vietnam War. As a pilot, he had witnessed firsthand how a rigid hierarchy with authority enforced through verbal abuse caused accidents in hazardous situations. When he left the navy and entered medical school, he found a very similar design in place.

During his training, the first intensivist noticed a sharp distinction between the bedside caregiver, typically a resident nurse who spends long hours monitoring individual patients or small groups of patients, and the physician, whose responsibilities include attending to a larger number of patients, with less time spent monitoring each individual patient. Because of their experience with individual patients over long periods of time, bedside caregivers such as nurses are often the first organizational members to detect slight changes in patient conditions that signal latent health problems. Therefore, while the information necessary to provide care for a child may come from advanced knowledge of disease processes or from discussions with other experts, it may also come from intimate knowledge gained by bedside nurses. The intensivist noted that physicians with whom he was familiar relied on information from laboratory values, radiographic findings, and physician colleagues as resources to make effective decisions, but often overlooked information from bedside staff.

The intensivist wanted to design a unit that avoided the mistakes of the U.S. Navy and departed from the worst aspects of organizational design in traditional medical units as he saw them. To this end, he believed that the unit's design should involve nurses and other support staff more equally in patient care decisions. When the PICU began admitting patients, the intensivist began asking nurses for their opinions on patient treatment options and inviting them to perform some tasks traditionally reserved for doctors. This approach was not well received at first. Accustomed to traditional roles, some nurses became resentful, suggesting that the intensivist was asking them to work too hard or to do his job as well as their own. Other nurses saw the intensivist's behavior as a sign of incompetence or lack of confidence and became concerned about his abilities as a physician. This initial reaction surprised the new PICU director and convinced him that instituting his desired participative organizational design in the unit would require a long-term commitment and evolving effort. He came to see that many of the nurses did not feel adequately trained to take on the added responsibilities he was offering them.

During the PICU's first months, nondedicated nurses and respiratory care practitioners worked some of their shifts in the PICU and others elsewhere in the hospital. On the basis of the resistance encountered to delegating some decision-making responsibilities to nurses, the intensivist decided that his design interventions could work only with dedicated support personnel. This was true for two reasons. First, because people resisted roles other than those to which they had become accustomed through training and experience, only dedicated staff members could accumulate enough experience with a new design to begin to trust it. Second, even if nurses could be convinced to participate in patient treatment decisions, they needed additional training to do so successfully. This type of training would be possible only with a relatively small number of dedicated nurses. Early in his tenure, the PICU director approached hospital administration to request a dedicated nursing staff. Administrators granted the request. Later, the director also asked for dedicated respiratory care practitioners. While initially resistant, administrators also eventually granted this request.

As the intensivist continued encouraging nurses to assist in making patient care decisions, many of the dedicated nurses (and later the dedicated respiratory care practitioners) began warming to his approach. At this point, participative decision making in the unit was quite informal and largely involved queries for staff members' observations about patients and requests for their opinions about appropriate treatment options. Several nurses and respiratory care practitioners working in the unit at the time report that the intensivist's approach made them feel valued, but that they did not feel qualified to offer suggestions on patient treatment options at that time. In response to this concern, the intensivist started teaching staff members about medical decision making. He introduced lessons through conversations with care staff and increasingly invited staff members to attend his physician's rounds.

Growth

The PICU director's inclination to involve the support staff in patient care decisions was reinforced by necessity. He made an early policy decision to not turn away any children referred to the PICU. This policy contrasted sharply with prior practices in the original adult ICU, which resulted in the admission of only 40% of referred children (the ICU turned away children that they could not treat with available equipment and also deemed some children to be in insufficiently critical condition for admission). The new PICU policy quickly raised the admission rate to more than 90% (and eventually as high as 99%) of referred children.

WHTCH's PICU admitted more than 500 children during its first year, while the PICU director was its only physician. This is a heavy workload for a pediatric intensivist. For reference, an average PICU has one physician for every 4–5 beds and roughly 200–300 admissions per year. The focal PICU, at 8 beds and more than 500 admissions, had roughly double this ratio in its first year. Thus, in addition to involving staff members to improve patient care, the intensivist realized that he simply needed their help.

Eleven months after the PICU's establishment, a second intensivist came to the unit as assistant director of critical care. The PICU director recruited him specifically because of his background in fire department emergency medical services. The second intensivist independently concluded that organizational structures in fire departments could handle emergencies more effectively than those in the medical centers with which he had experience.

Despite the addition of a second intensivist, the patient/physician ratio at the PICU remained high. The PICU admitted roughly 900 children in its second year, nearly 1,200 in its third, and 1,400 in its fourth. The unit's growth quickly outstripped its allotted 8-bed space in the adult ICU. During its second year, the PICU moved into a new building with 25 beds. A study published shortly thereafter found that 40% of PICUs in the United States have 4–6 beds, while those with more than 18 beds make up less than 6% of the national total. The latter averaged 1,277 ± 63 patient admissions per year. According to these numbers, WHTCH's PICU was one of the largest PICUs in the country by its third year. Part of this growth resulted from a pediatric critical-care transport system established by the second PICU intensivist in 1989, allowing the unit to transport and accept highly critical children from other less-equipped hospitals. WHTCH's pediatric critical-care transport system quickly grew into one of the largest of such systems in the country.

At the end of 1994, an intermediate ICU was established as a separate unit at WHTCH. The intermediate ICU served three purposes related to the functions of the PICU: It admitted children who required a high level of nursing attention, but not the same level of critical care as patients in the PICU; it took recovering PICU patients who no longer required intensive care; and it housed the WHTCH cardiothoracic ICU, where children with heart conditions were treated. The establishment of the intermediate ICU served to increase the severity of conditions treated in the PICU because the less critical patients were referred directly to the intermediate ICU.

Staff Training as Continuing Design

Because of his background, the second intensivist became an enthusiastic supporter of the PICU director's push to delegate care decisions and functions to nurses, respiratory care practitioners, and residents. The first intensivist's efforts had secured the unit a dedicated nursing staff, many of whom learned to enjoy taking an active role in treatment decisions. Yet nurses and other staff members still complained that they lacked the expertise to make important medical decisions. The PICU's emerging design required a high level of distributed knowledge and expertise, as well as distributed authority. As both intensivists wanted to further increase the level of bedside caregiver participation in the PICU, they made attaining this level of staff medical knowledge one of the major drivers behind their design efforts.

While the first intensivist previously conducted informal lessons, training became increasingly formalized after the second intensivist's arrival. The intensivists began teaching staff members how to identify medical problems that brought children to the PICU. They taught caregivers how to identify and treat complications that could arise because of disease or inappropriate medical care. The intensivists also gave staff members formalized decision-making aids to help them know when they could treat a patient themselves and when they should ask for help. They taught staff members to break down a patient's symptoms into categories, assess the severity of each category, and begin treating the most acute symptoms while calling for additional help if needed.

To further facilitate decentralized decision making, the intensivists emphasized that they would respond immediately to staff questions. They gave out their personal phone numbers and encouraged staff to feel comfortable calling them if they were not present and the attending physician could not assist.

Both intensivists continued to teach informally when opportunities arose, but they also initiated formal in-service training sessions for all staff members on duty. As part of the training, the intensivists encouraged staff members to read medical journals and textbooks to further educate themselves. Several former nurses and respiratory care practitioners report that they became so interested in what they were learning in these training sessions that they decided to return to school for advanced degrees.

Furthermore, all staff members regardless of position and disciplinary background were encouraged to attend the physicians' rounds on the PICU floor, and these rounds included an educational component to ensure that staff possessed the abilities necessary to function across roles. The intensivists took up the practice of wheeling a blackboard around the PICU during rounds so that they could write notes and draw diagrams to facilitate staff training.

While residents and fellows commonly take part in physicians' rounds at hospitals, the level of participation instituted at the focal PICU was extraordinary. Morning rounds routinely included all residents, the fellow (if on service), lead respiratory therapist, charge nurse, pharmacist, social worker, and the patient's bedside nurse and respiratory therapist. As PICU staff members became accustomed to participating in physicians' rounds, they undertook larger roles. Nurses began presenting patients and discussing treatment options with the physicians.

One intensivist notes that it took several years before staff members were trained well enough to implement his vision of an optimally decentralized PICU design. Prior to this time, staff members did not possess the knowledge to participate in medical decisions and treatments to the extent that he desired. Thus, the establishment of the PICU's decentralized design was a process rather than an event.

Supporting Staff Decisions

As staff members received more training, they began to feel comfortable accepting more responsibility, and the two intensivists increasingly delegated authority to them. However, specialists from other hospital departments were unaccustomed to such a degree of knowledge distribution and occasionally resisted decisions made by staff when treating PICU patients. The PICU directors developed a policy to always support their staff members' decisions in these situations. While staff members' decisions were not always right, the two PICU intensivists believed that their decentralized design improved response times and decision quality on average because staff with direct information about critical situations made important care decisions. Distributed decision-making authority reduced the need for information to flow up through the chain of command and back to the bedside caregiver.

The PICU directors also assigned bedside caregivers the role of ensuring common and consistent patient treatment plans. As situations developed and additional people and resources responded to critical events at the PICU, arriving members were trained to inquire about and use information from bedside caregivers to assess the situation and develop a common treatment strategy. This was one of the PICU's central design elements, and also perhaps the source of its greatest difference from other units in the hospital.

When the second intensivist arrived in the PICU, he brought the notion of postevent debriefings from his experience in emergency services, and frequent debriefings were quickly institutionalized in the unit. He routinely conducted debriefings open to all involved staff following major events. While most large healthcare organizations utilize some form of postcrisis debriefing, the intensivists believed that these meetings tended to be rare and typically restricted to physicians, residents, and hospital administrators. Debriefings at the PICU became unusual in their frequency and inclusiveness. The purpose of these debriefings was twofold: First, to encourage staff to learn from an experience while it was still fresh and second, to act as a form of therapy for staff members. These sessions allowed staff members to talk through their emotions and prepare themselves to return to work.

Resistance and Buffering

The decentralization and elevated educational focus designed into the unit encountered opposition from some staff members. As a result of their educational focus, some of the physicians' rounds lasted longer than normal. This was, and still is, one of busiest PICUs in the country, and some staff members considered the rounds a waste of time. Some resistance to the goal of increasing staff autonomy also arose. While most of the staff embraced or at least cooperated with the intensivists' push to delegate decision making, the approach required a significant commitment by staff members to learn how to perform new duties.

However, internal resistance to the decentralized design in the focal PICU was not nearly as strong as resistance from other departments in the hospital. Colleagues from other departments increasingly discussed the PICU's design and processes with the intensivists, at times to advise the intensivists of resistance from administration, and at other times to argue that staff members made poor care decisions. Hospital administrators and some physicians from other departments also saw the practice of staff members attending in-service trainings and physicians' rounds as a waste of time and resources.

To preserve their desired organizational design in light of these concerns, the PICU directors developed formalized protocols to constrain bedside caregiver discretion within certain boundaries. For instance, they created new rules that required bedside caregivers to first open the airways of new patients before beginning to design a treatment plan. This rule ensured that patients were stable before staff members began to think about appropriate treatments and gave staff members time to consult with physicians as needed. In addition, the new protocols required PICU staff to ask for assistance under specified conditions. When a patient exhibited one or more of a certain set of symptoms, they were required to get a second opinion from another staff member before proceeding with treatment; when a patient exhibited one of more of a second set of symptoms, they were required to ask a PICU physician for assistance; and when a patient had one or more of a third set of symptoms, they were required to call a specialist from another department in the hospital for a consultation.

By following these metarules for decision making, bedside caregivers maintained their ability to make decisions regarding routine patient care without consulting physicians while avoiding further conflicts with outside specialists. The metarules placated administrators and physicians outside the PICU by giving them indirect but formalized control over caregiver activities, because physicians could modify rules governing the breadth and scope of allowable discretion. While the PICU's initial design called for broad staff decision-making authority, the two intensivists realized that the new formalization created a superior organizational design. Not only did the institution of formal metarules placate hospital administration but it also helped some staff members feel more confident in their patient care decisions.

Despite this change, some physicians in the hospital remained uncomfortable. To minimize resistance from these physicians, the two intensivists moved to buffer the PICU from the remainder of the hospital as much as possible. Early efforts in this direction led to the assignment of dedicated nurses and respiratory care practitioners to the unit. Later efforts were aimed at increasing the unit's autonomy. Before the PICU's establishment, physicians from other hospital departments (pediatricians, surgeons, cardiologists, and others) came from their home departments and managed critically ill children in the original adult ICU as needed. This practice continued to an extent after the PICU's founding because critically ill children often required the care of medical specialists. The two intensivists came to see the porosity of the PICU's boundaries as a potential hazard to patient safety.

As their vision of an effective organizational design evolved, the two intensivists decided to minimize the unit's porosity by assuming primary responsibility over all ventilator patients. They became the main points of contact for specialists from outside the PICU to discuss patient matters and solicit advice regarding patient care within the unit. This simplified work for staff members but complicated the intensivists' responsibilities, because they now handled conflict with outside physicians. Discussions about appropriate care would occasionally arise between them and external specialists, diverting some of their time and attention away from responding to their own staff. The intensivists viewed the change positively, believing that staff members could operate more effectively when buffered from external conflict.

In addition to serving as gatekeepers between the PICU and the hospital, the two founding intensivists took steps to reduce the PICU's dependence on outside expertise. They each received additional training so that they could personally perform many of the functions that previously had required the services of a specialist. For example, at the beginning of the PICU's history, external ear, nose, and throat (ENT) specialists performed difficult intubations in the unit. When some ENTs voiced disagreement with practices in the PICU, the two lead intensivists began performing difficult intubations themselves and training their fellows to do them as well. They also requested that an anesthesiology fellow be assigned to the unit to reduce their dependence on outside anesthesiologists.

The intensivists argued that the changes improved patient care in the PICU because children's conditions often deteriorated while they were waiting for specialists to arrive. However, these moves also further buffered the PICU and its unique design from the rest of the hospital. The second intensivist took additional steps to make PICU admission through the pediatric critical-care transport system independent of the outside hospital by training transport paramedics and PICU staff to perform functions originally assigned to hospital triage staff. In addition, the intensivists gradually discontinued offering care outside of the PICU. While the high workload within the PICU itself often precluded the intensivists from responding to pediatric emergencies in other departments, the intensivists also felt that they could not maintain a consistent quality of care when working with resources and staff outside of the PICU.

Reliability and Outcomes

Compared to the other PICUs, the focal PICU had normal mortality rates for a PICU of its size during its first two years. After this period, however, its mortality rate began to decline, even while the unit was growing rapidly. By 1993, the focal PICU's mortality rate was 4.6%, compared to the average rate of $7.8 \pm 0.8\%$ for PICUs with more than 18 beds. Except for a brief increase in 1994, associated with the establishment of the intermediate ICU (which increased the average severity of the conditions of PICU patients), the mortality rate at WHTCH's PICU remained low. In 1999, the last full year that the original intensivists remained at the unit, its mortality rate was 3.5%.

Mortality rate is a poor indicator of healthcare performance, both because numbers are difficult to obtain and because it is notoriously difficult to control for the severity of a unit's caseload. We mention it here simply as an indicator that the PICU's design appears to have helped it perform well. Aside from mortality, several other indicators of patient medical outcomes also appeared to improve as the PICU's distinctive decentralized design was put in place. For instance, the unit's staff introduced several innovations that improved patient care. These innovations would not have been possible without the additional medical training and patient care discretion given to staff members in the PICU. In one case, respiratory care practitioners changed the blend of helium and oxygen when administering gas to patients with severe asthma. The innovation gave children on ventilators increased energy, allowing them to play for longer periods. In another case, resident nurses began placing the children on their stomachs during a period when the unit experienced a higher incidence of acute lung disease. They discovered that children had better lung function in this position, with oxygen entering the blood more easily. In a third case, some respiratory care practitioners began setting ventilators to higher breath rates, sometimes reaching levels higher than those generally considered safe. Further study of the practice found that higher ventilator rates made some patients more comfortable and alert and did not cause adverse health outcomes.

The design instituted by the two managing intensivists also led to higher satisfaction and lower turnover among staff members in the unit. The PICU's founding director saw one of his primary responsibilities to be creating a supportive environment. As a consequence of this effort, the PICU had an extremely low turnover rate for nurses and therapists, much lower than is common in intensive care generally. Several former residents reported the PICU residency to be the most difficult but most enjoyable of their residencies.

Culture Clash

In 1993 the PICU brought in an additional pediatric intensivist fellow to assist the original two intensivists. As the unit grew, others were hired and the number of doctors (including fellows) in the unit soon stabilized at five. Until 1997, the only physicians assigned to the PICU were the original two intensivists, their fellows, and intensivists who had received their fellowship training in the unit. As a result, the unit's physicians strongly agreed that its decentralized design, although unorthodox, was effective.

Beginning in 1997, intensivists trained elsewhere were hired into the unit. The PICU's continuing expansion and the departure of intensivists trained in the unit for leadership positions elsewhere created vacancies. The PICU's high utilization demanded that vacancies and new positions be filled quickly, and the founding intensivists eventually turned to externally trained intensivists to expedite staffing needs.

A few of the externally trained intensivists did not see the value of the PICU's approach and believed instead that the unit's design might constitute malpractice because physicians in the unit did not always control patient treatments. The new intensivists introduced notions of strict physician authority and one-way, downward communication. Although the protocols allowing staff to exercise discretion remained in place, staff members learned that the new doctors interpreted them differently than the original two intensivists did. In fact, during this period, staff members began to refer to cultural differences between "PICU north" and "PICU south" because the founding intensivists' offices were located on the south side of the unit. Concerns of malpractice liability from physicians inside the PICU resonated with negative feelings about the unit held by some physicians elsewhere in the hospital. Physicians from other departments saw the growing rift within the PICU and became more outspoken about their disagreement, often refusing to let the two founding intensivists treat their patients even within the PICU. Some hospital administrators, never completely comfortable with the level of autonomy at the PICU, used these concerns to argue against providing dedicated resources or supporting the unit's continued expansion. In this environment, both of the original intensivists chose to leave WHTCH and accept positions elsewhere in 2000.

According to staff members who remained at the PICU, the design features of the unit changed following the departures of the two original intensivists. Physicians began to assert their authority over patient care decisions and ignore suggestions from bedside staff members. Staff turnover in the unit increased and staff members who remained learned to follow physician instructions and largely keep their opinions to themselves. Although the PICU retained some procedures allowing staff discretion and might still have been considered "participative," its staff no longer enjoyed broad decision-making autonomy. Furthermore, procedures put in place to support staff autonomy were gradually discontinued. The new physicians did not encourage staff members to participate in rounds and no longer used rounds as a training opportunity. Similarly, the practice of holding postevent debriefings was all but discontinued and, when debriefings were held, staff members were not encouraged to participate.

Although current staff members believe that the new PICU intensivists are skilled doctors and that the PICU remains a relatively safe unit, they suggest that its health outcomes are not as good as they once were. The annual mortality rate at the unit has increased since its low in 1999. Finally, as noted previously, staff turnover has increased during the same period. WHTCH's PICU remains a good unit, but has lost its distinct design and may be less reliable than in its previous form.

Discussion

The design of WHTCH's PICU evolved over time in response to environmental and technological demands, resulting in an extremely decentralized decision-making structure for an industry where strictly enforced hierarchical relationships are more often the norm. The PICU also became unusually self-sufficient in an area in which organizational boundaries are typically porous or unidentifiable.

The PICU's experience provides several implications for organizational design theory and practice. The case draws a connection between organizational design and leadership. The coincidence of the founders' departures and design changes at the PICU suggests the alternative explanation that good leadership rather than organizational design led to the PICU's performance. It may have been that the charisma and personal leadership qualities of the two head intensivists motivated staff members to achieve high performance independent of any design interventions that were introduced. According to the PICU members with whom we spoke (including the two intensivists), this was not the case. Neither intensivist claims extraordinary leadership qualities, and other staff members do not attribute such to them. In fact, while most of the PICU staff accepted and came to agree with the intensivists' approach, others did not—some harboring personal dislike for the intensivists themselves. Furthermore, current staff members are quick to point out that the intensivists who headed the PICU after 2000 are neither poor leaders nor poor physicians. Rather, several of them emphasized that the reason for the PICU's success stems from the fact that its design differed from those of other ICUs.

Despite these assertions that the PICU case is a design story and not a leadership story, the case seems to suggest a closer connection between the two explanations than previously acknowledged. Organizational design is often seen in terms of impersonal structural characteristics: span of control, levels of hierarchy, formalization of rules, and so on. The PICU case instead suggests that organizational design exists at least as much in designers' visions as in organizations' formal structures. For example, the PICU director's vision for the unit was continuity of high-quality care through a highly knowledgeable, motivated, and involved support staff. While this vision did not change during the PICU's growth and evolution, many of its structural characteristics did change as the unit met new challenges. For example, when the first intensivist arrived at the unit, he did not fully appreciate the amount and formality of staff education necessary to fulfill his goals for the unit. Similarly, the two intensivists originally sought to minimize formal boundaries on staff decision-making authority, but later decided that encasing staff authority in formalized metarules actually created a more effective design in line with their original vision.

The PICU's design was an ongoing effort, and its most stable components centered on a vision of distributed knowledge and decentralized intensive care. To the extent that this vision existed largely in the minds of the two PICU directors, the unit's design cannot easily be separated from its leaders. Many (perhaps most) of the design features that eventually came to characterize the PICU were not planned from the foundation of the unit. Rather, they were instituted in response to new challenges or unanticipated consequences of the unit's evolution. For example, neither of the two intensivists anticipated the lengths to which they would eventually go to isolate and buffer their unit from the broader hospital. Their buffering efforts were necessitated by unexpected hostility to the PICU's design from other hospital units. The case highlights the cyclic nature of organizational design. Organizational leaders put a design in place, observe its effects on the organization, adjust the design, again observe the effects, and so on.

In another vein, the PICU experience shows that a design's origin may be as important as its content. While much work examines the adoption of legitimized forms and increasing conformity among organizational designs in a field, few perspectives address the motivation to search for alternative designs when commonly accepted forms exist. The PICU story highlights the idea that organizational leaders with diverse prior experiences can introduce this form of divergent change. Many of the unit's design features were based on organizational designs employed by fire department emergency medical service organizations. However appropriate these designs may have been to pediatric intensive care, they were unfamiliar to nurses, therapists, and physicians. Unfamiliarity led many members of WHTCH and the PICU itself to distrust the new design. Much of the ongoing design effort undertaken by the two PICU intensivists was devoted to combating this distrust.

Similarly, the PICU case also illustrates some of the unique challenges of designing an organizational subunit to operate much differently than does its parent organization. Any organizational design that differs from an accepted, institutionalized model in its industry is necessarily fragile. However, the PICU's design was even more tenuous because it was at odds with accepted designs in its parent organization. While the PICU directors succeeded in implementing such a design, the unit's design required constant and effortful maintenance. The PICU's director quickly discovered that his unique design was difficult for many physicians and staff members to accept. He responded by taking steps to buffer his unit from its parent organization and associated designs. He obtained dedicated nurses and respiratory care practitioners, unified the unit's contact with other departments through himself and his associate, and limited the need for outside specialists to enter the unit.

The PICU case suggests that buffering subunits with unique designs from their environments is important to their operation, but also raises specific challenges. Much prior work focuses on organizations naturally buffered from outside pressures and lacking exposure to market or competitive forces. Indeed, many such organizations may be conceived of as "total institutions," as they achieve strong cultures by largely removing their members from outside society. The present examination reveals that such isolation takes considerable effort in multiunit organizations. While such a subunit may need to distance itself as much as possible from its parent organization, the case illustrates that resistance may develop from members of other organizational subunits and organizational leaders who perceive such buffering as a threat to their power. Without continuous buffering efforts, the unit may easily be overrun by the culture of its parent organization or its industry at large.

The case also suggests that several characteristics of the PICU's design evolved in direct response to challenges posed by the unit's technology and environment. There are many examples of organizations facing similar hazards that have attempted but were unable to reach goals for safety and operational reliability. There are several differences between the PICU and designs at these other organizations. Specifically, the PICU was highly decentralized, as its founders delegated authority through the organization. Organizations desiring consistent performance under hazardous conditions indeed must be designed to give frontline employees tremendous levels of decision-making authority and flexibility. The relationship between complex organizational environments and decentralized decision-making authority has long been acknowledged by contingency literature on organizational design. While many organizations distribute knowledge and delegate decision-making authority during periods of abnormal operations or crises, they normally display high levels of centralization and formalization during more routine periods. However, the decentralization of decision making at WHTCH's PICU was broad based and not confined to emergency situations, suggesting that decentralized decision making need not be coupled with periods of strict hierarchy.

The PICU experience also reinforces the assertion that decentralization requires distributed knowledge. The founding intensivists devoted a great deal of time and attention to training staff members about how to make treatment decisions. Their experience shows that frontline employees cannot be expected to effectively shoulder decision-making responsibilities without sufficient knowledge and training. Some prior studies suggest that the high levels of training required to create such knowledge distribution may be too costly for organizations in most environments. However, the focal PICU functioned quite efficiently with such a structure in spite of the training requirements. Indeed, the unit's low doctor/patient ratio was one of the conditions that necessitated decentralization.

The PICU experience also lends support to a growing recognition that even generally successful organizations make mistakes and must learn from them to maintain their consistency. Behavioral perspectives argue that organizations and the people in them often learn through performance shortfalls, interpreting successes as a sign that change is not needed and learning only in response to failure. Crises inevitably arise in any complex healthcare setting. Postcrisis debriefings provided opportunities and time for the staff and founders to learn from failures, and because PICU leaders did not search for "responsible" parties to blame for poor outcomes, unit members were able to learn from their experiences without fear of retaliation.

A recurring question for the founders, however, was whether an organization can be designed to operate reliably in some more benign way than waiting for lessons learned in blood, as failures are costly and often difficult to learn from. In fact, the leaders of the PICU did not wait for a serious accident before delegating authority, developing structures to distribute knowledge, and creating other conditions that they believed would lead to enhanced learning and performance. Rather, in designing the unit, they drew on the failures and successes of other organizations with which they had been associated. As a result, their design interventions sought to avoid strict hierarchy, absolute physician control over patient treatment, and strict individual accountability (or blame) for adverse patient outcomes.

Discuss:

- How did the PICU directors continually readjusted their design to meet internal and external challenges?
- Do you believe that the PICU's design resided perhaps more in its leaders' vision than in its structures and processes?
- What difficulties did the PICU directors encounter while attempting to institute unique designs within their subsystem of a large organization?

SOURCE: "Mitigating hazards through continuing design: the birth and evolution of a pediatric intensive care unit," by P. Madsen, V. Desai, K. Roberts, and D. Wong, 2006. *Organization Science, 17*(2), pp. 239–248. Reprinted with permission.

REFERENCES

Alvesson, M., & Willmott, H. (2002). Identity regulation as organizational control: producing the appropriate individual. *Journal of Management Studies, 39*, 619–644.

Berwick, D. (2002). Quality chasm factors. *Health Affairs*, 21(5), 301–302.

Bolton, S. C. (2004). A simple matter of control? NHS hospital nurses and new management. *Journal of Management Studies, 41*, 317–333.

Burton, R. M., DeSanctis, G., & Obel, B. (2006). *Organizational design: A step-by-step approach.* New York: Cambridge University Press.

Clegg, S. (1981). Organization and control. *Administrative Science Quarterly, 26*, 545–562.

Daft, R. L. (2007). *Organization theory and design* (9th ed.). Mason, OH: Thomson South-western.

Deloitte Health Care Review (2004, July/August). *Decentralization, consistency, and concentration on delivery and quality account for ProMedica's rapid rise to fourth most integrated U.U. health system, CEO says.* Available at: http://www.deloitte.com/dtt/cda/doc/content/us_healthcare_hcr_0904(1).pdf.

Evans, M. (2008). Integrating efficiency: Verispan's annual ranking of the top integrated health networks shows improved operating margins along with expanded service. *Modern Healthcare, 38*(5), 26–29.

Fayol, H. (1949). *General and industrial management.* London: Pitman.

Friedson, E. (1984). The changing nature of professional control. *Annual Review of Sociology 10*, 1–20.

Friedson, E. (2001). *Professionalism: the third logic.* Chicago, IL: University of Chicago Press.

Hage, J., & Aiken, M. (1969). Routine technology, social structure, and organizational goals. *Administrative Science Quarterly, 14*, 366–376.

Hall, R. H. (1962). Intraorganizational structural variation: Application of the bureaucratic model. *Administrative Science Quarterly, 7*, 295–308.

Hall, R. H. (1996). *Organizations: Structures, processes, and outcomes* (6th ed.). Englewood Cliffs, NJ: Prentice Hall.

Halvorson, G. (2007). *Health care reform now: A prescription for change.* San Francisco: Jossey-Bass/John Wiley & Sons.

Hickson, D. J., Pugh, D. S., & Pheysey, D. C. (1969). Operations, technology and organization structure: An empirical reappraisal. *Administrative Science Quarterly, 14*, 378–397.

Hodgson, D. (2002). Disciplining the professional: The case of project management. *Journal of Management Studies, 39*, 804–821.

Institute of Medicine (2001). *Crossing the quality chasm: A new health system for the 21st century.* Available at: www.nap.edu/books/0309072808/html/.

Kast, F. E., & Rosenzweig, J. E. (1985). *Organization and management: A systems and contingency approach.* New York: McGraw-Hill Book Company.

Katz, D., & Kahn, R. L. (1966). *The social psychology of organizations.* New York: John Wiley & Sons.

Kleinke, J. D. (1997, November 5). The industrialization of health care. *The Journal of the American Medical Association, 278*, 1456–1457.

Larson, M. S. (1977). *The rise of professionalism: A sociological analysis.* Berkeley, CA: University of California Press.

Madsen, P., Desai, V., Roberts, K., & Wong, D. (2006). Mitigating hazards through continuing design: The birth and evolution of a pediatric intensive care unit. *Organization Science, 17*(2), 239–248.

Marcus, A. A. (1985). Professional autonomy as a bias of conflict in an organization. *Human Resource Management, 24*(3), 311–328.

Meyer, P. G., & Tucker, S. L. (1992). Incorporating an understanding of independent practice physician culture into hospital structure and operations. *Hospital & Health Services Administration, 37*(4), 465–476.

Miller, D., & Friesen, P. H. (1984). *Organizations: A quantum view.* Englewood Cliffs, NJ: Prentice Hall.

Miner, J. B. (1973). *The management process: Theory, research and practice.* New York: Macmillan.

Miner, J. B. (2002). *Organizational behavior: Foundations, theories and analysis.* New York: Oxford University Press.

Mintzberg, H. (1979). *The structuring of organizations.* Englewood Cliffs, NJ: Prentice Hall.

Monteiro, M. (2002). Outline of organizational designs and structures and linkage to innovation. *Businessgyan,* Available at: http://www.businessgyan.com/content/view/180/434/.

O'Connor, S. J., & Lanning, J. A. (1992). The end of autonomy? Reflections on the postprofessional physician. *Health Care Management Review, 17*(1), 63–72.

Parsons, T. (1968). Professions. In D. L. Sills (Ed.), *International Encyclopedia of the Social Sciences, Vol. 12* (pp. 536–547). New York: Macmillan.

Philip, M., Padsakoff, L., Williams, J., & Williams, D. (1986). Effects of organizational formalization on alienation among professionals and nonprofessionals. *Academy of Management Journal, 29,* 820–831.

Porter, L. W., & Lawler, E. E. (1964). The effects of tall versus flat organization structures on managerial job satisfaction. *Personnel Psychology, 17,* 135–148.

Raelin, J. A. (1986). *The clash of cultures: Managers and professionals.* Boston, MA: Harvard Business School Press.

Ravenscroft, E. F. (2005, June). Access within a fragmented healthcare system: A nurse's perspective on Romanow. *Nursing Leadership—Online Exclusive,* Longwoods Publishing Company. Available at http://www.longwoods.com/product.php?productid=19031&cat=252.

Scott, W. R. (1982). Managing professional work: Three models of control for health organizations. *Health Services Research, 17,* 213–240.

Scott, W. R., Ruef, M., Mendel, P. J., & Caronna, C. A. (2000). *Institutional change and healthcare organizations: From professional dominance to managed care.* Chicago, IL: University of Chicago Press.

Sharma, A. (1997). Professional as agent: Knowledge asymmetry in agency exchange. *Academy of Management Review, 22,* 758–798.

Tannenbaum, A. S. (1968). *Control in organizations.* New York: McGaw-Hill Book Company.

Taylor, F. W. (1911). *The principles of scientific management.* New York: Harper and Brothers.

Thompson, J. (1967). *Organizations in action*. New York: McGraw Hill Book Company.

Tolbert, P. S., & Stern, R. N. (1991). Organizations of professions: Governance structures in large law firms. *Research in the Sociology of Organizations, 8*, 97–117.

Weber, M. (1947). *The theory of social and economic organizations* (A. M. Henerson & T. Parsons, Trans.). New York: Free Press.

Weisz, G. (2006). *Divide and conquer: A comparative history of medical specializations*, New York: Oxford University Press.

Woodward, J. (1965). *Industrial organization: Theory and practice*. London: Oxford University Press.

OTHER SUGGESTED READINGS

Best, R. G., Hysong, S. J., Pugh, J. A., Ghosh, S., & Moore, F.I. (2006). Task overlap among primary care team members: An opportunity for system redesign. *Journal of Healthcare Management, 51*(5), 295–307.

Bohmer, R.M.J. (2005). Medicine's service challenge: Blending customer and standard care. *Health Care Management Review, 30*(4), 322–330.

Gerardi, D. (2005). The culture of health care: How professional and organizational cultures impact conflict management. *Georgia State University Law Review, 21*, 857–890.

Hearld, L. R., Alexander, J. A., Fraser, I., & Jiang, H. J. (2008, June). How do hospital organizational structure and processes affect quality of care? A critical review of research methods. *Medical Care Research and Review, 65*, 3, 259–299.

Vera, A., & Kuntz, L. (2007). Process-based organization design and hospital efficiency. *Health Care Management Review, 32*(1), 55–65.

Closing Remarks

Nancy Borkowski, DBA, CPA, FACHE

In the proceeding 22 chapters, we have examined the multiple theories and concepts relating to organizational behavior and organization theory. I hope that you have gained a greater understanding of how individuals' behaviors affect organizations and how organizations are affected by individuals' behaviors.

The role of today's healthcare manager is complex and sometimes overwhelming. Not only are you motivating and leading diverse populations but doing so in a dynamic and complex environment. It was my goal that after reading this book, you will have gained additional knowledge and skills to effectively lead and manage your organizations.

In 1999, six professional associations came together to form the Health Leadership Alliance (HLA) to address the "things" healthcare executives ought to know. The alliance identified 300 competencies (either skills or areas of knowledge) that were sorted into one of five categories: (1) leadership, (2) communication and relationship management, (3) professionalism, structure and functions, (4) business knowledge and skills, and (5) knowledge of the healthcare environment.

This book has addressed all five categories. In the micro-level analysis section, leadership, communications, and relationship building were addressed. In the macro-level analysis section, structure and functions, business knowledge and skills, and knowledge of the healthcare environment were addressed. In addition, I hope that I was successful in demonstrating to you how these competency areas are not silos of information but each interrelate at all levels and that a manager needs to be proficient in all of these areas to be successful. For example, to achieve high performance, a healthcare organization needs to match its structure and design to its goals in order to successfully implement the entity's strategies. A manager will only be successful in this endeavor if the organization has the right culture with the right people in the right positions to motivate and lead to achieve the organization's goals . . . goals that are valued by the environment!

Please let me know if I have accomplished my goal! You may reach me at Nancy.Borkowski@fiu.edu.

Index

A

absenteeism
    attitude assessment and, 45
    resistance to change and, 358
    Satisfaction-Performance Theory and, 134
    work-related stress and, 227, 237, 239
acceptance
    of clinical practice guidelines, 360
    executive charisma and, 209
    joining groups for, 296–297
    in Maslow's Hierarchy of Needs, 107
    overcoming resistance to goal, 136–137
    of reality, in resilient people, 150
    of responsibility for delegated tasks, 193
    sought by behavioral-style managers, 279
    of stimuli, in perception process, 51
accommodation conflict-handling mode, 269
ACHE (American College of Healthcare Executives), 29–33, 218
achievement motivational need, 3-Needs Theory, 118–119
achievement-oriented style, Path-Goal Leadership Theory, 191
Action Research Model, 344–350
    comparing two models, 347
    diagnosis, 346–349
    entering and contracting, 346
    evaluating and institutionalizing change, 350
    overview of, 344–346
    planning and implementing change, 349–350

actions (behaviors)
    attitudes and, 42
    leaders in, 206
ad hoc committees, 314
Adams, J. Stacy, 131–134
adhocracy, 462
adjourning stage, group development, 316
Adler, Alfred, 43
adrenaline, stress response, 231
affective conflict, 260–263
affiliation needs
    Maslow's Hierarchy of Needs, 107
    McClelland's 3-Needs Theory, 118–120
    satisfying in employee, 109
age
    future workforce and, 36–37
    gender and, 21–22
    projected US population from 2000–2050, 19
    resident US population by, 18–19
ageism, 28
aggression
    attributions associated with, 150
    in desk rage, 229
    as undesirable motivational state, 148–149
aging population
    changes in US, 18–20
    within clinical setting, 27–29
    gender and, 21–22
    overview of, 20–21
    recruiting within, 37
agreeableness, Big Five personality framework, 62, 204, 214
alarm phase, stress response, 231